Data Base of Indian Economy, Volume IV

Social Statistics: Health and Education

DATA BASE OF INDIAN ECONOMY SERIES

Data Base of Indian Economy: Vol. I
Edited by C.R. Rao
and published by
Statistical Society, Calcutta, 1972

Data Base of Indian Economy: Vol. II
Edited by V.M. Dandekar
and published by
Statistical Society, Calcutta, 1974

Data Base of Indian Economy: Vol. III
Edited by Ashish Bose
Devendra B. Gupta
Gaurishankar Raychaudhuri
and published by
Vikas Publishing House

DATA BASE OF INDIAN ECONOMY, VOLUME IV

Social Statistics: Health and Education

Edited by

Ashish Bose
Devendra B. Gupta
Mahendra K. Premi

VIKAS PUBLISHING HOUSE PVT LTD

VIKAS PUBLISHING HOUSE PVT LTD
Regd. Office: 5 Ansari Road, New Delhi 110002
H.O. Vikas House, 20/4 Industrial Area, Sahibabad 201010
Distt. Ghaziabad, U.P. (India)

ISBN 0-7069-1083-4

1V2B3903

Printed at Roopak Printers, Naveen Shahdara, Delhi 110032 (India)

Contributors

C. Bal Krishna is working with the Indian Statistical Institute, New Delhi.

R.K. Bhandari is working with the Statistics Unit, Ministry of Education and Social Welfare, New Delhi.

Durgaprasad Bhattacharya is working with the Indian Statistical Institute, Calcutta.

Ashish Bose is Professor at the Demographic Research Centre, Institute of Economic Growth, Delhi 110007.

B.C. Das is Professor at the Biometry Research Unit, Indian Statistical Institute, Calcutta.

P.K. Devi is Professor of Obstetrics and Gynaecology, Post-graduate Medical Institute, Chandigarh.

Trilok N. Dhar is Joint Director (Education), Planning Commission, New Delhi.

S.N. Gandam is with the Gokhle Institute of Politics and Economics, Poona.

B.B. Gaitonde is with the Haffkins Institute, Bombay.

Shanti Ghosh is the Head of the Department of Pediatrics, Safdarjang Hospital, New Delhi.

Devendra B. Gupta is Associate Professor at the Institute of Economic Growth, Delhi.

Gopal Kadekodi is Associate Professor at the Institute of Economic Growth, Delhi.

A.R. Kamat is with the Gokhle Institute of Politics and Economics, Poona.

R.L. KAPUR is Professor of Community Psychiatry and Head of the Department of Psychiatry, National Institute of Mental Health and Neuro Sciences, Bangalore.

Q.U. KHAN is Head of the Research Division, Institute of Applied Manpower Research, New Delhi.

R.B. LAL is Deputy Registrar General, India, New Delhi.

F.E. MARKER is the Director, Medical Records Department, Sir J.J. Group of Hospitals, Bombay.

ASOK MITRA is Professor at the Jawaharlal Nehru University, New Delhi.

P.R. GOPINATHAN NAIR works with the Centre for Development Studies, Trivandrum.

S.K. NOORDEEN is Deputy Director, Central Leprosy Teaching & Research Institute, Tamil Nadu.

P.G.K. PANIKAR works with the Centre for Development Studies, Trivandrum.

H.N. PANDIT is Professor and Head, Policy Planning and Evaluation Unit N.C.E.R.T., New Delhi.

V.P. PATHAK is with the Directorate of National Malaria Eradication Programme, Delhi.

S. PATTANAYAK is with the Directorate of National Malaria Eradication Programme, Delhi.

MAHENDRA K. PREMI is Associate Professor at the Centre for the Study of Regional Development, Jawaharlal Nehru University, New Delhi.

K.V. RAO works with the National Institute of Nutrition, Hyderabad.

K. RAMACHANDRAN is the Head of the Biostatistics Unit, All India Institute of Medical Sciences, New Delhi.

D.M. RENAPURKAR is with the Haffkins Institute, Bombay.

BINA ROY works with the Indian Statistical Institute, Calcutta.

RAMA DEB ROY works with the Indian Statistical Institute, Calcutta.

BIKAS C. SANYAL is the Head of the Research Project on Higher Education and Employment, UNESCO, Paris.

A.S.R. SHARMA is Statistical Officer, Directorate General of Health Services, Ministry of Health and Family Welfare, New Delhi.

P. SINGHA is OSD, Department of Family Planning, Government of India, New Delhi.

S.G. SRIKANTIA works with the National Institute of Nutrition, Hyderabad.

Preface

The first seminar on Data Base of Indian Economy was held in 1972 under the auspices of the Indian Econometric Society. This seminar was devoted to a discussion on the deficiencies in the official statistics relating to some important sectors of the Indian economy and offered suggestions for their improvement. The second seminar in this series was held in 1973. The theme of the seminar was the role of sample surveys.

The third Data Base seminar was organised, jointly by the Indian Econometric Society (TIES) and the Indian Association for the Study of Population (IASP). The theme of the seminar was population statistics for planning and policy. The initiative for organising such a joint seminar by the two scientific associations was taken by Dr C.R. Rao, the then President of TIES and Dr Asok Mitra, the then President of IASP. This seminar was held in 1974 at the Indian Statistical Institute in New Delhi. The fourth Data Base seminar was also held under the joint auspices of IASP and TIES in 1976 at the Institute for Social and Economic Change in Bangalore. The present volume is the outcome of this seminar. A large number of papers were received. A selection of these papers were revised and edited by an editorial committee comprising Professor Ashish Bose, Programme Director of the Seminar, Dr D.B. Gupta, Co-Director of the Seminar and Dr M.K. Premi, Joint Secretary, IASP.

While planning the seminar, the organisers wanted to highlight two important but neglected areas of social statistics in India, namely health and education. It can be said about health statistics that it has been a neglected area of social statistics and there are large information gaps. The statistics on education, however, are not neglected in the sense of data collection. In fact, there is a massive data collection on education in routine manner, much of which is unimaginative and has not been put to any worthwhile use. One of the objectives of this seminar was to examine the present system of data collection through the offiicial machinery, identify the gaps in our information and make suggestions for streamlining the system of data collection as well as for including new items of data for more effective planning and policy making.

The organisers of the seminar invited contributions from eminent doctors, public health experts, educational administrators, statisticians, demographers and other social scientists. The seminar succeeded in getting a fairly representative participation from experts in the field of health and education, as will be revealed by the list of contributors.

The papers are presented into two parts, Part One comprising 16 papers is devoted to health statistics and Part Two comprising 12 papers deals with statistics on education.

An overall review of health statistics is given in "Health Statistics in India—An Overview" followed by some specific aspects of the quality of health statistics in A.S.R. Sharma's paper. As is well-known, Kerala has the lowest mortality rate and infant mortality rate in India. Incidentally Kerala has also the lowest birth rate in India. In fact, the Kerala 'model' has attracted world-wide attention. Panikar's contribution deals with the health statistics in Kerala. The next two papers are devoted to hospital records and hospital statistics. The important question of infant and child mortality statistics is handled by an eminent specialist on child health. This is followed by a paper devoted to the statistics of foetal mortality which is of very great importance in understanding the mortality pattern.

One of the most deficient aspects of mortality statistics relates to cause of death data. Singha comments on the statistics on cause of death while Asok Mitra gives in summary form a comprehensive paper on morbidity statistics which was presented at the seminar. For reasons of economy of space, the whole paper could not be reproduced. We then move on to communicable diseases. The return of malaria in India in recent years, when it was widely believed that malaria was on its way out, has been the cause of very great concern on the part of public health experts. Pattanayak and Pathak deal specifically with malaria statistics. Noordeen's paper is on leprosy statistics. The next paper gives an overview of the statistics on communicable diseases. Mental health statistics is as neglected as the question of mental health papers. R.L. Kapur makes an important contribution on the subject of mental health statistics in India.

The subject of community health attracted world-wide attention after the success of bare-foot doctors scheme in China. In India, the Community Health Workers (CHW) Scheme was launched on a pilot basis in 1977. Subsequently it underwent modifications and improvement, and currently it is known as the Health Guide Scheme. The development of methodology for the collection of community health statistics remains a neglected field. "Community Health Survey" deals with some of the methodological aspects of community health surveys.

India has a long history of collection of educational statistics through governmental agencies. A brief historical survey of this is contained in the paper contributed by Bhattacharya and Roy. This is followed by an evaluation of the statistics on education in India. The subject of elementary education in rural areas is considered in C. Bal Krishna's contribution and the statistics on vocational education is taken up in the next paper.

The next four papers deal with the appraisal of educational statistics, gaps in educational statistics, suggestions for improving the educational statistics and an appraisal of the available educational statistics in the Censuses and National Sample Surveys.

Manpower statistics in India has been assuming an increasing importance in the context of planning for higher education and also the brain-drain. A review of manpower statistics is given by Q.U. Khan. This is followed by a discussion of data needs on higher education contributed by an expert in this field working at UNESCO, Paris. The statistical needs for education planning in totality is discussed in the next paper.

The last paper deals with both education and health and is devoted to a very important topic of great concern to planners, namely the inter-state disparities. On the basis of the available data, the author brings out the inter-state disparities in the per capita expenditure on education and medicine in India. This has several policy implications.

On behalf of the Indian Association for the Study of Population and Indian Econometric Society, we wish to place on record our grateful thanks to the following organisations for their help in organising this seminar: Government of Karnataka for financial assistance; The Indian Council of Medical Research (ICMR) for financial assistance; The Institute for Social and Economic Change, Bangalore for playing host to this seminar and all the infrastructure facilities; The Indian Statistical Institute; The Institute of Economic Growth; and Jawaharlal Nehru University for academic collaboration in making this seminar a success.

We deeply regret that on account of unavoidable reasons, this volume could not be brought out earlier. Since this book is concerned with the statistical systems and not with data as such, the value of the papers presented here remains undiminished. We hope scholars in the field of health and education as well as the administrators, planners and policy-makers will find this volume helpful.

Delhi

ASHISH BOSE
DEVENDRA B. GUPTA
MAHENDRA K. PREMI

Contents

Part One: HEALTH STATISTICS

Part Two: EDUCATION

PART 1

HEALTH

Health Statistics in India—An Overview

K. RAMACHANDRAN

The planned development of a comprehensive, equitable nation-wide network of health services has been accepted as the goal of the Indian health sector since the submission of the Bhore Committee report in 1946. However, in spite of sustained efforts in this direction during the last three decades, a great deal remains to be done and the resource constraints continue to be severe. In fact, the Group on Medical Education and Support Manpower set up by the Centre, submitting its report in April 1975, observed, "... The entire programme of providing a nation-wide network of efficient and effective health services needs to be reviewed *de novo* to evolve an alternative strategy of development more suitable for our conditions, limitations and potentialities." The context is clear and the need for health statistics to effectively plan and deliver health services in the country can hardly be overemphasized.

Health statistics embrace almost all aspects of life, since the health of a population, in the ultimate analysis, is a consequence of their way of life. The 13th report of WHO Expert Committee on Health Statistics listed the type of statistics required for planning, administration and evaluation of health services. The following is based on that list:

(*i*) The population to be served and its composition at the national, state and local levels;

(*ii*) Statistics on vital events particularly births, deaths and migration;

(*iii*) Morbidity data of different types, including temporary disability;

(*iv*) Mortality data, including cause-of-death data;

(*v*) Data on the physico-medical status of the population, nutritional status of the population, its immunisation status, and data based physico-medical examinations;

(*vi*) Data on health facilities and their utilisation;

(*vii*) Data on health manpower and institutions for their training;

(*viii*) Data on physical and social environment;

(*ix*) Data on physical resources, both present and potential, production of drugs, medical supplies etc; and

(*x*) Information on financial allocations to health services and their relation to total governmental expenditure.

This present paper limits itself to a consideration of some aspects of items (*iii*) to (*viii*) in the above list and a brief consideration of some aspects of the health statistics system existing in India.

Morbidity Statistics

The three major sources of morbidity studies are notification statistics, hospital statistics, and statistics from surveys and special studies. None of these three sources gives data of quality in India as yet though a great deal of discussions about these have taken place during the last two decades.

(*a*) *Notification Statistics.* There still exists a wide variation in the list of notifiable diseases from state to state. In addition, the diagnostic facilities vary in quality from urban to rural areas, the latter often having very inadequate facilities, resulting in very poor quality data. Further, there is variation in terminology used. For example, some states report tuberculosis cases while others report pulmonary tuberculosis; some report typhus cases while others report them as louse-borne typhus.

The system of reporting also suffers from drawbacks. This system is often linked at the periphery to that of vital statistics registration in which usually an illiterate, unpaid person with diverse responsibilities is charged with reporting of events. The consequence is not difficult to imagine. Added to this is the reluctance, sometimes, of concerned medical officers to notify infectious diseases for fear of adverse remarks from higher-ups, resulting in a good deal of under-notification. No systematic attempt at the state or national level has been made to assess under-notification. General practitioners' and private health agencies' help in this area has not been actively solicited till now.

The existing provisions of law seem to be inadequate in this area. The following suggestions need careful consideration for affecting improvement in notification statistics:

(*i*) The list of notifiable disease should have a basic uniformity with option for states to add diseases of special significance to them;

(*ii*) The list for urban and rural areas may be different—for rural areas it would be adequate to include only the internationally quarantinable diseases, and for urban areas the list may include in addition the following diseases: tuberculosis, infective hepatitis, diphtheria, tetanus, measles, chicken pox, enteric fever and rabies. (The availability of diagnostic facilities has to be borne in mind in including these in the list of notifiable diseases);

(*iii*) There is a real need for clearly spelling out the symptoms of the notifiable diseases in the form of a manual to be available with all reporting agencies;

(*iv*) Notification by hospitals, dispensaries and other institutions with better diagnositc facilities may be treated separately from notifications from agencies without adequate diagnostic facilities;

(*v*) It is worthwhile to consider the possibility of coordinating in some way the Sampling Registration System of the Registrar General of India's office with the notification system in the rural areas; and

(*vi*) Systematic training and supportive supervision to workers in the rural areas needs attention.

(*b*) *Hospital Morbidity Statistics.* Proper maintenance and reporting of hospital statistics is an exception rather than the rule in the country. Even when data are reported, they lack quality and uniformity. A vast majority of hospitals lack a set-up for medical records, and hospital statistics are, therefore, neglected. Further, medical personnel do not generally appreciate the need for statistics in hospitals due to lack of proper orientation. In addition to these administrative difficulties, there are technical shortcomings. Uniformity in definitions to be used and procedures to be followed in compilation are absent. No manuals are available to the staff who are employed in collection and compilation of patient statistics.

Though the essential step for bringing about noticeable improvement in hospital statistics is the establishment of medical record departments in all hospitals; this can only be a long-term approach due to the existing financial constraints. The points that need immediate attention in this area are:

(*i*) To agree on a minimum uniform list of items on in-patient records. The following items have been suggested by NIHAE as a result of the seminar on Hospital Information System conducted by them in 1974: 1. Serial Number 2. Year 3. Name 4. Full Address

5. Sex 6. Age 7. Diagnosis—preliminary and final 8. Paying/free 9. Notifiable 10. Complaints/History/findings 11. Treatment (drugs/ operation) 12. Blood smear for Malaria—positive/negative 13. Date of admission 14. Date of discharge 15. Condition at discharge 16. In case of death medical certification of cause.

(*ii*) It is worthwhile considering the adoption of a centralised system of collection of hospital in-patient morbidity in all states so that individual hospitals are not burdened with coding and tabulation of these data. Tabulation should relate only to discharges and not admissions. Discharges should include deaths and transfers to other institutions.

(*iii*) To adopt the international classification of disease of WHO, as far as possible, for coding. Related to this is the preparation of a manual of instructions for ensuring uniformity.

(*iv*) To recognise the need for individual patient records for out-patients also and to implement this wherever feasible. Where not feasible, a register should be maintained with information on name, age, sex, diagnosis, distance from home and address.

(*v*) Attention be given to the training and orientation of staff involved in the work.

(*vi*) The in-patient statistics should be reported separately for hospitals with 20 beds or more, cottage hospitals with less than 20 beds and Primary Health Centre hospitals. The last is particularly important in view of the pivotal role PHCs are expected to play in country's health programme.

(*vii*) The lack of uniformity in the data on hospital beds and their utilization should be corrected. The hospital bed should be defined as "one which is properly equipped to take care of an in-patient for all 24 hours of the day. It does not include the improvised bed which is sometimes provided for an in-patient on the floor or cot."

Data on emergency and observation beds need to be reported separately. Maternity beds and their occupancy also need to be reported separately.

(*c*) *Surveys and Special Studies of Morbidity*. The inadequacies of the permanent system for morbidity statistics in India have long been realised and the need for special surveys recognized. At the national level, the National Sample Survey has carried out health interview surveys during its 7th to 13th rounds as well as in its 28th round. These surveys used investigators to collect data, but doubts have been expressed about the reliability of the data on causes of sickness.

N.S.S. Report (No. 49) on morbidity itself has said, "... it is believed that a diagnostic study with a fully equipped team would be required for clinical and laboratory examination to supply reliable information on causes of sickness."

In view of the important need for community based morbidity data (with information on related variables) in health planning, it seems essential to create the necessary machinery both at the national level and at state level; the national level machinery taking a leading part in the planning of the surveys and the state level machinery playing a leading role in the conduct of the surveys. As part of these surveys, sample studies of in-patient and out-patient morbidity may also be conducted. These may be periodic, say once in three to five years. Health examination may be carried out in sub-samples while interview survey is conducted on the entire sample.

It is worthwhile considering the possibility of associating the Sampling Registration System machinery and the National Nutrition Monitoring Bureau (ICMR) machinery in collecting communitywide morbidity data.

The question of macro versus micro level information also needs some consideration.

Mortality Statistics

The principal source of mortality statistics on communitywide basis in India today is the Sample Registration System and Model Registration Scheme. The former gives data on the frequency of deaths while the latter attempts to provide information on the cause of death. These systems were evolved because of the serious shortcomings of the civil registration system in the country.

The SRS based on a carefully selected sample is well established now and provides fairly reliable estimates of death rates at the state and national levels. However, there is still the need for pursuing the idea of establishing a full scale civil registration system properly so that micro level statistics on death becomes available throughout the country.

The MRS, which is a survey of cause of death by para-medical staff at the PHC, is not based on probability sample. Only PHCs with adequate para-medical personnel available for carrying out the fieldwork for the MRS have been included in the scheme and the sample largely covers only PHC headquarter villages. Though the scheme has provided some useful data on broad causes of death, it remains an unsatisfactory system. The survey expects ten per cent of the deaths reported by the para-medical staff to be checked by the medical officer in charge. This rarely is done in practice.

There is an urgent need to involve the health departments at the district and state levels more directly in the collection of reliable information on cause of death using lay reporters. Periodical sample checks by senior officers of health or some other independent machinery is desirable. Well planned analytical studies on a small scale need to be carried out to effect improvements needed in the collection of information on causes of death. Ultimately it is by streamlining and strengthening the PHC that one can hope to get reliable cause of death statistics based on lay reporting.

The hospitals, as is well known, cater to highly (self) selected groups of patients, hence mortality data from hospitals is unlikely to be of much use in the larger planning of health services. Nevertheless, it is of interest to have them since they are medically certified.

Agencies for Health Statistics

State Level. At present there is no uniform pattern for the organization of health statistics at the state level. In some states there is a division of statistics in the health department while in others the work is done by the Bureau of Economics and Statistics. Where the agency is outside the Directorate of Health and Medical Services, the work relating to health statistics usually suffers. Further, if the agency is located within the Directorate of Health and Medical Services, better utilization of such statistics for health planning and administration can be expected. It, therefore, seems that there is need for having divisions of statistics under a senior statistical officer within the Health Directorate in the states to collect/collate needed health statistics.

Further, at the state level, in at least some states, there is almost a complete lack of coordination even between different divisions within State Health Directorate. Added to this is the problem of data relevant to health services planning being collected by organization outside the health directorate. There hardly exists any coordination between these agencies and the division of statistics dealing with health statistics.

Finally, though there is a great deal of talk about evaluation of health services, there is virtually nothing being done in this respect in most States of the country. In fact evaluation is a word that is looked upon with suspicion.

District Level. There is generally no statistically qualified person assigned specifically for collection and supervision of collection of health statistics at the district level. There are usually two statistical assistants to collect statistics related to family planning and tuberculosis programmes. The creation of a health statistics cell attached to the district medical health officer, under the control of a qualified health statistician, is necessary. Two statistical assistants under the family planning and tuberculosis programmes should be posted in this cell and the cell should be charged with the responsibility of collection and supervision of all health statistics needed at the district level.

PHC Level. There is no person for looking after health and medical statistics. Only one computer is appointed to look after statistics concerned with the family planning programme. Usually, some stores clerk or some such person looks after the health and medical statistics at the PHC level. It is indeed unfortunate that health statistics from the PHCs covering nearly 80 per cent of the Indian population is so badly neglected. Strengthening the health statistics staff at the PHC by providing one more computer would probably contribute substantially to the improvement of the health information system of the country.

A related point needs to be considered here. This is with regard to the flow and utilization of health statistics from the PHC. At present the flow is one way from the PHC to the district and to the state levels. Consequently the PHC medical officers and other staff do not care very much about the quality of the information. If the PHC staff (in fact even the district health staff) is expected to take interest in health statistics it is absolutely essential that they become aware of the utility of the statistics they collect. There has to be a feedback of essential information to the PHC to indicate the progress they are making on different programmes, the progress made by other PHCs in the district and state etc. This feedback must be regular and periodic so that the PHC (and the district staff) can assess its own performance and have a sense of participation in the planning of activities as called for.

Another related but important point that needs consideration is about the multiplicity of records and registers that have to be kept by the PHC staff like the ANM. There are, often, as many as 14 registers to be maintained by the ANM with a great deal of duplication of information leading to a lack of interest and inefficiency in keeping records. Streamlining of records and registers needs to be undertaken urgently. Training of staff and manuals for them need attention.

Health Facilities and Their Utilization

Data on health care facilities like number of hospitals, dispensaries, primary health centres, clinics, voluntary organization, their geographic location, the resources at their disposal, the number of beds in them are all routinely collected at the district level and completed at the state headquarters.

However, data on the utilization of the health facilities, particularly, the hospitals and health centre facilities in rural areas are conspicuous by their absence. (Some independent studies in PHC areas—unpublished data—have indicated that hardly two to three per cent persons reporting illness in a health survey attend a PHC facility for seeking advice and treatment. Distance is, of course, one factor that stands in the way of persons attending a PHC. Possibly other factors also play a role. No information on this aspect is available at all.) Similar is the picture with reference to the details of services provided by voluntary bodies.

There is urgent need for carrying out studies on utilization of health facilities particularly in rural areas.

Some Aspects of Health Statistics in India

A.S.R. SHARMA

"Health Statistics" is a generic term covering different aspects of quantitative information needed for health planning and administration. Conceptually, this covers vital statistics extracted from vital records maintained for continuous and complete enumeration of vital events like birth and death etc. The other components of health statistics are medical care statistics covering health facilities provided by hospitals, dispensaries, primary health centres etc., and morbidity statistics which are generated in the administration of hospitals and other institutions. Public health statistics is yet another component which deals with statistics engendered in the operation of primary health centres essentially for preventive services for the community. It would be necessary to take a brief review of existing situation and to delineate the deficiencies both qualitatively and quantitatively.

VITAL STATISTICS

Vital statistics are linked with registration procedures which are statutorily controlled by different acts in different states prior to 1969, and, from 1969 onwards, by a central act, The Registration of Birth and Death Act, 1969. This act streamlines existing machinery and provides a uniform law for adoption by the state governments. Many governments have notified rules and regulations under the framework of the new act.

Vital statistics are known to be deficient, both quantitatively and qualitatively. Quantitative deficiency is in respect of under-registration which may be due to several factors, such as availability of doctors, health consciousness, utility of registration, etc. It has been estimated that under-registration is about 50 per cent for the country as a whole. Qualitative deficiency is mainly in accuracy of the causes of death.

The coverage of vital events, no doubt, differs from state to state, but in any state there is no satisfactory coverage of vital events useful for providing annual birth and death rates, the main components of population growth. No systematic evaluation has been done for the country as a whole in this respect probably for the reason it is expected that the new act, coupled with other measures, can provide stimulus, in the near future for better coverage.

The existing information on causes of death are recorded and tabulated according to cholera, smallpox, plague, fevers, dysentery and diarrhoea, respiratory diseases, etc. Due to active and sustained control and eradication activities plague and smallpox have been wiped out in this country. Cholera still remains to be fully contained. Consequently, the first three specific diseases of cholera, smallpox and plague have little or no relevance in this country. The information on the other three broad groups of diseases will not be useful for health administration.

It is likely that this rudimentary classification is to continue for some time to come. Consequently, the office of the Registrar General of India, during the mid-1960s, adopted a new procedure of recording the cause of death in their scheme known as "Cause of Death Survey," at present operated in headquarters' villages of primary health centres utilizing para-medical staff for post-mortem inquiry into the symptomology of causes of death. A short non-medical list and a check-list of symptoms is provided for the para-medical personnel to be followed in the field and to record probable cause of death. Accuracy of the information depends not only on the knowledge of para-medical personnel with symptoms and strict adherence to list but also on the cooperation of the public. The survey has been conceived of to get more reliable information on causes of death and to evaluate them, in broad groups to give indication of the health problems in the areas covered for practical action. Recently, an evaluation team has toured many states to examine the working of the scheme and has come to the conclusion that time is still not ripe for expansion of the scheme.

Simultaneously, a parallel scheme of medical certification of the cause of death has been initiated in selected hospitals. Under the scheme, death has to be certified in the international form prescribed by the World Health Organisation. This certificate has to be filled up by the physician who has attended the deceased during his/her last illness. The recorded underlying cause of death in the certificate is coded according to the rules prescribed therefor to the International Classification of Diseases. The same is used for mortality tabulations. The resultant data are published separately.

Another important scheme initiated in this country is a continuous demographic survey aimed to provide reliable estimates of annual birth and death rates at the state and the national levels. These estimates are, at present, being used, *inter alia*, for population projections and assessment of the impact of health services using the comprehensive indicator of crude mortality rate. This scheme has been in operation from the year 1966 and, at present, covers the whole country. The results are published regularly in the quarterly bulletin for the Sample Registration by the Office of the Registrar General of India.

To sum up, the registration system continues to suffer from inadequacies which render the vital statistics unreliable for planning purposes. However, improvement in the registration system is a long drawn affair. It would be useful to evaluate, periodically, the extent of under-registration to watch improvements. To improve statistics on causes of death and to provide birth rates and death rates, ad hoc measures have been taken up. These schemes need to be strengthened with periodic evaluation.

MEDICAL CARE STATISTICS

Medical care statistics include hospital, administrative, and morbidity statistics and resources statistics pertaining to the medical care administration. Hospital morbidity component is the most important inasmuch as they constitute the main source of morbidity statistics in India today. These are extracted from in-patient and out-patient records maintained in the course of rendering curative services to the community. Conceptually, these morbidity statistics are selective and biased in nature, however, giving a rough idea of the trend of diseases obtaining in the community.

It may be mentioned in this connection, the most conspicuous lacuna in the system of hospital statistics is lack of medical record departments at hospital level. India can only boast of few of centrally organised departments, in a few leading hospitals, the majority of them either in private and public sectors not possessing even skeletal staff for maintenance of medical records and for tabulation of the data. Consequently, records usually maintained by the para-medical personnel, such as, compounders or nurses, cannot be on scientific lines. Although medical records do exist in the hospitals and are useful as a good source of statistical information, it would be a difficult proposition either to retrieve medical records for research or to maintain series of statistics, pertaining to the hospital.

However, the statement on hospital morbidity is usually compiled and tabulated in the Intermediate List of the World Health Organisation by the para-medical personnel. They are consolidated at the district and the state level for onward transmission to the national level, giving information on the total number of in-patients and out-patients treated and the number of deaths among patients. Morbid conditions or causes of mortality are not coded to the International Classification of Diseases.

The data so obtained are published by some of the state governments in their annual reports of civil hospitals and dispensaries or sometimes in the State administrative departments with a good deal of time lag. The quality of data is far from satisfactory. Some of the states cover both private and public hospitals while some do cover only public institutions under control of the government and the same may also vary from year to year. In spite of the limitations, the available statistics on morbidity are used to determine the leading causes of sickness, since there is no other source of information on morbidity.

Hospital administrative statistics in medical records are neither fully tabulated nor published. Indices like bed occupancy, turnover interval, hospital fatality ratio, the gross and net death rates are useful for hospital administration, hospital planning and efficient medical care. The Directorate General of Health Services as early as in 1958 suggested to the state governments suitable tabulation of the data to evaluate the working of the hospitals.

Recently, the Directorate General of Health Services has been making an attempt to collect hospital morbidity statistics by age and sex from those hospitals where medical record departments exist. This would provide uniform coverage and uniform tabulation of data with application of concepts followed in tabulation of hospital data. It is suggested the unit of tabulation would be discharge and final diagnosis at the time of discharge.

The Indian Council of Medical Research is also making independently an attempt to collect hospital morbidity statistics in a few selected hospitals with provision to examine the deficiencies that occur due to varying coding practices. The data for 1973 from these hospitals were published. It is hoped that this survey would serve as a pilot survey to standardise the procedures in the collection of data from hospitals.

Simultaneously, the Directorate General of Health Services has made an attempt to publish annual inventory of hospitals, collecting information on basic items of information relating to the hospitals on facilities, staff etc. It is intended to cover both private and public hospitals in this inventory. A detailed analysis on facilities available will be made.

To sum up, for building up hospital statistics medical record department is an essential pre-requisite. Efforts are being made to persuade the state governments to establish them, providing simultaneously the consultative services from the World Health Organisation. The recommendations of the Workshop on the Hospital Statistics mentioned above, it is felt, will be most useful in standardisation of the procedures for tabulation and collection. Attempts are underway to collect information on age and sex classification, hitherto missing and to take annual stock of health care facilities.

PUBLIC HEALTH STATISTICS

Notification of communicable diseases is an important element of public health statistics. This is primarily meant for prevention and control of these diseases and is also a source of morbidity statistics. This system is usually operative through public health acts. Some of the state governments do not have any specific act except invoking the Epidemic Diseases Act, 1897 while in some of the states, executive instructions regarding control of epidemic diseases and prevention of an outbreak of epidemics are issued. The lists of the notifiable diseases vary from state to state and from rural to urban areas. The number of diseases show a large range sometimes with vague and undefined terms.

This system is linked with vital statistics machinery as reporter is often a village chowkidar or headman. The two officials of the Revenue Department being illiterate and ill-paid and burdened with many other responsibilities, show slackness in the reporting of these diseases unless epidemic diseases become of dangerous proportions. These personnel are supposed to intimate fresh infections. According to the law mentioned above, registered medical practitioners and heads of households are also responsible for notification.

However, in view of the fact that these acts have not been enforced seriously, under-notification of diseases is quite large and, in practice, the three diseases of cholera, smallpox and plague are usually notified and the other diseases on the lists do not usually get reported. The statistics on the international quarantinable diseases of cholera, smallpox and plague reported in a weekly telegram to the national level giving cases and deaths by the state health authorities/local health authorities are consolidated and sent to the World Health Organisation and State Health Directorates every Saturday. Thus, the time series on weekly basis is available for cases and deaths for these quarantine diseases. In view of what has been stated above, accuracy of this information is dubious; coverage is open to question.

The existing operation of the system reveals a few disquieting features. The lists are long and the disease entities not accurately defined. Short lists depending upon the facilities available in the rural and urban areas may be introduced. It will thus be quite possible to verify their accuracy and better coverage can be expected. Because of better coverage and accuracy publication of age and sex data can be attempted.

Compulsory notification needs to be backed by law enforceable throughout the country. The extent of under-notification for different notifiable diseases need be attempted from time to time. Vital registration needs to be coordinated with notification system for mutual benefit.

Another element of public health statistics is immunisation statistics. These have a crucial role to play in the control programmes for communicable diseases. In India, incidence of communicable diseases is still high. Eruption of these diseases is usually followed by immediate control measures including immunisation. National control programmes were initiated both for smallpox and tuberculosis. The smallpox eradication was started in 1962 and the BCG campaign in 1949.

Statistics available are presented on total number of anti-cholera inoculations, district-wise for cholera and smallpox. Age classification for smallpox is also adopted and it is as follows: Less than one month, 1-12 months, 1-4 years, 5-14 years, 15-29 years and 30 plus.

These statistics are presented separately for primary and re-vaccinations districtwise. In both the categories, total number for successful vaccinations and the percentage of success are also presented districtwise. These statistics published annually do not usually serve to indicate the protection through immunization enjoyed by the community covered.

Besides, the statistics of immunization on most other diseases like polio, typhoid, whooping cough and tetanus are presented in absolute numbers in public health reports. Again, these will be useful only to indicate the total work done by the public health personnel rather than immunity enjoyed by the community in different age groups. Regarding BCG, the programme is operated by special teams and the total number vaccinated in age groups of less than 1 year, 1-4, 5-14, 15-19 are published quarterly and annually.

It may be recalled that the Central Expert Committee for Control of Cholera and Smallpox of the Indian Council of Medical Research recommended that the villagewise registers containing data on family composition should be maintained at the primary health centres. If they are maintained properly, information on immunization can also be entered therein so as to enable calculation of percentage of the population protected through different types of immunizations in different age groups. Otherwise, the statistics available at present do not serve much purpose unless periodic surveys are conducted to assess immunization status of the population. Such surveys are conducted on ad hoc basis and, also, there does not seem to be any regular programme in this direction.

Mention may also be made in this connection of attempts in the Directorate General of Health Services to standardize the other items of information generated in the working of primary health centre. In 1967, a regional seminar of the World Health Organisation was held on the subject. This was followed up in 1969 by a national seminar in the Directorate General of Health Services. Proformae for in-patient and out-patient cards, epidemiological cards, mothers', children cards and in-patient and out-patient registers have been streamlined and have been given to the state governments for adoption. Not much progress seems to have been made in the adoption of these proformae.

Health Manpower Data

One of the most important areas of statistics for social planning is on health manpower. These are usually drawn from the licence registers maintained for a few categories of personnel namely, doctors, nurses, dentists, pharmacists, midwives, auxiliary nurse mid-wives and health visitors, by state medical and nursing and pharmacy councils. These statistics suffer from well-known deficiencies. They are not kept upto-date since there is no system of renewal of registration. The figures for doctors are published in the two categories of graduates and licentiates. Those for nurses and mid-wives, ANMs and health visitors are published annually with sex break-up.

Some states, union territories do not have their own councils and they are covered by the council of the adjoining states. These statistics although available regularly on annual basis, do not exactly correspond with the geographical area of the state and consequently, the statistics are not useful for calculation of doctor or nurse population ratios. The other important source of information on health manpower is the individual slip canvassed in the population census. These slips give information, *inter alia*, on sex, age and occupation. The data so obtained are published according to the National Classification of Occupations of the Directorate General of Employment and Training, with total and urban break-up. Since occupation is the main criterion, there is a possibility that unqualified might have been enumerated as practising doctors and indigenous practising midwives. Apart from this limitation of census figures, they are at a certain point of time. From what has been stated above, it can be seen stocks of doctors, nurses and other categories of registered personnel are not available annually.

If the licence registers are brought up-to-date by a system of periodic renewal this source could prove immensely useful for providing information on health manpower and renewal has to be incorporated in law.

The Institute of Applied Manpower Research attempted estimates for doctors, nurses, dentists and pharmacists. These estimates are available for different states.

The available statistics on health manpower are unsatisfactory and, at present, standard methodology for providing annual estimates at the state level for different categories of personnel needs to be developed.

SURVEYS AND SPECIAL STUDIES

The contribution of National Sample Survey for health statistics was by way of conducting health interview surveys for estimating prevalence and incidence rates for rural and urban areas with sex and age break-up. Average duration sickness per spell, expenditure on medicine per month per person, percentage distribution of villages having medical practitioners, average distance of the nearest hospital by population size for sample villages were the other characteristics analysed. Such surveys were conducted during the 7-13 rounds and analysis of the data were presented in the N.S.S. report 49 (report on morbidity) and 54 (vital rates). Attempt was made to collect data on cause of sickness too.

Besides, as part of consumer expenditure survey, information on expenditure for medicine categories by systems of medicine was collected. Unfortunately separate estimates for medicine were not presented and these were clubbed together under the broad group, "miscellaneous."

Nine surveys were conducted in community development areas by the D.G.H.S. These surveys were conducted as general health surveys collecting data on morbidity and other socio-economic characteristics such as income, housing conditions, nutrition etc. The reports of these surveys were published. Follow-up surveys were not done in these areas. Many other ad hoc surveys also were done.

As part of the sample registration scheme additional information is being collected for deaths on the type of attendance (institutional, at home by recognized and unrecognized practitioner or none).

This information especially in the rural areas is useful to indicate to what extent the facilities made available are adequate or not. Collection of statistics on cause of death was precluded from the purview of the scheme.

Until 1931, enumeration of physical handicaps was attempted in the censuses and it was discontinued thereafter due to unreliability. The N.S.S. conducted a survey in one round on the physically handicapped, giving statewise distribution.

As a part of the control programmes for leprosy, trachoma, filaria, goitre etc. a series of surveys for case detection has been under way. The data thrown up have great potentialities for calculation of morbidity rates for the specific diseases. But the data have not been fully exploited. Besides, a nationwide sample survey first of its kind in India was conducted for T.B. covering sex-defined zones round the tuberculosis centres. Children below five years were excluded from the purview of the survey. Accessible rural areas within half mile to which mass X-ray unit could be taken were also covered. The survey could not throw up national estimates.

Apart from what has been mentioned, all surveys conducted were mainly local surveys ad hoc in nature, incapable of throwing up estimates of morbidity for a state or the country.

Under the aegis of the Central Statistical Organization an interview-cum-diagnostic survey on morbidity has been attempted on a pilot basis in Rajasthan, Uttar Pradesh and Gujarat in three selected districts. This survey has adopted a new approach not only conducting a post-mortem inquiry through lay and trained investigators into the past sickness with a suitable recall period but also to get the current sickness diagnosed by the medical personnel available in the areas selected. The survey in Rajasthan and Uttar Pradesh have been completed and is awaiting analysis and evaluation. The survey in Gujarat is awaiting completion. With this survey it can be told that to the already available approaches of collecting data on morbidity either through health interview survey which is not diagnostic in nature and the purely diagnostic surveys conducted in the community development blocks by the Directorate General of Health Services mentioned above is added another dimension of trying to get the current sickness diagnosed by the medical personnel. If this pilot survey proves to be successful this methodology can be extended to the other areas employing the existing survey organizations to use.

Environmental Sanitation

Statistics on the number of villages and towns covered with protected water supply are collected annually statewise from Public Health Engineering Organisations of the State Health Directorates. Statistics on adequacy of water supply provision of drainge facilities, water and air pollution are not collected.

Mention may also be made in this connection of the important work that has been done by the Directorate General of Health Services in getting the staff employed in the field of health statistics trained. The courses available are for intermediate statistical personnel like assistants, computers, medical coders, health statisticians at the supervisory level, medical record officers and technicians. Four institutions have been working in this regard, one at Model Vital and Health Statistical Unit, Nagpur; and others at the Christian Medical College, Vellore, Safdarjang Hospital, New Delhi, and at the All-India Institute of Hygiene and Public Health, Calcutta. The course at Calcutta is for health statisticians, and is of one year duration while the course at the Christian Medical College, Vellore, is for medical record officers with one year duration. The course at Safdarjang Hospital, New Delhi, for medical record technicians, is of six months duration, and the courses at Nagpur are of an average of ten weeks duration. In this connection, the course for medical coders, available at Nagpur, is of a special significance in view of the fact that the medical certification of cause of death is acquiring more momentum in this country than ever before.

These training programmes are being conducted for quite a number of years and are quite popular. The courses are open to the employees of the state health directorates, local bodies and other institutions. The Government of India encourages the utilization of these courses with a suitable stipend and TA for coming and going. It is considered that these training courses fill up the important gap in the development of the health statistics in this country.

Health Statistics in India: A Case Study of Kerala

P.G.K. PANIKAR*

INTRODUCTION

Improvement of general health of the population is one of the avowed objectives of our five-year plans. Obviously, the formulation of a health plan would require a sound data base. But such a data base was not available in India at the time of independence, as pointed out by the Bhore Committee.[1] The Health Survey and Planning Committee (Mudaliar Committee), reporting a decade and a half later, noted some progress in the field of health statistics.[2] Broadly speaking, the data position has registered further improvement since then. But are the available health statistics adequate to meet the data requirements of health planning?

Ideally, public health and medical care programmes must be linked with the pattern of morbidity and mortality. Therefore, planning of health programmes would require detailed information on the nature and extent of morbidity and the rate and causes of deaths. What are the most prevalent types of diseases? What factors—inadequate nutrition, poor sanitation and hygiene—account for them? Data on available health care delivery system are also needed in greater detail than now available. It is not enough to know the over all hospital-population ratio, bed-population ratio, physician-population ratio, per capita expenditure, etc. The effectiveness of a medical care delivery system would depend upon accessibility of the facilities as determined by the distribution of the institutions and personnel

*Centre for Development Studies, Trivandrum.

[1]Government of India, *Report of the Health Survey and Development Committee*, New Delhi, 1946, p. 272.

[2]Government of India, *Report of the Health Survey and Planning Committee*, Vol. I, 1962, pp. 202-204.

between regions, between rural and urban areas, between public and private sectors, the cost of medicines and so on.

The coverage of health statistics would depend upon that of health infrastructure. This is exemplified by the record of Kerala. Side by side with the extension of public health and medical care delivery system in this region, a machinery was evolved for the collection of health statistics from comparatively early times. Hence a case study of health statistics in Kerala should be useful.

HEALTH STATISTICS IN KERALA

Historical Evolution of Health Statistics in Kerala. The remarkable achievements of Kerala in health, as reflected in the low general and infant mortality rates and high expectation of life in comparison with the rest of India, have attracted wide attention in recent times. As pointed out elsewhere, this fall in mortality rates in the major part of Kerala started way back in the early decades of this century and could be attributed to a balanced development of public health and medical care programmes in this region from early times.[3] Concurrently with the extension of public health and medical care in the erstwhile states of Travancore and Cochin, a system of collection and compilation of health statistics had gradually evolved from early times.

The Administration Reports of the Governments of Travancore and Cochin include a wealth of information on the number of hospitals and dispensaries, the incidence of contagious diseases, the number of patients admitted and treated classified according to diseases, etc. The Administration Report of the Government of Travancore for the period 1862-64, for example, contains information on the number of patients treated in the hospitals and dispensaries, the annual cost of the hospitals and dispensaries with the break-up into physicians' salaries, cost of medicines, etc.

As one moves along, one notices a progressive expansion in the coverage of the reports. The Administration Report for 1875-76 contains information on the number of in-patients in each hospital at the beginning of the year, the number died, the number discharged, etc., the report also gives information on the number of vaccinations, total receipts and disbursements of the medical department, etc. By the time we come to the end of the last century, the coverage

[3]P.G.K. Panikar, Fall in Mortality Rates in Kerala, *Economic and Political Weekly*, Vol. X, No. 47, November 27, 1975.

of the administration report is seen to be further enlarged. Thus, the report for the year 1899-1900 contains some data on the incidence of chief diseases such as cholera, small-pox and fevers; it is interesting to find that the authorities had attempted to figure out the coverage of medical facilities. "The ratio to area and population was one Government medical institution for every 140.2 square miles and 53,286 of the population. Taking into consideration grant-in-aid institutions, the total was 97, one hospital/dispensary for every 69.5 square miles and 26,368 of population."[4]

This year's report also included, besides the usual information on the number of in-patients and out-patients treated, total expenditure on the medical establishments, etc., with some break-up of expenditure like average cost on diet and medicines per patient.

A quarter of a century later, the administration report for the year 1925-26 incorporates more details, the number of in-patients and out-patients treated in government institutions and grant-in-aid institutions, the strength of the medical personnel in government hospitals and dispensaries, more detailed break-up of the expenditure of the medical and sanitary departments, number of deaths classified according to diseases, taluk-wise data on sanitation work, etc.

Public health surveys and investigation were launched from the beginning of the thirties. The authorities had recognised the value of health statistics sufficiently early, as is evident from an observation in the administration report for the year 1930-31: "As correct morbidity statistics are essential to the planning of public health work, it was decided to collect such statistics as an experimental work in one of the taluks, viz., Vilavancode. The epidemiologist and his field staff made house to house enquiries daily regarding the incidence of infectious diseases such as cholera, small-pox, chicken-pox, enteric fever, as well as chronic diseases like malaria, tuberculosis and leprosy."[5] A hookworm survey covering most parts of the state was completed during this year.

By the time of independence, we notice further widening of the scope of the annual reports so as to include details on the number of institutions, and persons treated under the western and indigenous systems of medicine, number of deaths classified according to causes,

[4]Government of Travancore, *Report on the Administration of Travancore*, 1075 (1899-1900), p. 94.

[5]Government of Travancore, *Report on the Administration of Travancore*, 1106 (1930-31), p. 185.

training of para-medical personnel, number of labour cases attended by medical officers and midwives, registration of practitioners under the different systems, etc. In the adjacent princely state of Cochin also similar progress is discernible over the years in the collection and reporting of health statistics. Thus, in brief, at the time of the formation of the state, Kerala had already a long tradition of a fairly comprehensive data base in the field of health. Currently, collection and compilation of health statistics in Kerala conforms to the all-India scheme laid down by the Directorate of Health Intelligence, Ministry of Health and Family Planning, Government of India. Such data have been published as an annual series, *Health Statistics of India.* In the following section we shall examine some of the salient features and limitations of these data.

Morbidity Statistics. In the nature of things, there cannot be complete and accurate data on morbidity in any community; this is especially so in a country like India where the infrastructure of health is underdeveloped. Information on the incidence of diseases in Kerala, as in other States, is being collected through a network of medical care institutions like primary health centres and hospitals and other reporting agencies. The data are compiled on a weekly or monthly basis in prescribed proformas and transmitted to higher authorities. Finally they are pooled together and published annually by the Central Bureau of Health Intelligence in *Health Statistics of India.*

Such statistics are characterized by incomplete coverage and low degree of reliability. Gaps in coverage result from two reasons: (*i*) A good proportion of the sick do not avail themselves of medical aid and thereby fail to register their morbidity, like the invisible portion of the proverbial iceberg this chunk of morbidity goes unnoticed, escaping the net of official data collection machinery, and (*ii*) the same is the case with a sizable number of persons who receive treatment in private hospitals and dispensaries or under indigenous systems of medicine like *Ayurveda* and *Unani.* Thus, only a portion, and this portion is apt to be small, which enters the portals of government institutions of modern medicine is captured in official statistics of morbidity.

True, thanks to a more even spatial distribution of medical care institutions in Kerala, a larger proportion of the population avail of the facilities.[6] This would imply that the coverage of morbidity

[6]Centre for Development Studies, *Poverty, Unemployment and Development Policy*, Department of Social and Economic Affairs, United Nations, New York, 1975, Chapter X.

statistics in Kerala would be more representative than elsewhere in India. But, the data is still incomplete in view of the fact that in Kerala both the Ayurvedic system, and private hospitals and dispensaries under the modern system of medicine are well established and widely resorted to.[7]

We will now turn to the question of reliability of the data. Published data on the subject appear under two heads: causes of mortality, and diseases of patients treated in hospitals and dispensaries. Presumably the former set of data is based on model registration scheme and the reliability of the reported causes of deaths is any body's guess. On the other hand, the morbidity data relating to patients treated in hospitals and dispensaries have a diagnostic base.

True, owing to the disproportionately large number of patients that any one physician has to handle in a typical institution in Kerala, where the daily turnout is quite heavy, the diagnosis cannot be sufficiently detailed or thorough. Novertheless, *prima facie*, the primary data may be expected to be reliable. However, there is many a slip between the cup and the lip; errors may enter into the final figures through the various stages of compilation. Thus, for example, according to the published data, the number of in-patients and out-patients treated for Kala-azar in Kerala in 1959 came to 10,613 and 40,611 respectively. Next year, the corresponding numbers were 7,379 and 3,39,402.

In the subsequent years also, the incidence of Kala-azar appears to be more or less of this order of magnitude.[8] But according to knowledgeable persons in the local medical profession, the incidence of this disease is usually brought to the notice of teaching hospitals and during the last two decades not more than two or three cases have been reported.[9] It is significant to note that the entry of this curious

[7]As of 1956-57, at the time of the formation of the state, there were 22 Ayurvedic hospitals and 97 dispensaries in Kerala, and the total number of patients treated in these Government Ayurvedic institutions stood at about 3.6 million. By 1967-68, Kerala had 37 Ayurvedic hospitals and 207 dispensaries and 8 special institutions; the total number of cases treated in these government institutions added up to about 9.4 million. See *The Kerala State Administration Reports* 1956-57 (p. 204) and 1967-68 (p. 192).

[8]Central Bureau of Health Intelligence, *Health Statistics of India*, 1959-60, 1961-62, 1964 and 1965.

[9]Kala-azar (Leishmania) is a parastic affection of human beings, the responsible parasite being Leishmania Donovan. The disease is relatively unknown in Kerala as the vector, sandflea (transmitting agent) does not occur in Kerala.

item figures repeatedly in a number of successive years and that the number involved runs into hundreds of thousands. If it is true that the incidence of this disease has been so rare as competent authorities assert categorically, this entry knocks the bottom out of the credibility of official morbidity statistics.

Then the question arises as to how such errors get into the final figures. As mentioned earlier, it is possible that the errors creep in at the various stages of compilation. Under the present scheme, every reporting unit like the primary health centre or hospital has to submit numerous statements on the incidence of various diseases within its jurisdiction. There are weekly, fortnightly and monthly statements to be prepared in the prescribed proformas.

In the case of certain diseases more than one proforma is to be filled up every month, if not every week. The officers in charge of these institutions have to attend to this type of chores in addition to their normal professional duties and without sufficient supporting staff. Usually such compilation work is done by L.D. Clerks, again in addition to their routine administrative jobs. With such a multiplicity of proformas and an overburdened staff who soon develop fatigue compilation of morbidity data is given a low priority. Errors and discrepancies may get in at subsequent stages, at the district level, at the state level and so on all along the line.

It is perhaps pertinent to ask whether any one carefully scrutinises these morbidity data before they are published. Do the planners and policy makers ever make use of these data? If the answers to these questions are in the negative, one wonders why do we go through the motion of collection and compilation of such data?

Health Services. "The main components of a total health service system are identified as personal health (or medical care) services, environmental health (or public health) services, and education and research. In addition to these service components, a component identified as resources provides the manpower, building space, technological equipment, and materials that are allocated to provide the three types of service.[10] For Kerala, as for other states, available data include the above-mentioned components. But the data are inadequate in coverage and detail.

(*i*) Published data on medical care services consist of the number

[10] Dr. H. Mahler, Report to the Regional Director (Background Paper for the Regional Meeting of Senior Medical Administrators from SEARO), W.H.O., New Delhi, Mimeographed, p. 4.

of institutions like hospitals, dispensaries and primary health centres, number of beds, specialised centres like maternity hospitals, tuberculosis hospitals, V.D. clinics, etc. Information is also available on public expenditure on medical subjects with some broad break-up like medical establishment, hospitals and dispensaries, medical colleges and schools laboratories, etc. However, as mentioned earlier, the official statistics do not include hospitals and clinics run by private organisations and individuals. As a matter of fact, the private sector of medical care is comparatively well developed in the State. No information whatsoever is available on private expenditure on medical care by way of doctors' consultation fees, hospital charges, medicines, etc.

(*ii*) The data on public health services in Kerala cover immunization against cholera, small-pox, plague and tuberculosis, malaria eradication programme and provision of protected water supply. Expenditure on public health by the government under broad heads such as control of epidemic diseases, bacteriological laboratories, establishment, etc. and per capita expenditure are published every year. No data are forthcoming on the availability of sanitary latrines, drainage and sewerage or other aspects of environmental sanitation, a crucial factor governing the incidence of communicable diseases which dominate the morbidity pattern in the developing countries.

(*iii*) The number of doctors, dentists, pharmacists and nurses registered with the State Medical Councils are published. Information on the number of institutions for the training of medical and para-medical personnel, their capacity and annual out-turn, and annual expenditure on the training programmes is also available. It would, however, be interesting to know the ultimate disposition of these personnel trained at considerable public expense. How many of them are absorbed in the government medical care and public health service? How many join private clinics or set up independent practice? How many doctors serve in the rural areas where the vast majority of the population live? How many migrate to foreign countries? As it is, no information is readily available to provide answers to these important questions.

An Overall Assessment of Data

In the foregoing sections we examined the categories of health statistics in Kerala, their coverage and reliability. True, the scope and coverage of the data have been widened over the years. Still it is pertinent to ask: do we know enough about this problem? The answer to this question would depend, in the final analysis, upon what we need the information for.

Health statistics are needed for empirical studies in the health field. Recent years have witnessed the emergence of health economics, a branch built upon the findings of empirical studies in this field. Studies relating to the demand for health covering the income and price elasticity of demand for health services and demand projections for various types of health servlces are one set of empirical studies.[11] Another set of studies deals with the supply aspects such as production function for hospitals, economies of scale in medical practice, analysis of costs of hospital service, etc.[12] These empirical studies seek to give a picture of the working of the health care delivery system, the inputs and outputs of the health sector, the efficiency, or lack of it, in the allocation of resources, the cost (and reasons for the rising cost) of medical care, its accessibility and rate of utilization of the facilities, etc.

By and large, the above may be described as positive studies, although the techniques and tools developed therefrom are highly useful for normative studies. A major development of this latter category, that is normative studies with applied orientation, consists of cost-benefit analysis and cost-effectiveness analysis. By their use it is possible to select an optimal approach from a group of feasible alternatives; with the use of these techniques it will be possible to maximise the efficiency of both the programmes which serve the people and the administrative procedures which these programmes dictate.[13]

[11]Morris Silver, "An Economic Analysis of Variations in Medical Expenses and Work-loss Rates," in Herbert E. Klarman (ed) *Empirical Studies in Health Economics*, Johns Hopkins Press, 1970; See also: Victor R. Fuchs "Growing Demand for Medical Care," in Victor R. Fuchs (ed) *Essays in the Economics of Health and Medical Care*, National Bureau of Economic Research, New York, 1972.

[12]Martin S. Feldstein, *Economic Analysis for Health Service Efficiency*, North-Holland Publishing Company, Amsterdam, 1967; Richard M. Baily, "Economies of Scale in Medical Practice," Empirical Studies in Health Economics op. cit.; Harold A. Cohen, "Hospital cost curves with Emphasis on Measuring Patient Case Output," Ibid; Edgar W. Francis, "Analysis of cost variation Among Shortterm General Hospitals," Ibid., etc.

[13]Royal A. Crystal and Agnes W. Brewster, "Cost Benefit and Cost Effectiveness Analyses in the Health Field—An Introduction," *Inquiry* Vol. 3, No. 4, 1966. See Also: C. Teeling—Smith, "Health-Economic and Cost-benefit Analysis" in *Health Planning and Organisation of Medical Care*, World Health Organisation, Copenhagen, 1972; Robert N. Grosse, "Cost-Benefit Analysis of Health Services," *The Annals of the American Academy*; "Cost Effectiveness and Cost-Benefit Analysis of Tuberculosis Programmes

Empirical studies of the above types require a great deal of data of considerable detail. For example, the empirical analysis of demand for health care would require detailed information on medical expenses, family income, cost of medical care services, etc. Economic analysis of the cost of medical care would involve data on direct costs such as medical, nursing, professional and technical staff and material resources like clothing, bedding, and laundry, drugs, surgical appliances and equipment, buildings, furniture, etc. Medical care also implies indirect costs by way of loss of income or production through sickness absence. The extent of coverage and details of the health statistics of Kerala available at present are clearly inadequate for carrying out such quantitative analysis.

CONCLUSION

To improve the data availability we would offer two suggestions. First we would propose more detailed compilation by interested researchers of the data presently buried in the hospital records. The nature of services provided by selected hospitals, pattern of morbidity, diseases which need hospitalisation, the relationship between distance from hospital and utilisation of the hospital services by the surrounding population, average length of stay of particular categories of patients, etc. can be collated from hospital records.

Second, community health surveys may be initiated to collect primary data on sanitation, vital statistics, prevalence of morbidity, the patterns of response to sickness, the preference pattern vis-a-vis different systems of medicine, expenditure on medical treatment, and various socio-economic characteristics. Needless to say, the quality of data would depend upon the extent to which they are used. The quality will improve when, and only when, planners and policy makers and social scientists start using the data.

---

in the Countries of South-East Asia," World Health Organisation, Regional Office for South-East Asia, August 1972.

Hospital Records In India

F.E. MARKER

Hospital records can be broadly divided into two categories: (*1*) Administrative Records, and (*2*) Patient Records.

Administrative Records

Administrative Records may be divided into: (*a*) financial, (*b*) material, (*c*) personnel, and (*d*) infrastructural requirements i.e., food, medical supplies, stores, laundry, water, ambulance, garbage, sanitation, etc.

Administrative Records represent a major neglected area of social statistics. The application of modern management techniques in the collection and use of this data can yield spectcular results in affecting savings and improving service.

Data on administrative records are submitted to the state governments in two statements annually.

Statement 'F' indicates the income and expenditure for the hospital. The items of expenditure include salaries, cost of medicines, expenditure on diet, operating theatres, ancillary services, capital expenditure on buildings and equipment and miscellaneous expenditure.

Statement 'A' refers to the type of hospital urban/rural and general/specialized.

Statement 'B' lists the number of personnel according to the different categories employed by the hospital.

Patient Records

Non-clinical

Statement 'C' shows the in-door and out-patient attendance according to male, female, and children. The deaths and deliveries are also shown on this statement.

INDOOR

Bed Strength. The bed strength of a hospital is the actual number of beds sanctioned for that particular hospital, by a specific order or Government Resolution. The bed strength must be clearly distinguished from the actual number of "bed-steads" that may be available in the hospital. The bed strength is a factor that is utilized in several calculations by the administration for framing the budget and analysing the facilities available. The total bed strength is distributed among the departments available in the hospital. Discrepancies arise when the administration adds to or increases the number of beds in a hospital in the absence of formal sanction. When this occurs, the figures for admission and occupancy of the hospital rise while the sanctioned bed strength remains unaltered. All calculations based on this bed strength are therefore rendered erroneous.

Bed Occupancy. The beds occupied on a particular day, may be in excess or may fall short of the number of "sanctioned" beds. The bed occupancy ratio

$$\frac{\text{Total number of occupied days}}{\text{Number of beds available for the same period}} \times 100$$

measures the utilization of bed facilities and will be affected if the sanctioned bed strength has not been correctly arrived at for reasons mentioned in the previous paragraph.

The figures for total admissions, discharges and deaths as they occur in a hospital may be taken as fairly reliable. The number of births and deliveries can also be taken as reliable.

Operations. The proforma on which the Operation Statement 'E' is compiled was drawn up about forty years ago and has not been revised since. The advances made in operative surgery over this period are so vast that a large number of operations performed today are not included in the list and have perforce to be entered in a miscellaneous group. For example, operations on the brain only show two sub-divisions (*i*) For abscess, tumour or cyst, (*ii*) Other operations; and operations on the thorax are sub-divided into (*a*) paracentesis of pleural cavity, (*b*) incision and drainage of pleural cavity, (*c*) artificial pneumothorax and (*d*) other operations.

Resection of brain tissue, ventriculography and stereotaxis cannot be accounted for nor is there any mention of operations on the heart and lungs.

The sub-division of operations into major and minor, has not been clearly defined and therefore comparisons from different groups of hospitals on this basis become meaningless.

OUT-PATIENT

New patients. There is no difficulty in collecting the attendance figures for new patients being registered in the out-patient department.

The difficulties arise in trying to list these cases by disease. This is partly due to the fact that the physician does not mention the diagnosis on the case paper and partly due to the fact that patients do not go through the complete set of investigations required, for the doctor to conclude a final diagnosis. Under the prevailing conditions in most general hospital out-patient departments, the patient rarely gets to see the same doctor again on a subsequent visit and the diagnosis remains unentered on the case paper.

In spite of the fact that the diagnosis is lacking on the case papers, the compounders working in the dispensaries are expected to return monthly and annual statements on the number of patients treated according to the various diseases. It is common knowledge that they do so on a purely arbitrary basis trying to match the figures of the previous report which was in all probability prepared in the same manner. Superintendents are submitting these reports under their signature without so much glancing through the figures to question or weed out obvious incongruities of relatively rare conditions like meningococcal infection being reported from a small non-urban hospital in several hundreds.

Statistics on diagnostic or disease data on out-patients should therefore be totally ignored from all except a very few institutions in the country.

Old patients. The method of counting the attendance of "old" or "repeat" patients in the out-patient department varies from hospital to hospital. In most hospitals the out-patient case paper is retained by the dispensary after dispensing medicines. In such cases the old patient is counted when he comes on a subsequent visit to collect his case paper before attending a clinic or requesting continuation of treatment.

In hospitals where the out-patient case paper is retained by the patient, the attendance is counted by each department he visits, or at the dispensary if he is renewing his prescription. Since some patients may not be counted at all, and others be counted more than once on a single day, these figures can only be taken as a rough estimate of the attendance in the out-patient department.

All out-patient figures are generally available in the format:

Old				New				Total			
Adults		*Children*		*Adults*		*Children*		*Adults*		*Children*	
M	F	M	F	M	F	M	F	M	F	M	F

Clinical: The Medical Record. The medical record is defined as a document containing the patient's identification particulars and in which are entered the history of his ailment, the clinical examination, investigations and sufficient data written in sequence of events to justify the diagnosis and warrant the treatment and end results.

Identification and Sociological Factors

The identification and sociological factors are used mainly for administrative purposes.

Age. While compiling statistics by age from hospital records, it must be borne in mind that a large number of patients seeking treatment in the general and public hospitals do not know their exact age, and it can only be arrived at to the nearest decade. It is not an infrequent occurrence to find that a patient gives his age to be less than that recorded during a previous admission.

We do find however that in the younger age group, there is a greater degree of accuracy and parents are able to produce the age or date of birth of their child from records of their delivery or from school health cards.

Occupation. Though diagnostic statistics by occupation are very relevant for certain diseases, currently only information on cancer is being requested according to occupation. The occupation of a patient requires to be enquired into in greater detail before entering words like "service" and "general worker."

Income. The correct income is not necessarily revealed by the patient for obvious reasons.

The declared income distribution for the year 1970 in a Government Hospital is given below:

Monthly Income:	*% of Total Patients*
Nil	40.18
Rs 0-150	50.86
Rs 150-250	7.06
Rs 250-500	1.46
Rs 500 and above	0.41

Address. Complete addresses are not always available. This is particularly so in cases when the patient resides in a temporary dwelling in a "bustee" "jhugi" or "hutment" and this factor has greatly hampered the conduct of follow-up studies.

Clinical Details

The clinical part of the medical record is deteriorating rapidly in quality, since the attending physician who is primarily responsible for an accurate and adequate medical record is not fulfilling this respon sibility. The administration is not specifically empowered or authorized to reject sub-standard records and has proved incapable of disciplining the attending physician who neglects the medical records of patients entrusted to his care.

The notes entered by the resident or intern should be carefully read through and signed by the physician incharge of the case, who thereby accepts the responsibility for the accuracy and adequacy of the medical record, an obligation which he should be assuming when he accepts the responsibility for the care of the patient. The notes entered by the resident or intern are not necessarily scrutinized by the physician incharge of the case.

Absence of attention to the medical record in a teaching institution is a sad reflection on the lack of supervised instruction being imparted to undergraduates and postgraduates.

The scientific value of a medical record is in direct proportion to the care with which it has been compiled. The present state of the medical record renders it quite invalid for purposes of retrospective research.

History. Histories of patients are inadequately entered and woefully lacking in pertinent data. Vagueness cannot be dismissed on the grounds of lack of fluency in the English language.

Physical Findings. Recording of the findings on physical examination of the patient often reveals that too little thought and time have been spent on this important aspect, and basic data on the patient's affliction is lacking.

Investigations. When an investigation is asked for it is the duty of the department conducting the investigation to see to it, that a written report of the investigation signed by a competent authority of the department, reaches the Consultant requesting the same within 24 hours of the investigation having been ordered.

The report of an investigation is as much an integral part of the medical record as the history, examination and treatment entered therein. Yet, we find that reports are removed from the case record by interested parties rendering it unusable by others for want of essential data.

Diagnosis. The diagnosis as set down on the case paper is far too frequently incomplete. The diagnosis must essentially indicate the system or part of the body affected with its etiology, and the site of the lesion should be indicated.

In the absence of a standard nomenclature being adopted for general use, the terminology employed in writing a diagnosis is too often, vague, incomplete or incorrect. A common example is "Blunt Injury." The instrument with which the injury was inflicted may be blunt, but the resulting injury should only be defined using terminology prescribed for describing traumatic lesions *e.g.* bruise, haematoma, abrasion, contusion, etc.

Diagnostic data from most institutions is being compiled according to the International Classification of Diseases (WHO).

The main drawback of this classification is that it is based on the selection of a *single* underlying cause, and though codes have been provided for certain categories of two or more conditions jointly reported *e.g.* 382 "Otitis media with mastoiditis," difficulties arise when a patient is suffering simultaneously from two or more unrelated diseases *e.g.*, pulmonary tuberculosis and diabetes mellitus.

The determination of which of two or more diagnoses is primary and which is secondary is influenced by the interpretation of the individual coders. No universal rule can be stated since a diagnosis which is primary in one situation may be secondary in another. This fact invalidates the statistics of primary and secondary diagnoses. Recognition of these facts has influenced many institutions to stop the cross-indexing of primary and secondary diagnoses and to record all conditions, whether primary, secondary, or associated on the appropriate disease-classification card without reference to their relationship.

Since the diagnostic index in a teaching hospital is used for retrieving material for study, in addition to providing a disease classification, symptoms and syndromes where the underlying cause is known are also coded additionally *e.g.* "Rheumatic Mitral Stenosis with Congestive Cardiac Failure" 394.0 and 427.0. While compiling a statement of diseases, the latter should be excluded.

A satisfactory classification for the multiple conditions arising during pregnancy, labour and the puerperium which affect the mother and the foetus in different ways has yet to be devised.

Operation Notes. Operation notes are often wanting in the details required. Lesions exposed during an operation and operative procedures are often sketchy and poorly described:

> "The area was cleaned, the part was draped, the tumour was exposed and the swelling excised. All bleeding points were ligated, and the wound was closed in layers."

It would be almost impossible to study the effect of changing methods of operative treatment from operation notes as they are entered today. On several occasions the operation notes have been found to be totally inadequate when a patient has been readmitted for post-operative complications. The insertion and removal of drainage tubes, the condition of the operation wound on discharge and removal of sutures are rarely entered on the case paper by the attending surgeons. The anaesthetist's record appears on the case paper only in a few hospitals.

Treatment. The treatment ordered for a patient is generally recorded on a separate order sheet or on the regular case sheet and signed by the physician.

However, the actual drugs and dosage given to the patient are often recorded only in the sister's day order book and not on the patient's case paper. In some institutions, the nurses' notes are available on the medical case record, while in others only injections are charted on the temperature chart.

This makes it very difficult to assess the total amount of medication given to a patient, either to gauge its efficacy or to determine the cost of treating certain selected conditions.

Progress Notes. It would appear from going through the majority of case records that the medical resident and intern has not been taught the purpose of or the method of making notes on the patient's progress in the hospital between admission and discharge.

Data in this part of the medical record are totally incomplete, inaccurate and unreliable, entries often being added retrospectively, when there is a sudden deterioration in the patient's condition.

Discharge Note. The condition of the patient at the time of being discharged from hospital is rarely recorded, much less, is it compared to his condition at the time of admission and a final assessment made of his progress.

Discharge Summary. The discharge summary serves two main functions. Primarily it aids the attending physician to obtain a quick and clear picture of the patient's previous illness, treatment and results in the event of a readmission.

Secondly, it is an invaluable tool for training the resident or intern, in the selection of the salient points of the case and presenting them in a concise manner for use by other persons who have not attended on the patient but require information regarding his illness.

Unfortunately the discharge summary is looked upon as an unnecessary "chore" rather than as an essential and logical conclusion to the medical record.

Major Gaps in Data Required for Social and Economic Planning

The major gaps in data collected from hospital records are qualitative rather than quantitative.

Though all the agencies mentioned earlier in this paper and others have held conferences, seminars and workshops to emphasize the need for good medical records and have made recommendations and passed resolutions regarding budget requirements, staffing patterns, standardization of forms and equipment required none of them has taken any positive steps to analyse or improve the quality of data being generated from the medical record.

The basic foundation of medical statistics, namely the quality of the medical record and the time taken to complete it has been completely and thoroughly neglected. No matter how detailed the items of data collected or how sophisticated the tools of compilation, the end result of any statistical tabulation can only be as accurate as the data from which it has been compiled.

That the medical profession practising in the hospitals is directly responsible for this state of affairs cannot be denied. This impasse will only be overcome when they accept and react constructively to the prevailing situation. Only then will medical statistics become meaningful. However, the statisticians and the agencies concerned with the collection and compilation of hospital data cannot remain aloof from this problem and ignore the quality of one of their basic tools.

Distribution of proformae for the required information by the agencies to the hospitals, followed by a bombardment of reminders will not yield the requisite results.

The time-lag for the completion of case records has in some cases exceeded one year.

It would not be out of order to quote here from the conclusions and recommendations of Miss Mary Sue Meads, short-term WHO Consultant in Medical Records requisitioned by the Office of the Directorate General Health Services in early 1974 to assist in the development of medical record departments in hospitals with particular emphasis on the essential information required for health and health administration.

> . . . The production of quality medical records has low priority when compared with the many other needs of the hospital . . . .
>
> . . . The impetus to begin keeping quality medical records and to establish medical records departments must come from the physicians not from statisticians, and therefore, until the doctors insist upon organized medical records departments the hospital authorities should devise other means of supplying the required statistics.
>
> . . . In the leading hospitals with organized medical records departments, attention should be given to raising the quality of diagnostic data.
>
> . . . Standardization of forms and procedures is not as urgent a need as are the standardization of data requirements and definition of terms.
>
> . . . An organized effort to acquaint the physicians of the country with the need for in-patient data and to solicit their cooperation at all levels should be initiated immediately. . . .

Implementation of these recommendations is long overdue, and if cooperation cannot be solicited, the requirements should be enforced by making the necessary provisions in the rules and regulations governing the conduct and performance of physicians in the hospital.

There is no forseeable reason as to why a beginning cannot be made in this direction by making it mandatory for the physician under whose care the patient has been treated to sign the medical case record within forty eight hours of the discharge of the patient and further to specifically empower the head of the Institution to reject substandard records.

The quality of the medical record in a teaching institution may be taken as a direct measure of the quality of the instruction being imparted. The medical record passes its own judgement on the author.

It is therefore doubly important and equally urgent that this situation be remedied without further delay and that the doctors graduating from these colleges each year be made to realize the importance and the value of complete, concise and accurate medical records.

A properly compiled medical record contains a wealth of information and an improvement in its maintenance would greatly enhance its utility. Simultaneously, greater utilization of the medical record would act as an added impetus to better record keeping, thus helping to break the vicious cycle of neglected records which cannot be utilized and lack of purpose causing a further deterioration in the character of the medical record.

Diagnostic Data

Another major point arising from the collection of diagnostic data from hospital records is discussed below.

Under the prevailing system of maintaining medical records, the case papers of all patients discharged from the wards do not necessarily reach the Medical Records Department.

For various reasons, they are either withheld in the wards or removed therefrom by the clinicians or the administration. Further, incomplete case papers are requisitioned from the Medical Records Department and are not returned to it.

The diagnoses from these incomplete and missing papers are therefore not posted on the diagnostic index, the use of which for the collection of morbidity and mortality data leaves a lacuna in the total number of cases to be covered for a particular period.

When the number of incomplete and missing case papers is large or when it affects one particular category of cases, the data produced will present a false picture.

The measurement of morbidity and mortality data as taken from hospital records would therefore be impaired at its origin, unless all entries in the sample are accounted for.

While tabulating morbidity and mortality data from hospitals, no check appears to be kept on or provision made for missing case papers. For a given period, a given number of cases are covered, the number is fixed according to the patients admitted during that period or the patients discharged and those who have died during that particular period. By convention, the latter is in general use.

At the end of the tabulation, one finds that the total number of cases reported upon fall short of the number of cases that should have been included for study, namely the total number of patients discharged and deaths occurring during the period under study.

Since no permanent record is kept as to which cases have been discharged during a particular period, it becomes impossible to check on this deficiency.

To maintain a separate list of the daily discharges would mean extra work for most of the poorly staffed hospitals in the country.

We should therefore consider an alternative base which is readily available against which the completeness of data collected can be readily checked.

The alternative which presents itself is the admission register in which the numbers run serially and in which the diagnosis is entered on discharge of the patient. The admission register affords quick and easy reference to the material contained in it. This method has been in use at the J. J. Group of Hospitals for over 16 years and yields very good results. Before compiling the diagnostic Statement we are able to account for every patient admitted during the calendar year under study.

The CBHI is collecting hospital data under the age groups:

(*i*) Under one year, single years 1 to 4 years, 5 year groups from 5 to 84 years, and over 84 years.

(*ii*) Under one year, 1-4 years, 5-14 years, 15-24 years, 25-34 years, 35-44 years, 45-54 years, 55-64 years, 65-74 years, 75 years and over.

Since 42 per cent of the population in this country is below 14 years of age, there should be greater emphasis on the younger age groups rather than on the age groups 55-65 years, 65·74 years, 75 years and over in a country where the expectation of life at birth is 45-47 years.

Furthermore, hospitals in India consider "children" as 12 years and under, while "adults" are considered to be 13 years and over. It would therefore be more practical to subdivide the age group of 5-14 years into 5-12 years and 13-14 years, to render the results more practical for use in our country.

Other suggested age groups are 000 years (still births) 1-7 days, 1-4 weeks, 1 month-1 year, 1-4 years.

SUMMARY

Statistics from Hospital Records cover a wide range of indices.

The maintenance of Hospital Records varies from the almost non-existent to the fairly well supervised ones in selected hospitals.

Sufficient attention is not being paid to the quality of the medical records and attention must be focussed on the medical profession to re-educate them in the art of history taking and the necessity for complete, concise and accurate medical records to serve the best interests of the patient, the doctors, the hospital administration and last but not least to render worthwhile the efforts of the statistician who is struggling with a mass of data trying to convert it into usable material for social and economic planning.

APPENDIX

Agencies Collecting Data from Hospital Records

I. International Statistical Organizations	World Health Organization	
	↑	
II. Government Agencies: Centre	Directorate General of Health Services (D.G.H.S.) and (C.B.H.I.)	
	↑	
State	Directorate of Health Services (D.H.S.) and (S.B.H.I.)	
	↑	↑
	Directorate of Medical Education	
	↑	
	Medical College Hospitals	District Hospitals
Special Agencies:	National Institute of Communicable Diseases, New Delhi	
III. Other Agencies:	Municipal Corporation Indian Council of Medical Research Indian Cancer Society Employees' State Insurance Scheme	

Hospital Records

- **Administrative**
  1. Financial
  2. Material
  3. Personnel
  4. Infrastructural requirements viz:
     - (*a*) Food
     - (*b*) Medical supplies
     - (*c*) Stores
     - (*d*) Laundry
     - (*e*) Water
     - (*f*) Ambulance
     - (*g*) Garbage
     - (*h*) Sanitation etc.
- **Patient Records**
  - **Non-Clinical**
    - **Indoor**
      1. Bed Strength
      2. Bed Occupancy
      3. Length of Stay
      4. Admissions
      5. Discharges
      6. Deaths
      7. Births
      8. Still Births
      9. Deliveries
      10. Operations
      11. Investigations
      12. Special Facilities
    - **Outdoor**
      - New patients attending
      - Old patients attending
  - **Clinical**

Medical Record

- **Identification and sociological factors**
  1. Name
  2. Age
  3. Sex
  4. Marital Status
  5. Occupation
  6. Income
  7. Religion
  8. Address
  9. Dates of Admission and discharge
  10. Mode of discharge
- **Clinical details**
  1. History
  2. Physical Findings
  3. Investigations
  4. Diagnosis
  5. Operation Notes
  6. Treatment:
     - (*a*) Drugs and Orders
     - (*b*) Physiotherapy
     - (*c*) Occupational Therapy
  7. Progress Notes
  8. Discharge Note
  9. Discharge Summary

Hospital Statistics

GOPAL KADEKODI*

The hospital system in India is a unique instance of demonstrating the classical Say's law that supply creates its own demand. With improvements and additions to our hospital facilities, the demand for hospitalisation has also been increasing markedly. This, however, cannot be taken for a measure of efficiency of any hospital system. Efficiency is to be measured by correlating the utilization of hospital facilities with costs and managerial improvements.

The hospital system in our country (as much as in many others) has some peculiar characteristics which make this system totally unidentifiable.

One of the first factors that distinguishes this sector from others is that medical profession and the associated hospital environment completely separates the information between a patient (consumer) and doctor (producer). Adam Smith's invisible hand does not work when consumer ignorance dominates. If only a survey or census data were available, we could show that almost 95 per cent of the patients do not know what they suffer from, what are the long-run or short-run effects of the disease, what are the medicines given, what for is the doctor a specialist etc. All that a patient knows is to trust the doctor. The patient ignorance clubbed with specialization in the profession and the referral system makes the system totally closed.

Needless to say that evaluation of any health system has to be based on the principle of "need" rather than standard principle of costing and pricing. Thus the concepts of efficiency for this industry have to be carefully defined and measured. Above all, health being both an investment (human capital) and enjoyment (personal consumption), evaluation of any health care system, either in a macro-economic model or in a micro-system becomes subjective. Peculiar to our health care system is the socialisation of the facility under the public health

*Associate Professor, Institute of Economic Growth, Delhi.

programme and facilities hence they are typically non-profit institutions in nature.

Many of the single or multi-purpose hospitals are also teaching hospitals. Thus the hospital systems can also be characterized as joint production units with the types of services being quite heterogeneous. In the absence of methods and data information to isolate the factors, functions and relationships between the multi-purpose units, evaluation of any hospital system has become a matter of judgement.

These are some of the major characteristics of a hospital system from the point of view of a social scientist that are distinct and make health economics a concern of social scientists.

Hospital Economics

There are a number of economic issues to be identified and analyzed for better hospital planning and administration. We only mention the major ones to strengthen our views on hospital statistics. Classically, most economists and hospital planners are, at one stage or the other, interested in the relation between the size of a hospital system and its efficiency. It has been found in the U.S., that the single speciality type of hospitals do really enjoy the advantages of economies of scale whereas the multi-purpose speciality hospitals are not found so economical.[1] Only next to this efficiency issue is a problem of allocating beds to different specialities in multi-purpose hospitals as in our country.

A recent study by a group of researchers from the National Institute of Health Administration and Education[2] has found that the allocation of beds to different specialities varied between hospitals and the variation could not be strictly linked to the occurrence of the types of diseases (requiring in-patient treatment) and the geographical and locational pattern of hospitals in the north zone.

Another important aspect of hospital management is the utilization of medical manpower. The manpower planning in hospital environment requires: integration and balancing, bed/doctor, patient/doctor,

[1]See Larry J. Kimbell and J.H. Lorant "Physician Productivity the effects of speciality, mix and scale" (mimeo) Human Resources Research Centre, University of Southern California, 1973.

[2]See T.J. Ramaiah, G. Radhaiah, M. Kataria and A. Timmappaya "Systems Analysis of Hospital Bed Utilization," NIHAE Research Report No. 23. 1974. They also note variations in bed utilization rates between specialities, between hospitals (state and other).

and equipment to doctor relationships and setting the relationships between doctors, nurses and other supportive staff. Thus the vertical and horizontal identification and the integration of personnel, equipment, bed and patient relationships call for a proper occupationwise manpower demand model. The projections of manpower for health services do require a variety of statistical information regarding population, hospital systems, diseases, personnel under training etc.

The utilization of hospital facility, though does not measure allocative efficiency, can reveal several issues like misuse of beds in certain types of facilities and the tendencies to lengthen the average length of stay (as related to hospital size, for the rural and urban population etc). The utilization of bed facilities can be studied using several factors like patient characteristics (income of the patient, distance, rural and urban based, family size, head of the household or not etc.) hospital and physician characteristics.[3] Often social scientists suggest evaluation methods like benefit-cost analysis, cost-effectiveness, PERT analysis etc. to examine the utilization issue. Even though, we do not agree on the application of such techniques in hospital economics, we do want to emphasize at least a cost-effectiveness analysis to derive certain basic parameters necessary for a thorough systems analysis (programming techniques etc).[4]

Hospital Studies in India

A number of valuable studies are available on the economics of hospital systems in India. Among various micro-level researches are the cost-effectiveness studies on the utilization of surgical wards, laundry facility, X-ray and other units etc.[5] The ICMP sponsored study on the hospital bed utilization is one of the major works in integrating patient, hospital and physician characteristics to examine

[3]See Appendix 1 for a list of types of characteristics associated with a hospital system. The NIHAE study mentioned above shows that average length of stay is increasing with family income whereas rural and urban population are found to be similar in their average length of stay.

[4]Ramaiah suggests simulation techniques for such allocative problems. See T.J. Ramaiah "Dynamic Scheduling Simulator of Patients in a Primary Care Clinic." Thesis Research, School of Hygiene and Public Health, The John Hopkins University, 1973.

[5]For a survey of studies on costing, utilization etc., see A.B.L. Srivastava and J.P. Gupta, "Review of Indian Studies on Cost Analysis in Health," NIHAE Bulletin, Vol. 7, No. 1, 1974.

the factors that are responsible for prolonging the average length of stay.[6] They find that among many other factors, the "number of changes in medication" and the "type of discharge" to be the most crucial variables that can be attributed for unnecessary prolonged stay in a hospital. Notice that these and such other factors are the result of interactions between patient, hospital, and physician characteristics (see appendix). Hence time and flow information like the "patient progressive care" report, "physician attendance" report etc. are the important sources of data to examine the factors affecting the length of stay, misuse of drugs, linen, food etc.

Need for Hospital Statistics

The WHO Expert Committee[7] on Health Statistics in its 13th report categorically identified the primary need for health statistics. They are (*i*) to assist in the administration and coordination of health services in any particular community, region, or country, and for the effective management of curative, preventive, and environmental health services, (*ii*) for the short-term and long-term planning of health services, both locally and nationally, (*iii*) for assessing whether health services are accomplishing their objective, *i.e.*, their effectiveness, and whether they are doing so in the best possible way, *i.e.* their efficiency, (*iv*) for the study in depth of particular problems of health and disease and their effect on the administration of health services, *i.e.* for research purposes, (*v*) to provide background data that may be required from time to time by the administration, by legislative bodies, and by members of the public.

Over and above what WHO, CBHI and other organizations have been emphasizing on the necessity of hospital statistics, I am tempted to go into the nature of available hospital statistics in India.

The Central Bureau of Health Intelligence publishes a skeleton of hospital statistics in the annual reports. Currently much of the coverage is on the statistics of a number of hospitals, dispensaries, primary health centres and beds in the hospitals.[8] The bed capacity in India has increased from 0.24 per thousand population in 1946-47 (pre-independence period) to 0.57 in 1971-72. However, the variation in the bed population ratio over the states, between the districts, between

[6]NIHAE, op. cit., Research Report No. 23.

[7]WHO Technical Report Series No. 429. Geneva, 1969.

[8]Appendix 5 lists some of the major hospital data published by the Central Bureau of Health Intelligence.

zones of developmental and geophysical configurations are striking.[9] It is logical for a social scientist to attempt to identify factors that can determine the bed capacity given socioeconomic and health factors associated with a hospital environment. For want of data on such characteristics, health economics remains limited to the estimation of utilization rates and comparison between hospitals. We have listed some of the major socioeconomic factors in Appendix 1.

Another major area of data is on cost informations. Except for budgetary costs at the hospital level, no further details are available on a regular basis. Even information on the number of doctors-nurses and the supporting staff are hard to come by. One can not go by the budgetary provisions on staffing, just as, it is difficult to evaluate an educational system from the enrolment statistics.

The patient progressive care reports are valuable sources of information on expenditure on the patient, the progress and satisfaction of the patient etc. Such reports should be made available either on a sample basis well spread over the year, or intensive reporting on all patients during few randomly selected months. Such data are quite relevant in both cost effectiveness studies and peak load problems of the hospital systems.

WHO in their Technical Report Series No. 429 also stress the need of data on capital resources and human resources.

SUGGESTIONS

There is a prime need to restructure the accounting methods in hospital environment to obtain economic and sociological data like costs, patient characteristics, flow of resources to related health facilities and programmes etc. Appendix 4 lists some of the pertinent cost data that are traceable from an improved accounting system. Performance Budgeting also be introduced in the hospitals.

Hospital services are essentially flows with, over the time peaks and slacks in demands. Since need is the criteria for an evaluation the

[9]As shown in appendices 2 and 3, bed population ratio is as low as 0.34 in the state of Bihar and Madhya Pradesh and as high as 4.51 in Andaman Islands; in a state like Orissa with a low state average (0.4), the variation among the districts is still alarming. In a study by Timmappaya and Ramaiah, the variation with Delhi among for hospitals and within in each hospital, among specialities are examined. They also have related this capacity variation to the utilization rates. See A. Timmappaya and T.J. Ramaiah "Utilization of services in four general hospitals in Delhi—a preliminary study" *NIHAE Bulletin* 11, No. 3, 1969.

planning be based on a peak-load method. This requires special data information on the patient progressive cares and time and motion data on physician and staff attendants.

Socioeconomic and health characteristics of patients and hospitals be published on hospital basis at regular intervals of time. Even once in two years information will be a major breakthrough in health statistics.

One way to streamline the data collection and analysis of the hospital systems is to set up a well defined functional unit or division in the health ministry. Such a division should be a part of the Central Bureau of Health Intelligence. Its objective be specific to collect hospital level informations and process them regularly.

Such an agency of hospital statistics should standardize the terms, definitions and formats of data information. In order to facilitate the recording system, the cross tabulation of various data be properly formated and such norms be used in all hospitals uniformly.

APPENDIX 1

Important Characteristics Associated with a Hospital System

Patient Characteristics	*Hospital Characteristics*	*Physician's Characteristics*
Disease	Bed capacity	Qualification
Age	No. of doctors	Experience
Sex	No. of nurses	Origin (rural or urban)
Education	No. of launders	Family background
Occupation	No. of food specialists	
No. of family members	Diagnostic facilities	
No. of earners		
Patient's income		
Family income	No of admissions	
Place of origin	No. of patient days	
	No. of discharges	
Distance from hospital	Average length of stay	
Date of last visit		
No. of times admitted		
Mode of admission		
Out-patient or in-door (type of bed)		
Surgical or non-surgical		
No. of Investigations		
No. of changes of medication		
Result after discharge		

APPENDIX 2

All India Hospital Bed Facility

State/Union Territories	*Hospitals** *No.*	*beds*	*Dispensaries**	*Total No. of P.H.Cs. functioning*	*Bed/popl. (per '000)*
Andhra Pradesh	417	28610	691	415	0.66
Assam	85	7266	429	106	0.49
Bihar	117	19041	1049	587	0.34
Gujarat	131	11068	1466	251	0.41
Haryana	76	5644	160	89	0·56
Himachal Pradesh	39	2139	425	75	0.62
Jammu & Kashmir	34	3531	603	76	0·76
Kerala	119	19603	431	162	0.92
Madhya Pradesh	203	14152	482	451	0.34
Maharashtra	414	38035	997	388	0.75
Manipur	13	733	61	14	0.68
Meghalaya	—	+	+	9	—
Karnataka	190	23534	1021	265	0.80
Nagaland	29	900	79	10	1.74
Orissa	214	8987	331	313	0.41
Punjab	126	8253	338	127	0.61
Rajasthan	423	13970	638	232	0.54
Tamil Nadu	326	22888	536	379	0.56
Tripura	11	796	100	23	0.51
Uttar Pradesh	842	31992	438	818	0.36
West Bengal	310	36072	521	286	0.81
A. & N. Islands	12	529	52	1	4.51
Arunachal Pradesh	17	1180	80**	79	2.52
Chandigarh	1	200	12	1	0.78
Dadra & Nagar Haveli	1	30	2	2	0.41
Delhi	55	10146	248	5	2.50
Goa, Daman & Diu	48	2264	31	15	2.64
Lakshadweep	2	50	—	7	1.56
Pondicherry	8	1212	22	11	2.57
Mizoram	3	234	27	—	—
Total (India)	4266	313059	11270	5197	0.57

\+ Data not available.
* Figures are provisional and likely to undergo changes.
** Including P.H.C's.

Source: Annual report 1971 and 1972. Directorate General of Health Services, Ministry of Health and Family Planning, New Delhi, issued by Central Bureau of Health Intelligence.

Appendix 3

Districtwise and Regionwise Variation in Hospital Bed Jacility

	District	*No. of hospitals and dipensaries per lakh of popl.*	*No. of beds per thousand of popl.*
O	Balasore	2.24	0.21
	Balangir	1.58	0.26
R	Cuttak	1.88	0.69
	Dhankanal	2.47	0.34
I	Ganjam	2.40	0.58
	Lajajamdo	1.72	0.50
S	Keonjhar	3.35	0.38
	Koraput	2.55	0.41
S	Mayurbhanj	1.60	0.35
	Phulbam	3.05	0.66
A	Puri	3.03	0.48
	Sambalpur	2.76	0.65
	Sundargarh	5.14	1.00
	Orissa	2.47	0.51
U.	Eastern Hill	—	0.31
			1.01
P.	Bundelkhand	—	0.34
	Central	—	0.49
	Western	—	0.40
	Uttar Pradesh	—	0.41

Sources: (1) Directorate of Health Services, Orissa.
(2) Directorate of Medical and Health Services, Uttar Pradesh.

APPENDIX 4

Typical Hospital Cost Informations.

The following diagram illustrates the sources of costs in a hospital environment.

BLOOD LAUNDRY DIET STORES HOUSE KEEPING
B (ADMINISTRATION) C
HOSPITAL

P A
A OUT-PATIENT IN-PATIENT DOCTORS
T UNIT UNIT NURSES
I STAFF
E CLINIC E
N
T
S D
PHARMACY BUILDING LABORATORIES LIBRARY

The type of cost data are listed below:

A. *Salaries and Social Allowances*
1. Medical
2. Nursing
3. Medical technicians
4. Kitchen, domestic, maintenance, porters
5. Clerical and administration
6. Special allowances for vacation
7. Special allowances for transport fares
8. Special allowances for technical books
9. Superannuations

B. *Administration Expenses*
1. Transport (contract)
2. Travel expenses
3. Mileage
4. Transport (own)
5. Transport drivers' salaries
6. Printing and stationery
7. Postage
8. Telephone
9. Rent
10. Electricity and water
11. Municipal taxes
12. Cleaning materials and maintenance of gardens
13. Uniforms
14. Contribution from outpatient clinic
15. Contribution from Laundry

C. *Running Expenses*
1. Catering
2. Dressings, drugs and X-ray films
3. Salaries of chemists and assistants
4. Laundry
5. Heating
6. Consultants (only for odd session)
7. Occupational therapy materials (net cost)
8. Recreation and entertainment (patients)
9. Patients' pocket money
10. Orthopaedic appliances material
11. Orthopaedic workshop salaries
12. Contribution from Outpatient Clinic
13. Contribution from Laundry

D. *Equipment and Maintenance Expenses*
1. Maintenance (buildings, etc.)
2. Minor development (alterations)
3. Medical equipment
4. Fire extinguishing equipment
5. Medical Library
6. Contribution from out-patient clinic
7. Contribution from Laundry

E. *Out-patient Clinic*
1. Medical salaries
2. Nursing salaries
3. Medical auxiliaries salaries
4. Clerical and administration salaries
5. Drugs, dressings and X-ray films
6. Contribution to administration expenses
7. Contribution to running expenses
8. Contribution to maintenance expenses

F. *Laundry*
1. Salaries
2. Electricity and water
3. Fuel
4. Chemicals
5. Transport
6. Maintenance
7. Equipment
8. Contribution to administration expenses
9. Contribution to running expenses
10. Contribution to general maintenance expenses

Source: C. Montacnte "*Costing and Efficiency in Hospitals*" Oxford University Press, 1962.

Appendix 5

Types of hospital information available in *Annual Report*, Central Bureau of Health Intelligence: No. of hospitals, No. of beds, No. of clinics, No. of wards in selected hospitals, Hospital staff—Doctors, nurses, tech. staff, No. of Speciality, No. of students, trainees.

Infant and Child Mortality Statistics

SHANTI GHOSH*

The historical record of the vital registration system in India began under the British rule in 1850s down to the comprehensive all-India Registration of Births and Deaths Act, 1968 (enacted by the Indian Parliament in 1969) which came into force from 1 April 1970—covering a period of 120 years of search for better and more complete registration—is not without interest. It reveals the countless drawbacks and weaknesses of the system, the attacks and criticisms to which it was subjected throughout the years, and the reforms and reorganization which the system has undergone.

The entire procedure of vital registration as in the census organization resembles a pyramid and the worth and reliability of the nation's vital statistics rest entirely on the validity of the information supplied by the base, the village functionaries and the municipal sanitary departments. Rural India, which accounts for a majority of the country's births and deaths has the weakest system of registration. The rural agent—the *patwari* or the village headman who is used for recording and reporting all vital occurrences—is often illiterate, ill-paid and has to attend to his permanent and more important job of being the administrative functionary of the village, who usually has to travel a considerable distance to make his report. He in turn depends on the report of a sweeper, barber or the village *dai*. Since none of them realizes the importance and utility of this data, human factors of carelessness and disinterestedness creep in and make matter worse.

From time to time various high powered committees have been set up in India since 1939 which have made recommendations for bringing about qualitative and quantitative improvement of the registration system, such as the report of the Central Advisory Board of Health of 1939, the Bhore Committee of 1946, the Vital Statistics Committee of

*Head of the Department of Pediatrics, Safdarjang Hospital, New Delhi.

1949, the Registrar General's Scheme of 1952, the report on the Pattern of Statistical Units for Health Department 1960—all pointing to the fact that setting up an efficient registration system is a long and slow process.

During the last two decades, there has been a phenomenal rise in population which has become the concern of planners and administrators. Census is an important piece of information on enumeration but it is taken once in 10 years. The rates calculated from the dicennial Census data cannot give a measure of change from year to year.

In 1961, a conference on improvement of vital rates recommended a short term scheme of sample registration. This aims at providing reliable estimates of birth and death rates (without giving the cause of death) separately for rural and urban areas at state and national levels. The sample for rural areas usually consists of 150 units in a state, the unit being either the whole village or a segment if the village had in 1961 population of 2,000 or more. In the case of urban areas, the sample varies from 60 to 100 blocks. A part-time enumerator, usually a teacher, or a full time enumerator maintains a continuous record of births and deaths as they occur, information being provided by a midwife, washerman, barber, sweeper, etc. once in six months, the supervisory staff conducts a retrospective survey to arrive at an independent set of vital events. The two matched on a unitary basis and unmatched and partially matched events are verified in the field. Thereafter, an unduplicated count of births and deaths is derived from which the vital events are calculated.

It is postulated that the system has been able to measure the birth rate at the national level with a coefficient of variation of less than one per cent. S.R.S. was tried in Kerala on a pilot basis in 1964-65 and a full scheme came into force from July 1965, since then annual rates on birth and death have been regularly published.

The main purpose of the scheme is to provide reliable estimates of birth and death rates by states and all India, both urban and rural. Statewise data are necessary because of vast differences between states.

The model registration scheme—survey of causes of death—fills an important gap in the health statistics system in the country by providing data on the causes of death for the rural areas. In the urban areas this gap is meant to be filled from compilations from hospital and other medical records, however, unsatisfactory they might be.

In the scheme all deaths occurring in the selected village of the primary health centre are covered and an investigation of the cause of death is made by a para-medical person employed at that centre.

This person, called the "field agent," follows a procedure based on prescribed symptoms and conditions, anatomical site and duration of the disease. The current list comparises a set of nine major cause-groups (including conspicuous symptoms) sub-divided into several probable specific diseases. The manual of procedure lays down a number of synoptic questions as well as associated symptoms attending upon each cause to facilitate the identification of probable causes.

In order to achieve qualitative accuracy and quantitative completeness, the collected data are retreated through a process of inspection and detection by an independent agency. All the events collected by the field agent in a month are forwarded in the form of a statement to the recorder attached to the primary health centre. The recorder is required to check the consistency of this statement. Doubtful cases are referred back to the field agent. This checking may involve clerical correction of the causes of death recorded. After this first check at the recorder's level, the medical officer in charge of the primary health centre scrutinizes the causes of death. He is supposed to investigate at least one-tenth of the total deaths by personally visiting the households. Such types of rechecking promote the accuracy of the statistical data and also instill a sense of discipline and responsibility among the field agents.

The field agent and/or recorder is required to visit every household in the area once in a quarter or, if that is not possible at least once in a half year. This visit is meant to net events which might have been missed by the field agent during his earlier visit to the village. The two sets of figures when matched for numerical correctness also bring out the type of events which are usually missed by field agents. While the plan is a reasonably sound one, there are often lapses at almost every level and the gap between the occurrence of an event and its final record and check is so large that the correctness of the event cannot be verified.

The primary health centres were not selected on the basis of any established statistical procedures. The main consideration in the selection of units was that adequate para-medical personnel should be available at the primary health centre to carry out the basic tasks envisaged in the scheme. Generally, the Headquarter village of the primary health centre was selected but in a few cases an adjacent village was chosen for the sake of convenience. This produces a bias because of the village being within the out-reach of the health centre and its expected effect on the health services available there. The statistics of causes of death although representative of the area, are not usable for calculation of vital data, which indeed is not the purpose of the Scheme. The data highlight the predominance or otherwise of the various causes of death in the state and in its regions.

One major drawback of the Scheme of model registration is that very little actual supervision or check can be instituted to verify the information obtained and recorded by the field agent, in spite of the check points described earlier and the gap between the occurrence of an event and its final record and check is very large.

The causes of death are enumerated under nine heads—violence or injury, child birth and complications, diarrhoea, cough, swellings, fevers, other infant deaths, other clear symptoms, extreme old age and the rest.

The age grouping is 0-1, 1-4 and 5-14 years. There is no separation of perinatal or neonatal deaths and indeed most of the etiological factors for these are missing from the list of nine. Violence and swellings are very vague descriptions and combine a host of problems with different etiology and the services needed for their management.

There have been attempts at correlating the data for National Sample Survey and model registration. The periods referred to are usually different and so comparisons are difficult. NSS conducts only sample surveys. It is felt, however, that there is a great deal of sampling error. The incidence in NSS surveys is also lower.

Apart from the carelessness and the indifference of the reporting agent in any one of the schemes, the community itself has not developed enough civic consciousness and feel under no obligation to furnish the reporting agent with the necessary information. It is, however, not uniformly true that rural returns are less accurate than the urban returns which are under the care of the relatively more enlightened municipalities and corporations of towns and cities, and are equally defective. The indifference and apathy on the part of the people added to the insufficient and inefficient organization results in under registration.

The vital statistical information sought by these government agencies includes particulars of births (Live and Still) and deaths, by sex and religion. Attempts are usually made to obtain the following particulars from parents or guardians within a prescribed period of the vital occurrence. In case of births, the date of birth (sometimes according to the Hindu calendar, and calendars differ with different linguistic and religious groups) sex, name of the child (invariably a difficult proposition, for the children are not named immediately after birth), name of parents, age of mother, religion, history of previous children and number of deaths. The death registers have name, sex, date of death, religion, age and occasionally the cause of death to the best knowledge of the informant. Information on other aspects such as sickness, employment, income, marital status, details such as separation or divorce, nubility, fertility, legitimacy, dependency are not available for the total population even today.

It is generally true just as in other countries that statistics of deaths are more reliable than statistics of births. Death is a sad event and arouses sympathy all around and seldom escapes the notice of the community. The death rites are also attended by the neighbours and friends. As for births they are natural and happy events, and nobody bothers to take notice of them in any special sense. And when it is a case of illegitimacy the recording of the vital occurrence is understandably and intentionally avoided. This trend is exaggerated in India, for omissions in recording births are definitely greater than the omissions in recording deaths. When time is limited and there are more pressing demands on the workers the vital statistics registration is a casualty. This has happened at times because of the efforts of the staff of MCH Centres to fulfil the family planning targets.

Accurate information is necessary for vital statistics to formulate public health programmes. Unless it is known at what age men and women marry, their fertility, health and ailments, their deaths and their causes, no government can intelligently formulate an effective public health policy. Accurate statistics are necessary to formulate and evaluate the effects of a family planning programme. Formulation of National Public Health Policy can be possible only on the basis of a large body of reliable knowledge of births, sicknesses and deaths in the country. The problems arise first from omissions to record deaths and second from inaccurate causes of death, the ages at which they occur and the associated factors which might have contributed to it. Since the birth registration is unreliable, even the age of death is a guess and is not cross checked with the date of birth.

The following are the main sources of data collection in India:

(1) Records of the Registrar General of India—(*a*) Census, (*b*) Sample registration, (*c*) Model registration.

(2) National Sample Survey records,

(3) Municipal birth and death records,

(4) Hospital records, and

(5) Small projects, surveys and research data from time to time, such as Mysore Survey 1952, Khanna Study 1956-59.

The objectives of any analysis of vital statistics should be:

(1) To relate mortality to biological and other factors in which considerable information will be required regarding the home environment, parents, practice of breast-feeding and provision of health care;

(2) Age of the mother, birth order of the deceased, the previous reproductive wastage and evaluation of characteristics of those who died in early life and those who lived;

(3) Relationship of maternal health and antenatal care to birth weight and its relation to perinatal and neonatal deaths;

(4) Urban and rural differentials;

(5) Deaths during school years and their relationship to nutrition and school health services;

(6) Educational level of the mother and its influence on child mortality;

(7) Relationship to medical and health care and certain other environmental factors that influence deaths; and

(8) Accuracy of the cause of death from death certificates and autopsy reports, so that remedial measures may be instituted.

Since infants more than any other section of the population depend on the environmental conditions for their survival, it would not be wrong to say that the death of an infant in most cases is due to a poor environment. Infant mortality rate may be taken as a reliable and sensitive index of the total health condition of a community or a country. An adequate knowledge of the complex biological, economic, social and cultural factors affecting the health, morbidity and mortality of infants is necessary.

The government, which is anxious to lower the death rate, must know what conditions and diseases are responsible for a high death rate which they are seeking to reduce. The disadvantages of a new born infant in a poor insanitary and unhealthy environment and the family's poverty and inability to afford even a modicum of adequate nutrition and medical assistance coupled with ignorance, prejudices and taboos are obvious.

The information regarding socio-economic factors which influence infant and child mortality is not available in a manner that can be linked with mortality rates. In a vast country like India with vast differences in social and economic structure and various cultural, religious and ethnic groups, this assumes great importance for any purposeful planning.

High income, better education and better housing etc. go together, each one having its influence on the quality of life, death or survival and even the causes of death. Usually a lower fertility and lower mortality go together.

VARIABLES AFFECTING CHILD SURVIVAL

The variables of health and social environment that influence the child survival and on which information is needed are several.

Biological Factors. At least five factors are associated with infant mortality: Level of fertility, Level of mortality, Mother's Age, Birth Order, and Past pregnancy experience.

Levels of Fertility and Mortality. These are inter-related and a sustained low mortality results in low fertility. With a reasonable assurance that the children born will survive, acceptance of a small family norm does not seem difficult or remote.

Age of the Mother. This has relevance to perinatal mortality the incidence being higher at both extremes. This would have a correlation with the age of marriage and the fertility rate and thus influence Family Planning services.

Parity. Parity, just like maternal age, has its hazards at both extremes second order being associated with lowest perinatal mortality. The incidence is high after 4-5th parity.

Birth Intervals. Several small studies have shown that the mortality of the child is correlated with the birth interval, the rate being lower when the birth interval is between two to three years. The family planning programme could be channelled in this direction which would in turn reduce fertility.

Birth Order. This again is related to the nutritional status of the infant as well as the mortality rates. Malnutrition and mortality are higher after fifth order. This again is related to the acceptance or otherwise of family planning practices.

Past Pregnancy Experience. Past fetal losses as well as neonatal deaths have a relationship with the outcome of pregnancy. Perinatal mortality is higher among the mothers, who have had a bad past pregnancy experience and is a pointer to the need of efficient maternal health and obstetric services.

Gestation. Importance of gestation has been emphasised by several studies. Not all low birth weight babies are premature. In India about 25 to 30 per cent of babies weigh below 2500 g and as many as 8-10 per cent weigh very much less than that. Among these more than half are full-term but small for date babies, and not pre-term babies. Many interrelations have now been studied regarding maternal factors and low birth weight. These include maternal nutrition, adverse environmental factors, socio-economic status, maternal infections etc. Toxaemia has particularly been correlated with small for date babies. This would have implication in prenatal care of the mother.

Birth weight is also dependent on whether the birth is single or multiple. Majority of multiple births in India do not survive because of low birth weight. This record hence becomes very important.

Socio-Economic Factors

Education of the Mother. Even though higher education and higher economic status go together, several studies have highlighted the important relationship of maternal education with child survival. Maternal education in turn is related to a higher age of marriage and lower fertility all having their impact on child survival. This has been brought out in many reports from Kerala.

Per Capita Income. A direct relationship has been found in several reports between economic status and child survival, even though as mentioned above other factors like education and adequacy of health facilities and their acceptance may be as important as economic status per se.

Occupation and Education of Father. Father in general being the head of the household, his attitude and awareness depend to a major extent on his occupational and educational status and these variables need to be studied in the context of child mortality.

Influence of Maternal Health and Prenatal Care. Perinatal deaths both still births and live neonatal deaths are affected by antenatal and obstetric care both having their influence on the child before, during and after birth. The services necessary for providing this care would emanate from a meaningful information on these points.

Nutritional Deficiencies. These are grossly under-recorded because the immediate cause of death is some respiratory or intestinal disorder. Malnutrition and a high infection rate are interrelated but in labelling the cause of death the former is ignored, and so malnutrition as a cause of death is under-recorded.

Impact of Breast-feeding. Child rearing practices particularly breast-feeding are closely related to infection rate and malnutrition in the first year of life. This information should be available on all infant deaths. A change from breast to bottle particularly in the urban slums is a dangerous trend.

Communicable Diseases. Diseases such as whooping cough, measles, mumps etc. are grossly under-reported. Even though these are notifiable diseases, the attending physicians or hospitals seldom take the trouble to notify them. In case of death, the immediate cause of death such as pneumonia or some other complication is recorded and the underlying disease which is preventable, is lost sight of. Diphtheria is better reported because of admission of the infectious diseases hospital. In the past even deaths due to smallpox of children not admitted to infectious diseases hospitals were not notified because of various beliefs and prejudices.

Immunization Status of the Child. In India apart from smallpox vaccination, the rates of other immunizations are very low particularly in the rural areas. The cause of death if accurately recorded would ascertain how many children died of the preventable causes such as whooping cough, diphtheria, tetanus, typhoid, cholera etc. Measles vaccination is not available in India so far. The incidence of tuberculosis can be linked with BCG vaccination even though there is some controversy as to the duration of efficacy of BCG vaccination. The immunization programmes for children should be linked with the epidemiology of the diseases, the age, incidence and the mortality rates.

Exact Age at Death. Intrauterine adverse effects continue into the first week of postnatal life and may result in a still birth or a live perinatal death. The common causes are low birth weight, asphyxia and other birth problems. The remedial measures such as prenatal and natal care are also similar. Deaths up to four weeks after birth (neonatal) are continuation of the perinatal problems, with the addition of infections. Deaths between one month and one year are due to causes resulting from a combination of malnutrition, non-availability of breast milk and infections, mainly respiratory and gastrointestinal. It is important, therefore, to ascertain the age at death carefully for any future planning of health services.

In India deaths continue to be high up to the age of five years and account for almost half of the total deaths. However, they go on decreasing with each year of child's life, even within this period. While the high infant mortality has attracted the attention of medical profession and planners for some time, the high mortality between the ages of two to four years was somewhat ignored. It is important to identify the extent of mortality for every year of child's life up to the age of five so that the vulnerable group can be identified and the services geared to the population in that age group. The causes of death in the second and third years are mainly infections and malnutrition, the latter due mainly to ignorance of the nutritional requirements of young children. Infections are mainly waterborne resulting in diarrhoeas and intestinal infections. Planning, therefore, would have to emphasize the importance of health and nutrition education as well as giving priority to environmental sanitation and protected water supply. The present grouping of deaths between one to four years is hence unsatisfactory.

Sex. This is important because of the demographic trends and ratio.

Classification of Causes of Death. This will have to be looked at from the point of view of the prevalence of malnutrition and communicable diseases as the underlying cause of death. The exact diagnosis of the cause of death is very unreliable because most deaths are not certified by medical practitioners and hence the cause of death is at best a guess. Very often the person making the report just fills in this column according to his own whims or fancy. To achieve a medical certification of deaths when even the elementary health facilities are not available in the vast areas of the country seems an impossibility.

However, efforts should be made wherever possible. Pathological cause of death which would require an autopsy is much more reliable than the clinical one. This, of course, is only possible in bigger hospitals where adequate facilities exist for performing autopsy and studying the pathological material. Even from hospitals this data is very meagre because of the prejudice against autopsy by the community and lack of motivation of the medical and nursing staff. Sometimes it is due to lack of time because of the great pressure of emergency work.

In our experience, however, it has not been difficult to get autopsy permission in the newbron deaths. That has highlighted the main causes of death which are asphyxia and problems related with labour and pinpoints to the areas where remedial attention should be focussed.

It has to be remembered, however, that data from hospitals by its very nature do not accurately reflect the problems in the community. Only the acute problems are admitted to the hospitals and these are drawn from a large area. In the case of the obstetric and newborn problems also, there is a bias in favour of serious problems because these tend to go to a hospital. The hospital data should be linked with the place of residence of a particular person.

Availability of Health Services and Alternate Approaches. If a record is available of the relationship of death to the nearness or otherwise of health facilities it will help in planning the health services and ascertaining the worker population ratio as well as the radius within which the health workers can function effectively.

Some studies have shown that the outreach of a Primary Health Centre is about four to five km. with the result that the infrastructure available at the moment is not able to deliver even the minimum health services to a large section of population. This has relevance both in terms of numbers as well as training of the workers who are being used for health delivery. It also focuses attention on the usefulness or otherwise of existing resources like the Dais and practitioners of indigenous system of medicine who are already in the rural areas and community seems to accept them.

There is considerable interest at the moment in identifying a first contact person in the village itself who can be trained in promotive, prevention and simple primary medical care and act as a link between the community and the existing health infrastructure.

Suggestions for Collection of Data on Infant and Child Mortality Statistics

(1) *Standardization of Definitions.* It is essential that the various terms used are clearly and unambiguously defined so that the people who collect the information know what they are trying to collect and so reliable data is available for analysis. Unless the data base is clean it is impossible to achieve anything in the way of factors contributing to child mortality. The classification should be 0 to seven days, seven to 28 days, birth to one year and yearly thereafter till five years. After that the present grouping of four years is adequate. Still births and live births should be clearly defined.

(2) *Training to the Investigators.* After defining the technical terms used in the study it is also essential to train the workers regarding the methodology of data collection and a clear understanding of the technical terms. The investigators should also be trained in proper recording of the data without confusion.

(3) *Survey Period.* The data on infant and child mortality should be made available annually for different regions by the related factors and variables. It is essential to develop an organization permanently engaged in collection, compilation and analysis of these data and make it available in a way that it can be correlated to the factors mentioned earlier.

(4) *Unit of Data Collection.* The civil district or a Block is recogniz-

ed as a basic unit of planning in India. All the information in the other related disciplines is being made available at the civil district level. If child mortality statistics are also made available within the same area the entire structure can be viewed before allocating funds for various aspects of service and development for that region.

(5) *Computerized Data Base for Efficient Processing.* In view of the vast amount of data and the multiplicity of the factors involved in analyzing it, it is essential that one should have an approach, which brings about results accurately and efficiently without a great time lag, so that the information collected can be readily made available in a presentable and understandable form to the planners to act upon. Suitably precoded proforma should be designed and efforts should be made to create a Data Bank on Infant and Child Mortality Statistics in India.

Statistics on Foetal Mortality

P.K. DEVI*

This presentation is an attempt to review the existing systems of data collection in relation to the subject of foetal mortality including abortions, miscarriages and still births. The term "pregnancy wastage" is wider in concept as it includes still births and the term "reproductive wastage" covers even perinatal deaths. In this paper only statistics in relation to abortions and still births are discussed.

A confusing number of definitions related to abortion and stillbirth is the first aspect to be considered. A WHO group, which considered this question in 1970 in view of the practical difficulty of determining gestational age due to lack of accurate dating of the last menstrual period, suggested to classify both live births and foetal deaths as follows:

	Live Births	*Foetal Deaths*
Group I:	Upto and including 500 gms	Early foetal deaths
Group II:	Over 500 gms upto and including 1000 gms	Intermediate foetal deaths
Group III:	Over 1000 gms	Late foetal deaths

The situation thus is somewhat easier but still not realistic or practical unless the baby can be weighed soon after birth. To define foetal death, one has to examine the definition of live birth accepted internationally. "A live birth is the complete expulsion or extraction from its mother of a product of conception, irrespective of the duration of the pregnancy, which after such separation, breathes or shows any other evidence of live, such as beating of the heart, pulsation of the

*Professor of Obstetrics and Gynaecology, Post-Graduate Medical Institute, Chandigarh.

umbilical cord or definite movement of voluntary muscles, whether or not the umbilical cord has been cut or the placenta is attached; each product of such a birth is considered liveborn." The signs of live birth according to this definition can sometimes be present in very small babies who are incapable of survival because of extreme immaturity. Hence a viability criterion of 500 gm was added in 1970 for the recording of a live birth.

As used by the medical profession, the term "abortion" denotes the termination of a pregnancy before the foetus has attained viability, that is, before it has become capable of surviving (with appropriate care) and eventually maintaining an independent extrauterive life. According to medical tradition, viability is said to be attained after 28 weeks of gestation (counting from the first day of the last period) with a foetal weight of around 1000 gm. This definition is based on the experience that below this weight, chances of survival are small, though advances in the care of premature infants in recent years has led to survival of many infants born earlier than 28 completed weeks of gestation or weighing less than 1000 gm.

There are two major categories of abortion, the induced and the spontaneous—the distinction between these two categories is important for several obvious reasons. Induced abortions include legal or illegal types as determined by the laws of the country. The term "therapeutic abortion" is sometimes used in place of legal abortion and "criminal" abortion instead of illegal abortion. It is often not possible to distinguish between spontaneous and illegal abortions as history is unreliable and evidence of manipulations may not be present.

A major obstacle in the study of foetal death is the difficulty in detecting early pregnancy. Even the sensitive immunological tests detect pregnancies reliably only 10 to 14 days after the missed menstrual period. In India, this testing reagent is not available easily even in research centres and teaching hospitals. Even if made available, the test can only be performed if the woman presents herself after first suspecting that she is pregnant and that depends on her concept of her own normal menstrual cycle.

The highest risk of foetal death is actually in the first three months of pregnancy, precisely the same period when correct information is difficult to obtain. Also in a substantial proportion of early pregnancies which end as abortions, fertilisation is followed by some bleeding at the time of expected period and thus even the history of a missed period may not be available. It is well documented that a large proportion of early spontaneous abortions are associated with chromosomal or developmental anomalies and a high foetal loss in this period will indicate the extent of genetic, environmental, or chromosomal damage in the early embryo in the sample of population studied.

Apart from real problems for the woman on her medical attendant in identifying early pregnancies and foetal deaths, underreporting of foetal deaths by 30 to 40 per cent in retrospective studies are due to failure of 'recall', such recall lapses increase with the number of pregnancies.

Because of the fallacies inherent in the assessment of foetal deaths in the general population, the reported incidence varies from 25 per cent in the most conservative to 76 per cent in a most liberal estimate. This large variation can be minimised only if precise methods for reporting foetal deaths in the first trimester of pregnancy can be evolved. It should then be also possible to estimate the degree or extent of unreliability of such data.

Status of Data at Present

(1) *Traditional Approaches.* Such sources are the census, the vital registration system and the sample registration scheme. These are not geared to meet the requirements for obtaining data on foetal losses or pregnancy wastage. The sample registration scheme involves semi-annual house to house surveys and the range will have to be extended to detect pregnancy losses not subject to errors due to recall lapses.

(2) *National Sample Survey.* This is a multi-purpose survey covering a wide range of items and the data collection is staggered over a number of sub-rounds. The subject and item coverages are extended to meet the needs of different government departments. The samples are taken on all-India basis and the figures for States are obtained by post sampling grouping. This data source has great potential for supplying information on birth order, birth interval, still birth and death rates.

(3) *Standard Fertility Surveys.* Such surveys are sponsored in several countries to obtain reliable information on all aspects of fertility by observations on selected number of women over a number of years. The methodology used in most surveys is retrospective, investigating the total or the recent past history of the woman, though some may

be quite comprehensive, including detailed pregnancy and contraceptive histories obtained through structured questionnaires administered through personal interviews at regular intervals. Longitudinal and prospective studies are few in number, in which monthly, quarterly or six monthly interviews are conducted to collect on going information.

Among these surveys, there are differences in definitions, criteria for including woman (only married or all women), methodology used, and techniques of data analysis and presentation of results. Reports of such standard fertility surveys are available from several countries such as Latin America, USA, Taiwan, and several Asian as well as European countries. In India, the FPCARE-sponsored prospective standard fertility surveys are in progress at six centres and it is expected that reliable estimates of not only birth and death rates but also of several other sensitive indices for detecting small changes in fertility will be available in the near future. No comments are offered on this project because of the lack of access to the reports.

(4) *Ad Hoc Surveys and Research Studies.* A good deal of statistics on foetal deaths and still births is available from hospital settings from different parts of the country from among selected samples of women attending hospital departments for contraceptive devices. In countries where registration of abortions and still births is compulsory, data is available on extent of reported foetal loss and their causes; and profile of the women with reference to age, parity, occupation, income etc. (Abramson's study at New York 1973). The Latin American Study of Gaslonde (1976) emphasizes the methods of data analysis *e.g.*, the advantages of determining the proportion of abortions per 1000 pregnancies (emphasizes extent of unwanted pregnancies) or the rate of abortions per 1000 women (important as this relates to demand for services and supplies particularly).

Other types of prospective studies and their peculiar problems are illustrated by that of French and Bierman (1963) who used seven pregnancy detection procedures in their study at Hawai and still found that one third of foetal deaths were discovered after termination had already occurred. Awan (1974) from Pakistan stressed the need for reliable data on foetal loss as planned parenthood should assume the safety and survival of a planned and wanted frequency and so there is need for better understanding of the extent of the problem of frequency wastage and the factors associated with it.

The study carried out at Lahore by Awan involved a prospective follow-up of a sample of 1447 married women identified to be pregnant at the time of the survey. A life table method was used for the computation of pregnancy wastage and infant deaths (Reproductive Wastage). This study illustrates a different and simpler methodology. The field study carried out in Khanna in Punjab in the sixties is easily the best qualitatively from India. (Potter *et al.* 1965). The methodology was the familiar prospective field study employing trained investigators to collect information required through personal interviews.

(5) *Other Advances in Research Methodology.* The use of computers and innovative techniques of data analysis enable a large number of variables to be handled simultaneously in research surveys. Application of models to study real processes in the abstract has been used in demography over the past half a century. Model building stimulates precise thinking about the determinants of the process under study and locates areas in which better information is crucial. As a result, there have been notable extensions of models of reproduction, both stimulation and analytic, some more complex than the others. Illustrations are well known models of Ridley and Sheps (1966), Potter (1966), Barrett (1971), Holmberg (1972) and Horwitz (1971). The construction of more elaborate models is costly and time consuming and not worthwhile except as academic exercises unless some new and crucial aspect of reproduction in the human is uncovered in the near future.

Suggestions for Future Study

In India, the problems and fallacies in obtaining a reliable estimate of foetal loss through abortions and still-births have yet to be tackled in a purposeful and realistic manner. Information already available on reproductive wastage should be compiled and examined critically so that mistakes made in the past are not likely to be repeated in the future. The extent of coverage has to be improved to detect early pregnancies between six to eight weeks by suitable methods. The standard fertility survey can be suitably modified and restructured to obtain data in prospective studies in different regions of the country. Visits to target populations have to be at shorter intervals of time so as to avoid recall lapses. Model reporting areas on regional basis could be set up alternatively where well-coordinated long-term studies can be set up. Special emphasis is required on the quality of data collected and hence quantity or number of items should be selectively curtailed so that quality can be maintained.

Looking at the change in attitudes towards induced abortion in recent times, it is not expected that there will be large-scale under-reporting as in the previous decades. The analysis of the data collected has to be expeditious, using new technology so that the results are available to the planners in time.

When the data on the extent of foetal wastage and the factors related to it becomes available, one can legitimately ask as to what use is likely to be made of it. There are several questions for which one can seek the answers from the results of these studies—

(1) What are the social and other circumstances under which unwanted pregnancies occur?

(2) What are the annual rates of planned and unplanned births in the types of population studied?

(3) What are the changing trends and implications of specific policies and programmes in liberalizing the availability of abortions in terms of social costs and benefits?

(4) What is the real extent of mortality and morbidity among women as a result of induced and spontaneous abortions?

(5) How often is the period of susceptibility or non-susceptibility between births affected by abortions?

(6) Is it a fact that the practice of contraception will decrease as a result of a permissive policy of induced abortion?

(7) Can percentage of spontaneous abortions in the early weeks be used to identify and monitor environmental hazards and special genetic risks among the target population?

In conclusion, it is emphasized that the study of foetal deaths should be looked at from a proper perspective as only part of the complex and dynamic process of human reproduction under the influence of a number of physical, psychological, economic, political and sociological factors.

References

ABRAMSON, F.B., (1973), Soc. Biol. 20: 375-403.

AWAN, A.K., (1974), Amer. J. Obset Gynec 119: 525-532.

BARRERT, J.C., (1971), Demography 8: 481-490.

FRENCH, F.E. and BIERMAN, J.M., (1962), Public Health Rep. 77: 839.

GASLONDE, S.S., (1976), Studies in F.P. Aug. 1976: 211-217.
HOLMBERG, I., (1962), Demographic Institute Reports, Gothenberg.
HORWITZ, D.U., *et al.* (1971), Carolina Pop. Centre Monograph: 45-63.
POTTER, R.G., *et al.* (1965), Human Biol. 37: 262-273.
——, and SAKODA, J.M. (1966), Demography: 3: 450-461.
RIDGEY J.C. & SHEPS M.C. (1966), Population Stud. 19: 297-310.
WHO, Tech. Rep. Series No. 461 (1970), Spontaneous and induced abortion.

Nutrition Statistics in India

K. VISWESWARA RAO and
S. G. SRIKANTIA*

Nutrition has a vital role in the health of a community and profoundly influences socioeconomic and cultural development. Malnutrition leads to deterioration of physical fitness and can adversely affect mental efficiency. In addition, it can reduce work capacity. For the malnourished child, mortality and morbidity are extremely high, and common infectious diseases more often fatal. In many developing countries malnutrition continues to be one of the major public health problems.

Although malnutrition affects all segments of the population, certain specific groups are more vulnerable to its effects. The infant, the pre-school child, the pregnant woman and the nursing mother constitute such groups. A proper appreciation of the extent, nature and geographical location of the problem of malnutrition and a proper understanding of the aetiological factors are prerequisites for the planning and implementation of the most effective and most appropriate control and preventive measures where they are most needed.

In our country, energetic attempts are already being made to improve the situation. These need to be intensified. The results of the chosen methods need to be continuously monitored and adequately evaluated and these can be done only when adequate information on various aspects is available from the very beginning.

As with other aspects of public health, in nutrition too, it is necessary to have numerical measurements which can quantify not only the extent of the problem, but also the extent of changes arising as a result of specific interventions. Nutrition statistics are, therefore, necessary to map out the magnitude and geographical distribution of malnutrition as a public health problem and to discover and analyse

*National Institute of Nutrition, Hyderabad.

the ecological factors that are directly or indirectly responsible. Nutrition statistics will help to develop short-term and long-term plans for existing nutritional problems at the community level, the state level and the national level. A brief review of available nutrition statistics, the actual data requirements and the lacunae in the existing statistics are presented here.

As indicated earlier, in undertaking ameliorative nutrition programmes, the basic steps are to assess the existing situation, to define precisely the magnitude of the problem to monitor future trends, and to assess the impact of programmes at periodic intervals. There has been a growing interest among nutritionists in identifying and developing simple indicators which can reflect the health and nutrition situation of a community with a reasonable degree of precision. The use of such indicators could help to broadly identify areas where malnutrition is likely to exist and a closer look might then be taken in these areas by means of more detailed survey procedures. As can be expected, the use of just one or two indicators is unlikely to be reliable, but it has now been possible to suggest the use of a set of indicators—some direct and some indirect, which provide useful information on the nutritional status at the community level. These include indicators related to agricultural statistics as well as to social statistics.

Availability of Nutrition Statistics

The available nutrition statistics in our country can broadly be classified under the following categories:

Statistics available through clinical nutrition surveys which include nutritional anthropometry;

Statistics available through dietary surveys and food consumption surveys;

Statistics available through food balance sheets; and

Statistics available from current ameliorative measures.

Because of the close association known to exist between nutritional status on the one hand and morbidity and mortality on the other, statistical data available through vital and health statistics, agricultural and food production statistics and hospital statistics have often been used in the interpretation of nutrition problems.

SOURCES OF NUTRITION STATISTICS

Indian Council of Medical Research and Directorate-General of Health Services (1-15; 21)

Most States have a nutrition department which is expected to carry out studies related to the nutritional problems of that State. The results of diet and nutrition surveys carried out by nutrition departments were compiled annually by the Indian Council of Medical Research and made available in the form of the Report of Nutrition Work Done in States until 1967. Some details on family food consumption pattern and prevalence of nutrition deficiencies existing in the different segments of the population according to age, sex, socio-economic status and occupation were provided in these reports. Data on food consumption are available through reports brought out by the Indian Council of Medical Research since 1935. Since the formation of the Nutrition Cell in the Directorate-General of Health Services, the reports from the State nutrition departments are being compiled and brought out by the Nutrition Cell. The latest report available is for the year 1970-71.

These reports contain the results of diet surveys, nutrition surveys, laboratory and field investigations, information on ameliorative measures in progress and nutrition education and publicity in each State. It must, however, be pointed out that the data presented in these reports suffer from several serious limitations. Among the important drawbacks are the following.

(*i*) There was no uniformity among the States with regard to the procedure used for the collection and presentation of the data. In addition, selection of the sample on which dietary and nutrition surveys were conducted left much to be desired. In some states, all family members were covered, while in others, only school children were studied. Some States confined their surveys to either the rural or the urban areas, while others covered both rural and urban populations in small numbers. Data obtained from different socio-economic strata were pooled and presented, thus making the data extremely difficult to interpret, since social and economic factors are the well known variables which influence nutritional status. Thus, data from one State to another could not be compared; also data from two areas within a State could not be compared.

(*ii*) In most of the reports available, the basis on which the samples for the survey were selected has not been indicated.

(*iii*) Only a few States collected data on anthropometric measurements and even these have not made this information available.

(*iv*) In many States, no data were collected on dietaries and prevalence of nutrition deficiency signs.

There are some exceptions to these generally unsatisfactory reports. These refer to surveys conducted to assess the prevalence of specific endemic nutritional diseases such as goitre, fluorosis, lathyrism and beri beri which have a circumscribed distribution.

Ministry of Agriculture and Irrigation, and the Food and Agricultural Organisation

The statistics of food availability through food balance sheets are prepared by the Central Ministry of Agriculture and Irrigation and the Food and Agriculture Organisation of the United Nations. These data are available through publications of the Ministry of Agriculture and Irrigation and the publications of the FAO (20, 24, 25, 26 and 33).

The food balance-sheet is recognized as a macro-method of assessing the food consumption level. It shows food supply in a country at the retail level (as "purchased" or as "brought into the kitchen") as measured by the total production of individual commodities, adjusted for in-and-out movements of trade, for changes in stocks and for any quantities used for animal feed, seed and manufacture for purposes other than food and the amounts wasted during distribution up to the retail level. From this can also be calculated the nutritive value of food supplies expressed in terms of calories and other nutrients on a percaput basis at the retail level.

It is thus clear that this approach to the measurement of the average national calorie and nutrient supplies per head is only indirect, the food supplies available for human consumption, commodity by commodity, being estimated as residuals.

Thus, the estimate of calorie (or nutrient) supply per person per day at the retail level derived from the food balance sheets is given by

$$C = \Sigma \frac{(P+I+T_1-E-T_2-S-F-W-M)\ R.N.}{(\textit{Mid-year population})\ (365)}$$

where T_1 and T_2 represent the stocks at the beginning and at the end of the consumption year; I and E represent the imports and exports respectively during the consumption year; P represents the production during the year; S, F, W and M represent non-food utilisation, standing for seed, feed, waste and amounts used in manufacture for purposes other than food respectively.

R represents the extraction factor appropriate to the forms in which the commodity is measured at the retail level and *N*, the corresponding content of calories (or nutrient) per unit of quantity.

The statistics on food availability by this food balance sheet technique has been available since the 1940s in publications brought out by the Ministry of Agriculture and Irrigation, and the FAO.

It needs to be emphasised here that the information these statistics provide is of a very gross nature and variations in food consumption from one region to another, which arise as a result of maldistribution due to a number of factors, are completely masked.

Accuracy of the food balance sheets. The accuracy of the food balance sheets is dependent on the accuracy of statistics of food production, the accuracy with which the statistics of trade, stocks and those non-food utilisation are collected. The accuracy is also dependent on conversion factors and estimates of population that are available. Of all the statistics used, those of trade are of acceptable accuracy. Figures of stocks relate to stocks with the States and the Centre, while those held by the trade and producers are not accurately known.

The basis for adjustment of stocks can be improved. The statistics of seed rates and of areas sown and, in consequence, the amounts used as seed are known fairly accurate for most crops, but the amounts used for seed, losses in storage and transport between farm gate and retail level and used in manufacture, have to be more accurately estimated.

The proportion of foodgrains used for seed is sizeable. Up-to-date estimates for each item of food are necessary for the improvement of food balance sheet statistics.

Food losses, during storage and transportation of crops such as rice and wheat, are based on marketing survey reports. Depending upon the nature of the food, variable allowances are made for losses. Thus, in the case of potato, seed and wastage alone are estimated at a third of the total production.

For determining the extraction rate (R) for different commodities, one needs accurate estimates. These rates vary from one part of the country to another. A single commodity may reach the retail level in different forms. The extraction rates for rice, for example, can vary from 62 to 75 per cent. Estimates of proportion of rice consumed in different forms are lacking. A better estimate of 'R' may be expected to improve the accuracy of estimation of food availability.

The accuracy of the food balance sheet depends upon the accuracy with which the production of foods is assessed. Production statistics are based on the reports of areas utilised for crops and yield rates of different crops. Improved methods of estimation of food production in comparison with those based on conventional 'patwari' system will be of use in improving the accuracy of data. The yield rates are accurately estimated through crop cutting surveys in randomly selected fields.

There has been considerable progress in the availability of accurate statistics on milk production consequent on the series of random sample surveys conducted throughout the country. The estimates of fish catch have also been more accurate. Estimates of fruit, vegetable, meat and egg production are, by and large, not very accurate. Detailed and accurate estimates of production of meat and leafy vegetables are also not available.

Food balance sheets for states. Recently, the Centre for Development Studies located in Trivandrum (Kerala) has made available estimates of food availability for Kerala (27 and 28). Reporting of such data from other states as well will be of considerable use for planning purposes in all the states.

There have so far been no attempts to test the accuracy of the food balance sheet data either at the Central or at the state level. A method that may provide such information at the state level, though admittedly difficult, would be to compare data obtained from estimates of food consumption by dietary survey technique in the state with that obtained by the food balance-sheets of that state. The validity of the food balance sheet could then be assessed.

Nutrition Statistics from Research Organizations

A large body of statistics on the pattern of food and nutrient intake, prevalence of nutrition deficiency signs and growth status measured in terms of anthropometric measurements like height, weight, arm circumference and fat fold at triceps, are available through investigations carried out by several research institutions, notably the National Institute of Nutrition, Hyderabad, the All-India Institute of Hygiene and Public Health, the All-India Institute of Medical Sciences, New Delhi and the Christian Medical College, Vellore. These studies have mostly been done with the assistance of grants from the Indian Council of Medical Research and international organisations (4, 9-15).

The nutritional status studies undertaken by the research organisations were meant to evaluate the nutrition and health of populations in relation to their diets and modes of life. The studies covered either the whole population in a given area or a carefully defined segment identified by race, sex, age, physiological state, location of dwelling, occupation, income, social customs, environment and other characteristics. The basic information collected includes quantity and quality of food actually consumed through diet surveys either by the weighment method or by the oral questionnaire method, estimates of calorie and nutrient requirements through the use of food value tables and evaluation of physical status through clinical examination and anthropometry. Other useful data also collected include methods of food preparation and food processing, social and economic factors, incidence of various kinds of diseases, life expectancy and death rates from various causes.

It is necessary to point out here that the data collected on food and nutrient intake from diet surveys have certain limitations due both to sampling and non-sampling errors irrespective of the method used. Similarly, the use of food tables to obtain the nutrient intake from food items has certain limitations. It should, therefore, be recognised that properly collected diet survey data are applicable to a community and not to individuals.

The uses to which data obtained through nutrition and diet surveys can be put are obvious. These include comparison of one area with another with respect to diet and nutrition situation, identification of priority areas for intervention, determination of the type of intervention needed and evaluation of effectiveness of corrective measures that are implemented.

Although, as a rule, the quality of data which have come from these research studies is generally satisfactory and is a vast improvement over that of the data which were earlier reported from the nutrition departments of the various states, there is still considerable scope for refinement. In view of the known fluctuations in food availability during different seasons and in view of the known seasonal variations in disease patterns in a community which can influence nutritional status, it is desirable that these variables are taken into consideration in the collection and interpretation of nutrition statistics. A few but not all research studies have this factor built into them. The main reason for this is perhaps that it is time-consuming and expensive, since it would involve the same community being studied over at least a continuous period of 12 months, but the additional effort would be rewarding since the data would permit more accurate assessment of the situation.

National Sample Survey (NSS) Food Statistics

Statistics related to food consumption and consumer expenditure figures on food are available from some of the reports of the National Sample Survey. In these studies, data on food consumption were obtained by the oral questionnaire method for thirty days using comprehensive schedules. In most of the rounds, the monetary values of the food consumed for thirty days were collected and tabulated by monthly percaput expenditure classes and family size for each State as well as for the whole country. The NSS data will be of use for interpretation of consumer preferences to foods and the proportion of total income spent on food.

The direct assessment of dietary intake by either the weighment method of diet survey or by the oral questionnaire diet survey method has not been adopted by the NSS. Data from the NSS, therefore, suffer from certain limitations, because memory lapses are likely to be high if dietary intake of families is assessed over a period of thirty days in a retrospective manner.

There have been some "All-India Consumer Expenditure Surveys" conducted by the National Council of Applied Economic Research, New Delhi, which have limitations similar to those of the National Sample Survey.

Data Requirements at the National Level

At a conference of Asian Statisticians (29-31, 34, 35, 36 and 38), it was recommended that the following five indicators can be used to measure nutritional status:

(*i*) Percaput daily consumption of calories;

(*ii*) Percaput daily consumption of proteins;

(*iii*) Percentage of households with aggregate calorie intake below the minimum required;

(*iv*) Percentage of households with aggregate protein intake below the minimum required; and

(*v*) Percentage of first level new entrant school children considered under-weight.

All-India statistics or state-wise statistics concerning the nutritional status of the population with the above set of indicators of nutritional status are not at present available. Estimates of the per-caput availability of calories and proteins are available from the food balance sheets prepared by the Ministry of Agriculture and Irrigation and the FAO, but as indicated earlier, they cannot be construed as indicators of consumption.

It must also be recognised that these are indirect indicators of the nutrition situation. Although a large mass of data on consumption has been collected by the National Sample Survey, nutritional analysis of the data has not been feasible. However, some data using the first four indicators are available from limited studies conducted on households by the National Institute of Nutrition and by the Maharashtra Association for the Cultivation of Science, Poona (16-19).

Prevalence of Protein Calorie Malnutrition

Although among the poorer sections of our population a variety of deficiency diseases exist as a result of inadequate dietary intake of a number of nutrients, the major problem appears to be inadequate intake of food leading to intakes of calorie and protein below the recommended levels with consequent sub-optimal growth during infancy and childhood and low body weights during adulthood. Calorie-protein malnutrition thus is a major public health problem in our country. Until recently, intake of protein and calories used to be viewed independent of each other, but now it is recognised that the inter-relationship between these two nutrients is so close that they must be considered together.

A method of quantifying the prevalence of calorie-protein inadequacy in a community has, therefore, now been developed (P.V. Sukhatme, 16-19). As a result, it is now possible to classify families in a population as belonging to one of the following four groups:

(*i*) Households having inadequate intake of both calories and proteins;

(*ii*) Households having inadequate intake of calories with adequate intake of proteins;

(*iii*) Households having inadequate intake of proteins with adequate intake of calories; and

(*iv*) Households having adequate intake of both calories and protiens.

This must be considered as an improvement over earlier attempts to assess the quantum of calorie-protein adequacy in a community. There is, however, a need to assess the validity of this method by actual comparison of these data obtained in a community with the prevalence of clinical calorie protein inadequacy in the same community.

Indicators of Health and Nutrition for Developmental Planning

Existing survey methods for gathering information on general trends of nutrition and health status, though fairly satisfactory, are expensive, time consuming and very difficult in most developing countries including ours. The matter is further complicated for nutrition assessment by the fact that mild and moderate degrees of calorie protein malnutrition do not have specific clinical signs, unlike the very severe forms which are easily recognised as either kwashiorkor or marasmus.

A large number of anthropometric measurements have been used to assess the extent of the mild and moderate forms of malnutrition and tested to ascertain their utility, either individually or in combination, as reliable and sensitive indicators of nutritional status. It is possible to have a package of indicators selected from the following categories:

(*i*) Vital statistics or demographic indicators;

(*ii*) Anthropometric indicators reflective of growth and development;

(*iii*) Housing and environmental indicators;

(*iv*) Socio-economic indicators; and

(*v*) Morbidity and nutrition indicators from hospital admissions.

Many combinations of indicators are possible from each of these categories. A list of some indicators suggested by the National Seminar on Social Statistics held in 1975 (22,23,29-38) and by international organisations of the U.N. is presented in Table 1.

Though the necessity of using a variety of indicators for the evaluation of health and nutritional status has been recognised, attempts at assessing the inter-relationships between demographic, economic, agro-economic, health and nutrition indicators have so far been few due mainly to lack of such comprehensive data.

The results of analysis of limited data by the National Institute of Nutrition have shown that all these are, in fact, well correlated. Housing conditions, environmental sanitation, availability and prices of staples may be expected to be indicators of nutritional status, as is the age specific mortality rate, particularly in the 0-1 and 1-5 year age groups. There is thus a need to establish more precisely the value of each of these categories of indicators in predicting nutritional status.

Sources of Basic Data

Nuturition, health and social statistics derived from census and sample surveys and from administrative records are the main sources of data in constructing indicators of health and nutrition. In addition, data derived from opinion surveys and consciousness surveys are useful to assess the degree of consumer-satisfaction and efficiency of services offered. Social statistics are relatively less developed for various reasons in many developing countries including India, and the reliability of even the limited data collected and reported is often open to question. These pose problems in any attempt to develop integrated social, health and nutrition indicators.

Hospital Statistics

Hospitals are very good sources of valuable data on morbidity and mortality related to health and nutrition. Unfortunately, in our country, information available through publications on hospital statistics is extremely unsatisfactory. Some of the existing limitations are:

(*i*) Non-availability of certain basic data on morbidity, cause of specific mortality, manpower and cost, etc.;

(*ii*) Lack of reliability and incompleteness of coverage in the availability of data;

(*iii*) Lack of qualified statistical staff; and

(*iv*) Time lag in the publication of the data.

National Nutrition Monitoring Bureau (NNMB)

While there have been several studies in the past aimed at determining the nutritional status and dietary intakes of population groups in our country, there has so far been no organised study to determine the effects of changing environment on the nutritional status of the people and their dietary intakes. There have been several nutritional programmes in operation in various parts of the country, and it is to be expected that these programmes will bring about changes not only in the way of life, but also in the pattern of expenditure and food intake. The impact of these programmes on the nutritional status of the community has, however, not been properly evaluated so far.

Because of these considerations, the need was felt for a continuous nutrition monitoring service to study the nutritional status, dietary habits, food availability and the effects of changing social and environmental factors on the health of the population. The results of such a study, carried out on a representative cross section of the population in various parts of the country, would provide information and useful guidelines not only for food policies of the country, but also for the assessment of the impact of nutritional programmes currently in progress and for future planning.

With these objectives in view, a national agency, *viz*., the National Nutrition Monitoring Bureau (NNMB) was recently set up by the Indian Council of Medical Research at the National Institute of Nutrition, Hyderabad. There are nine units of the NNMB, one at each of the following states: Andhra Pradesh, Gujarat, Karnataka, Kerala, Madhya Pradesh, Maharashtra, Tamil Nadu, Uttar Pradesh and West Bengal. These units are under the administrative control of the State Nutrition Officer, but financed by the Indian Council of of Medical Research. They thus represent a State-Centre collaborative effort. The units function under the technical supervision and guidance of the National Institute of Nutrition.

The Plan of Work

The plan consists of monitoring the dietary and nutrition situation among various population groups in selected states. For this purpose, the following studies are carried out:

(*i*) Clinical nutrition survey;

(*ii*) Anthropometric survey—with measurements of height, weight, arm circumference and fat fold at triceps;

(*iii*) Dietary surveys—of families and individual members of the families; and

(*iv*) Collection of relevant background information associated with nutritional status and dietary habits.

A sample of 650 households consisting of 400 households in rural areas and 250 households in urban areas has been fixed for each State per year for dietary and nutrition survey. The sample design is a stratified three-stage random sampling and the total sample for each state is to be covered in a period of three years.

The NNMB surveys help to provide a national estimate of the nutritional status and it is hoped that valid comparisons will be possible between States and between different time periods.

At the present moment, the period over which baseline data are collected is long and this may vitiate the interpretation of changes taking place in the dietary habits and nutritional status of the population groups as a result of changing environment. Reducing the survey period to a shorter period with equal coverage of samples in all the regions may be expected to minimise the deficiencies. Also, the states so far not covered need to have regional units located in them, so that a truly national estimate of nutritional status and dietary habits can be obtained.

As indicated earlier, the results of studies conducted in India and elsewhere have shown seasonal variations in the prevalence of nutritional defiencies, dietary intakes as well as growth and development An attempt to provide corrections for seasonal variations and to facilitate inter-regional comparisons can be made in the results of the NNMB surveys.

Suggestions for Improvement of the Availability of Statistics of Nutrition

(1) There are good sources of data at the national level for assessing economic and social development. The development of an organisation such as the NNMB is a necessity for monitoring the diet and nutritional situation in India. Extension of the activity of the NNMB to all the States is necessary for a continuous flow of nutrition statistics.

(2) Various sources provide information which is necessary for assessing the nutritional status of communities or of the country as a whole. In aiming at national planning for nutritional improvement, it is necessary to have a variety of data (Tables 1 and 2) on direct and indirect indicators of health and nutrition. Compilation of these indicators state-wise in a single publication at periodic intervals will be a useful step.

(3) The details of anthropometric measurements and prevalence

of nutritional deficiency signs by age, sex, occupational status, monthly percaput income and expenditure levels in both rural and urban areas will aid future planning. Data on intake of both foodstuffs and nutrients by all these classifications need to be included.

(4) In all reports dealing with nutritional status, it is desirable to include the percentage distribution of households and population by levels of nutrient intake as percentage of recommended dietary allowances.

(5) A food balance sheet should be prepared for each state and district. This will provide information which can be used to anticipate scarcity periods, so that necessary preventive measures can be taken.

(6) The classification of population by adequacy of calories and proteins in comparison with the recommended allowances as indicated below, will be of use to indicate the percentages of populations with various combinations of adequacy or inadequacy of the two major nutrients, and such information is vital to recommend the nature of dietary changes called for.

	Protein deficiency (PD)	*No protein deficiency (NPD)*
Calorie deficiency (CD)	—	—
No calorie deficiency (NCD)	—	—

(7) Development of a manual for use by research and field workers who are concerned with collection of health and nutrition statistics may be expected not only to improve the quality of the data collected but also reporting and interpretation. This manual should contain information on the methodology, sample selection, filling up of schedules, definition of terms, etc. both under field and hospital conditions.

(8) An investigation assessing the extent of agreement between the estimates of food consumption by diet survey techniques and food balance sheet needs to be carried out by research organisations, the results of which will be useful in assessing the utility and validity of the food balance sheet technique.

(9) A sizable proportion of hospital beds, even today is occupied by frank nutritional deficiency diseases. A proper maintenance of

records of all such cases, which include anthropometric measurements, will provide valuable data not only for the proper interpretation of research findings but also serve as useful nutrition indicators.

Availability of reliable nutrition statistics of the type suggested here at the community, state and national levels may be expected to help in the proper planning for the improvement of nutritional status of population groups and to maintain effective surveillance of the situation.

TABLE 1: *Direct and Indirect Indicators of Nutrition and Health*

I. Vital Statistics

1. Birth rate
2. Death rate
3. Growth rate
4. General fertility rate
5. Net rural-urban migration rate
6. Percentage of urban population
7. Age specific mortality rates by sex:
   0-1 year 6-14 years 46 years and above
   1-5 years 15-45 years
8. Proportional mortality rate by age and sex:
   0-1 year 6-14 years 46 years and above
   1-5 years 15-45 years
9. Proportion of births by age of mothers:
   <18 years 19-25 years, 26-35 years, 35-45 years and 46 years and above
10. Proportion of births by parity:
    <3, 4-6 and 7th parity and above
11. Proportional mortality by parity:
    <3, 4-6 and 7th parity and above
12. Sex ratio
13. Sex ratio by age:
    0-1 year, 1-5 years; 6-14 years; 15-64 years and 65 years and above
14. Maternal mortality rate
15. Neonatal mortality rate by sex
16. Post-neonatal mortality rate by sex
17. Expectation of life by age and sex
    Ages: at birth: 3rd year; 5th year; 10th year; 15th year; 25th year; 35th 45th year; 55th year and 65th year
18. Age specific mortality rate from infectious diseases like diarrhoea, measles, etc.
19. Wills-Waterloo index-Ratio of deaths in children of ages 1-4 years to that of infants aged 1-11months.

II. Health and Nutrition

(*A*) *Indicators of dietary adequacies: Family diets and dietaries of vulnerable groups by ages*

Nutrients

1. Percaput daily intake of calories
2. -do- Total protein
3. -do- animal protein
4. -do- vitamin A
5. -do- vitamin B complex
6. -do- vitamin C
7. -do- iron
8. -do- calcium
9. Percentage of families with aggregate calorie intake below the recommended allowances
10. -do- protein intake " "
11. -do- calorie intakes and protein intakes below the recommended allowances
12. -do- calorie intakes and protein intakes above the recommended allowances
13. -do- calorie intake below the recommended allowances and protein intake above the recommended allowances
14. -do- calorie intake above the recommended allowances and protein intake below the recommended allowances

Dietaries

Percaput intake of foodstuffs:

1. Cereals and millets,
2. Pulses and legumes,
3. Milk and milk products,
4. Flesh foods: fish, meat and eggs,
5. Vegetables: leafy, roots tubers and others,
6. Oils and fats,
7. Condiments

(*B*) *Food Balance Sheets*

1. Percaput food available for consumption by item of foodstuffs
2. Percaput calorie content of national food supplies
3. Percaput total protein content of national food supplies
4. Percaput animal protein content of national food supplies
5. Percaput fat content of national food supplies

(*C*) *Prevalence of clinical forms of malnutrition*

(i) Percentage prevalence of nutrition deficiency signs by sex, age, socio-economic status

(ii) Percentage prevalence of nutrition deficiency signs by parity and sex in 0-5 year age group children

(iii) Percentage prevalence of nutrition deficiency signs by gravida in women of child bearing age

(iv) Percentage prevalence of water borne diseases by age and sex

(*D*) *Indicators of Growth and Development*

(i) Mean, S.D. & C.V. values of height (cm), weight (kg), arm circumference (cm) and fat fold at triceps (mm) by age, sex and socio-economic status.

(ii) Percentile values of height (cm), weight (kg), arm circumference (cm) and fat fold at triceps (mm) by age, sex and socio-economic status. Percentiles 3rd, 25th, 50th, 75th and 97th

(iii) Percentage of population by various grades of malnutrition (Jelliffe classification)

(iv) Percentage prevalence of normals and chronic current forms of under-nutrition in pre-school children

(v) Percentage of preschool children with weight/height^2 index less than 1.35; 1.35-1.50; 1.50-1.65 and above

(vi) Percentage prevalence of overweigt and obesity by age, sex and socio-economic status.

III. Hospital Nutrition Statistics

1. Percentage of 0-5 years' children admitted with mild or severe forms of malnutrition
2. Percentage of 0-5 years' children attending hospital with specific signs of malnutrition.
3. Percentage of hospital beds taken over by children of 0-5 years age with severe forms of clinical protein calorie-malnutrition, anaemia, vitamin A and B-complex deficiencies.
4. Mean, S.D. & C.V. values of height and weight measurements of pre-school children admitted for treatment—Initial: Final (at discharge)
5. Mean, S.D. & C.V. values for duration of treatment (in days) by specific forms of malnutrition
6. Number of hospital beds per 10,000 population
7. Number of days treated as percentage of total days of sickness by age, sex and social classes
8. Medical expenditure per day per patient treated in the hospoital: Inpatient and out-patient
9. Number of patients per day per medical or dental doctor or per medical personnel
10. Percentage of newborns with birth weight below 2.5 kg, by socio-economic status and sex
11. Percentage of newborns with birth weight below 2.5 kg. by parity (<3 and 4or more and Primipara and multipara).

12. Percentage pregnant women with haemoglobin levels below or equal to 10 g/100 ml by age and order of pregnancy
13. Foetal death rate and neonatal death rates per 1,000 hospital deliveries by socio-economic classes
14. Prevalence of tuberculosis in undernourished hospital admitted population by broad age groups and sex.

IV. Housing and Environment

(1) Percentage of households with out homes
(2) Percentage of households in permanent or semi-permanent dwellings
(3) Percentage of households with access to safe drinking water or piped water service
(4) Percentage of households using electricity for domestic purpose
(5) Percentage of households with more than two persons per room
(6) Percentage of households in densely populated areas
(7) Percentage population living in areas with sewerage system (or service)
(8) Percentage of population living in houses which do not require repair
(9) Number of telephones per 10,000 population

V. Income and Consumption Expenditure

(1) Per capita available income per household at constant and current prices
(2) Per capita household consumption expenditure at constant and current prices
(3) Percentage of household consumer expenditure on food by items of food intake
(4) Twentyfifth percentile and 75th percentile values of consumption expenditure on food as percentage of total consumption expenditure
(5) Per capita expenditure on health and medical care
(6) Per capita mean savings per household

VI. Other Indicators

1. Percentage of population who are literate by sex
2. Percentage of population with elementary school education by sex
3. Percentage of population with high school education by sex
4. Percentage of population with graduate degree or above by sex
5. Percentage of population owning cultivated land
6. Percentage of land owned by non-cultivators
7. Percentage of population—the top 5 per cent of land owners (arranged according to the size of land owned)
8. Doctor-population ratio in rural areas; tribal areas and urban areas.
9. Hospital bed population ratio in rural areas, tribal areas and urban areas
10. Average amount insured of life insurance per household/person

TABLE 2: *Information needed*

S. No.	*Source of information*	*Name of information obtained*	*Nutritional implications*
1.	Agricultural data and food balance sheets	Gross estimates of agricultural production, soil fertility, agricultural methods	Approximate availability of food to a population
2.	Socio-economic data, information on marketing, distribution and storage	Purchasing power, distribution and storage of foodstuffs	Unequal distribution of available foodstuffs between socio-economic groups and within a family
3.	Food consumption pattern, anthropological and cultural data	Lack of knowledge, prejudices, indifferences etc.	Adequacy of nutrient intake
4.	Diet surveys	Food consumption	Adequacy of nutrient intake
5.	Vital and health statistics	Morbidity and mortality data	Extent of risk to community identification of high risk groups
6.	Anthropometric studies	Physical development	Effect of nutrition on growth and physical development
7.	Clinical nutrition	Physical signs	Deviation from health due to malnutrition
8.	Biochemical studies	Levels of nutrients, metabolites and other components of body tissues and fluids	Nutrient stores in the body Impairment of biochemical function
9.	Additional medical information	Prevalent disease patterns including infections and infestations	Inter-relationships of state of nutrition and disease

REFERENCES

INDIAN COUNCIL OF MEDICAL RESEARCH, New Delhi, Special Report Series No. 22, "A Review of Nutrition Studies in India," 1951.

——, New Delhi, "Report of Nutrition Work done in States," 1948 etseq.

——, New Delhi, Special Report Series No. 36, "Review of Nutrition Surveys Carried out in India" 1961.

——, New Delhi, Special Report Series No. 32, "A Review of Work done on Infant Mortality" by Dr D.M. Satur and S. Bhatia, 1957.

——, New Delhi, Special Report Series No. 20, "Results of Diet Surveys in India 1935-48," 1951.

——, New Delhi, Speeial Report Series No. 37, "A Review of Nutrition Studies in India 1951-56," 1962.

——, New Delhi, Special Report Series No. 21, "A note on the Management and Technique of Diet Surveys in India," 1951.

——, New Delhi, Special Report Series No. 25, "A supplement to the Results of Diet Surveys in India 1935-48" by Dr. K. Mitra, 1935.

——, New Deihi, Technical Report Series No. 18, "Growth and Development of Indian Infants and Children," 1972.

AYKROYD, W.R., "Note on the results of Diet Surveys in India," Indian Research Fund Association, Special Report Series No. 3, 1939.

——, "Summary of the Findings of Investigations into Causes of Maternal Mortality in India," Indian Research Fund Association, Special Report Series No. 17, 1948.

PANDIT, S., "Summary of the findings of investigations into causes of maternal mortality in India," Indian Research Fund Association, Special Report Series No. 17, 1948.

PANDIT, C.G. and RAO, K.S. ' Nutrition in India (1946-58)." Indian Council of Medical Research, New Delhi, 1960.

GOPALAN, C., BALASUBRAMANIAN, S.C., RAMASASTRI, B.V. and VISWESWARA RAO, K., "Diet Atlas of India," National Institute of Nutrition, Hyderabad, 1971.

GOPALAN, C., and RAGHAVAN, K.V., "Nutrition Atlas of India," National Institute of Nutrition, Hyderabad, 1971.

SUKHATME, P.V., "Human calorie and protein needs and how they are satisfied today," In Eugenics Society Symposium on Population and Land Use, London Academic Press, 1973.

——, "Feeding of India's growing millions" Asia Publishing House, Bombay, 1964.

——, "The World's Hunger and Future Needs in Food Supplies (with discussion)" J. Roy. Stat. Soc. Vol. 124, No. 4, pp. 463, 1961.

——, "The World's future food supplies" J. Roy. Stat. Soc. Vol. 129, No. 2, p. 222, 1966.

DIRECTORATE OF ECONOMICS AND STATISTICS, Ministry of Agriculture, Government of India, New Delhi, "Bulletin on Food Statistics," 1972.

DIRECTORATE-GENERAL OF HEALTH SERVICES, Nutrition Cell, New Delhi, "Annual Report on Nutrition activities," 1968, 1969-70 and 1970-71.

JELLIFFE, D.B., "The assessment of Nutritional Status of the Community," W.H.O. monograph series No. 53, 1966.

——, and JELLIFFE, E.F.P., The arm circumference as a public health index of protein-calorie malnutrition of early childhood. Journal. Trop. Pediat. 15: 177-260, 1969.

F.A.O. OF UNITED NATIONS, "Freedom from Hunger Campaign Basic Studies, No. 11 and 12." Rome.

UNICEF, "Statistical Profile of Children and Youth in India," New Delhi, 1974.

WHO OF U.N., Technical Report Series No. 485 and 340, Geneva.

RAJ, K.N., "Extent of undernourishment in Kerala," Yojana Vol. XVI No. 9, p. 785. 1972.

PANIKAR, P.G.K., "Food Balance Sheet of Kerala" Working paper No. 6, Centre for Development Studies, Trivandrum, 1972.

RAMAIAH, T.J. and SRIVASTAVA, A.B.L., Review of the current status of health statistics in India and the needed improvements. National Seminar on Social Statistics, New Delhi 17-22 March, 1975, organised by the Central Statistical Organisation, Government of India, New Delhi (SSS/C-8), 1975.

DIRECTORATE-GENERAL OF HERLTH SERVICES, Government of India, "Statistics of Health and Nutrition," Paper presented at the National Seminar on Social Statistics, New Delhi, 17-22 March, 1976, organised by C.S.O., Government of India, New Delhi (SSS/B-3-1), 1975.

VISWESWARA RAO, K., "Availability of statistics of Nutrition and data requirements," paper presented at the National Seminar on Social Statistics, New Delhi, organised by the C.S.O., New Delhi (SSS/C-9), 1975.

VISWESWARA RAO, K. and SINGH, D., "An evaluation of the relationship between nutritional status and anthropometric measurements," Amer. J. Clin. Nutr. Vol. 23, No. 1, pp. 83-93, 1970.

United Nations Statistical Year Book, 24th issue, pp. 510-524, 1972.

RAO, N.V.S., Socio-economic indicators for developmental planning, paper presented at the National Seminar on Social Statistics, New Delhi, 17-22 March, 1975 (SSS/C-2).

KRISHNAMURTHY, K G, and DHRUVASAN, A.R., "Social Development Indicators," paper presented at the National Seminar on Social Statistics, 17-22 March 1975, New Delhi (SSS/C-3), 1975.

YUK MIURA, Measurement of National Welfare in Japan—"Net National Welfare and Social Indicators." presented at the National Seminar on Social Statistics, 17-22 March, 1975, New Delhi (SSS/D-3).

FAO OF U.N., "Short-term programme of Social Statistics and Indicators," paper presented at the National Seminar on Social Statistics conducted by the C.S.O. New Delhi, 17-22 March, 1975 (SSS/A-4).

CENTRAL STATISTICAL ORGANISATION, Government of India, New Delhi, "Data requirements of the proposed U.N. System of Social and Demographic Statistics" presented at the National Seminar on Social Statistics conducted by the C.S.O., New Delhi, 17-22 March. 1975 (SSS/B. 01).

Statistics on Cause of Death

P. SINGHA*

The scope and emphasis of public health programme are determined to a great extent by current relative significance of cause-of-death statistics in the absence of illness statistics. Cause-of-death statistics serve a variety of useful purposes, including medical, sociological, pharmaceutical and demographic researches. Yet, of all the items in the vital statistics system in India, perhaps cause-of-death statistics have received least attention.

There have been many attempts to improve the coverage and completeness of vital events but very little has been achieved to make the quality of cause-of-death statistics consumable for health administration and planning. Since the planned development programmes started, there has been a growing awareness for the need to improve the quality of data on cause-of-death in this country. The subject of vital statistics passed from the Ministry of Health and Family Planning (DGHS) to Registrar General, India in 1960. Since then various measures for the improvement of vital statistics system in India are being made. Some schemes have been initiated to improve the cause of death statistics also.

Quality of Cause-of-Death Statistics

Apart from incompleteness, the registered deaths in bulk of the cases do not have specific description of cause in diagnostic terms meaningful for any medical or statistical interpretations. Most of the registered deaths, specially from rural areas have their causes reported in symptomatic conditions like heart failures etc. Because of the statutory international obligations for reporting quarantianable diseases, three diseases smallpox, cholera and plague receive attention.

The list of causes of death, so far used as a result, consists of seven

*PSD. Department of Family Planning, Government of India.

conditions—cholera, smallpox, plague, dysentery and diarrhoea, respiratory diseases, fever, accidents and injuries and other diseases. This list which has been in vogue for long time is based mainly on non-specific conditions like fever, diarrhoea. This makes it worthless for any purposeful uses. The cause of death as reported by laymen is accepted as such. The reports usually consist of conditions present apparently with deceased mostly in terminal situation. Cause-of-death even reported from the qualified physicians conveys in most cases nothing more than a terminal condition or a mode of dying without mention of any specific diagnostic situation that causes the former. For this, physicians are scarcely to be blamed as there seldom exists any standard procedure as to how a cause-of-death is to be certified and even where a procedure exists in some areas, no machanism is there to prevail upon the doctors to follow it. Medical certificate in specific terms is insisted only in medico-legal cases, even through post mortem diagnosis by autopsy.

Let alone the deaths that occur without medical attendance, the large number of deaths that take place in hospitals or attended by private physicians, may very well have their cause specified in acceptable diagnostic term if a workable procedure is instituted for the purpose.

REGISTRAR-GENERAL'S SCHEMES FOR IMPROVEMENT OF CAUSE-OF-DEATHS

Ever since the responsibility for organizing vital statistics system has been taken over by the Registrar-General, India, attempts are being made in this direction to improve the cause-of-death statistics. At present two schemes have been introduced by Registrar-General of India throughout the country. The schemes are:

(1) Medical Certification of causes of deaths according to international procedure for the deaths attended by physicians.

(2) Under Model Registration Scheme (applicable to rural areas only)—Survey of cause of deaths.

Medical Certification of Cause-of-death

The first scheme relates to those deaths which were medically attended. It is by and large limited to the hospitals and medical institutions in the beginning with a scope to expand its coverage to include the deaths attended by private medical practitioners.

The scheme of the medical certification of causes of death is, at present, in vogue in hospitals and medical institutions of Andhra Pradesh, Assam, Haryana, Kerala, Madhya Pradesh, Maharashtra, Karnataka, Nagaland, Orissa, Punjab, Rajasthan, Tamil Nadu, Tripura, Uttar Pradesh, West Bengal and Union Territories of Arunachal Pradesh, Delhi, Goa, Daman and Diu and Lakshadweep.

Beginning with teaching hospitals the coverage gradually extends to the government hospitals. However, there is a variable coverage of the hospitals between states.

The percentages of deaths for which causes of deaths have been certified during 1969 and 1970 are given below:

	1969		*1970*		*Percentage coverage*	
	Total deaths registered.	*Deaths certified/classified according to ICD*	*Total deaths registered*	*Deaths certified/classified according to ICD*	*1969*	*1970*
Andhra Pradesh	244511	4027	252129	6739	1.7	2.7
Haryana	84000	NA	74983	2621	NA	3.5
Karnataka	163695	NA	162363	9478	NA	5.8
Punjab	111670	7278	110044	NA	6.5	NA
Rajasthan	28602	7603	27183	5958	26.6	21.9
Goa, Daman & Diu	7688	7688	7418	7418	100.0	100.0
Madras Corp.	39220	12248	35305	NA	31.2	NA
Greater Bombay	54831	54831	55898	55898	100.0	100.0
Nagpur Corp.	9382	9382	9011	9011	100.0	100.0
Poona	9819	9819	9875	NA	100.0	NA

Only three to four per cent of the total deaths are covered by the scheme. Thus much efforts are still needed to extend the coverage of medically attended deaths.

The ultimate goal of this scheme is to provide a meaningful data on causes of death. The procedural steps essentially consist of:

(1) Certification of cause of death by the attending physician in the international form of medical certification of cause of death in

which he indicates which morbid condition led directly to death and states the antecedent conditions, if any, which gave rise to this cause, with underlying cause stated last.

(2) Coding of underlying cause of death according to the WHO regulation by means of international detailed list of causes of death. The general rule for coding is to code the underlying cause of death which was the starting point in the sequence of events leading up to the direct cause. Exceptions to this general rule are given in the WHO International Statistical Classification of Diseases, Injuries and Causes of Death. The primary object of such rules is to obtain consistency and uniformity when certification is made faulty, ambiguous or inverted in assigning the conditions and diagnostic descriptions.

(3) Finally, tabulation of coded certificates into disease categories by age, sex and other relevant items.

It is advisable always to have separate tabulation for the data whose accuracy and validity are ensured. Medically certified deaths should have separate tabulation and should not be mixed with the data accrued from other sources.

This scheme has been introduced, it appears, with no proper spadework. The value and significance of the data accrued so far from this scheme have been assessed in an earlier paper 'Cause of death statistics in India' by the author. In this paper various types of errors that vitiate the data have been identified. These errors crop up through faulty certificates, wrong coding and irrelevant tabulation. Quality of cause of death statistics could be improved by minimising these errors. These could be easily accomplished if the scheme is implemented with adequate ground work, careful planning and effective control and direction.

The first step towards the introduction of medical certification of cause of death is the careful campaign of education and training in international procedures. Introduction of medical certification in hospitals should be preceded by thorough training of medical house officers, medical officer-incharge of wards and departmental incharges. There is good literature available in this regard. The WHO pamphlet in medical certification of cause of death is a very useful material containing the instructions and guide lines to the doctors as to how to certify cause of death Once the rule for completing international form of certificate and its purpose is understood, the certifiers require explanation and practice.

Teaching is not complete unless it is followed by a system of referral. This is lacking in the present scheme. The errors in certification that are committed could be minimised gradually through this system. The teaching paves the way for introduction, to achieve the quality of certificate, the programme of routine referral of the quality of certificate, the programme of routine referral of faulty and incorrect certificates is of supreme importance.

Routine referral is an effective supplement to education. Usually the method of referral consists in referring a copy of the original certificate to the certifying doctors of institution pointing out the error or ambiguity committed by the certifier. It may be emphasised that referral programme, however, costly is sine qua non in the process of adaptation. The author's experience in Nagpur in coping with the problem may be relevant to quote here. A study was undertaken by checking the completed certification with the case histories maintained in hospitals. Four types of deficiencies were detected—(*i*) omission of underlying cause, (ii) omission of maternal condition (*iii*) sequence not in order, and (*iv*) omission of external cause of injury.

To build up a tradition of good certification the instructions for all medical students are essential. Medical colleges may in their curricula include medical certification of cause of death. Such instructions may be reinforced to house staff by the trained registrars through supervised practice on actual death certification pending formal placement in the ward.

Cause of death coding procedures are a discipline in itself. It is a skilled job for which adequate training is necessary. Apart from the usual selection rules, understanding of the content as well as the intent of the international classification of causes of deaths is of supreme importance for medical coder. At present Health Statistics Unit at Nagpur runs a twelve week course on medical coding. Full advantage should be taken of this course to train coders. If need be more such centres may be opened under the directions and control of Registrar General, India. Coding of the certificates should be entrusted to trained coders and not to amateurists.

Lay Report of Cause of Death

It has been already mentioned that bulk of these reports on cause of death come from lay people. These reports are nowhere comparable to the medical certificates. The value and significance of these reports in deriving a meaningful mortality picture are dubious. However, some attempt has been made in the past to collect lay reports of 'cause of death' and make them useful for the purpose of health planning and administration.

Mention may be made of Yves Biraud's nod-medical list of 21 causes. This non-medical list (NM list) is devised for a system of recording of vital events and crude cause of death by lay man. It is a system on which current events should be recorded chronologically in specially designed proforma to include only age, sex and conditions as reported. This proforma is so designed that it covers 21 causes of death defined by symptoms of anatomical sites or duration of illness or combination of them. The idea is that such record in the context of the local conditions and seasonal variation may provide more clue to the prevalence of health conditions and health requirements of the population concerned. The information in this regard may be collected by non-medical investigators from the relation of the deceased.

Yves Biraud's non-medical list is reproduced: accidents, attacks from venomous and other animals, injury by other person (homicide), suicide, death of women in child birth, bellyache with diarrhoea, bellyache without diarrhoea, cough with short illness, cough with long illness, shortness of breath with swelling of legs, sudden death, difficulty or pain in passing urine, yellow skin and eyes with long illness, lumps, yellow skin and eyes with short illness, fever with skin eruption, fever with headache and stiff neck, fever with repeated attack, fevers—other (unqualified), other known causes of death, unknown causes.

Trial was given to examine the suitability of this list in some selected areas. The author was concerned with a trial made in Kalmeswar Health Centre near Nagpur. The Kalmeswar trial showed that Biraud's list does not provide any meaningful statistics consumable by the health department. Of the 1038 deaths recorded and tabulated in the list, heavy concentration was seen only in a few categories like "bellyache and diarrohea," "fever unqualified," "cough with short illness" and the residual category namely "other known causes of death." The "unknown causes" also accounted for large number of deaths. Judged from all those Biraud's non-medical classification as it stands does not very well suit to the data to serve any useful purpose.

The Registrar-General's survey of cause of death, under Model Registration Scheme, is but an extension of this attempt. This scheme, which was taken up first on pilot basis in 1965, is in operation in rural areas of the country. The scheme is at present functioning in almost all the major states. It envisages a systematic programme of collecting statistics on mortality by causes through lay reporting by the use of para medical staff functioning at the PHCs in rural areas. On the whole, one PHC for every million of population has been taken for each state. The field agent in his course of duty visits PHC villages and enquires about the cause of death from the household of members where a death has occurred and lists it in accordance with a non-medical list (NM list) prescribed by Registrar-General for the purpose. Information is collected about the symptoms, conditions, anatomical site and duration of illness from the deceased's relation in order to arrive at the probable cause of death.

A manual of instructions has been prepared by the Registrar-General, for its use by the field agents. The manual outlines the procedure for singling out the probable cause of death from the reported symptoms. The list comprises a set of eleven major cause group subdivided into numerous probable specific diseases. These groups are: Accidents and injuries, Child birth and pregnancy, Fevers, Digestive disorders, Cough (disorders of respiratory system), Disorders of the central nervous system, Diseases of circulatory system, Other clear symptoms, Causes special to infancy, Senility, the Rest.

The data collected through the scheme are published in special report. Latest available is the report for 1972. The report gives the causes of death as covered under the scheme.

The report provides commentaries on findings generalising observation on infant mortality, maternal mortality, mortality by age and sex, and leading causes of death for individual State. A number of tables further provide data showing inter-State variation. The data collected in 1971 comprise of only 16,824 deaths on the all-India level. However, 1972 commentaries are somewhat restricted; they refrain from making bold generalisation at least for individual States. The data collected in 1972 total only 16,104.

Most disquieting features of the tables is that they seldom show absolute number but provide only percentages, perhaps to avoid to show insignificant frequencies. No attempts are so far made in the report to assess the reliability and degree of acceptability of the conditions reported as cause-of-death by the investigator. Lacking this, data provided carry a little or no utility for whatever purpose and the generalisation made carries no much sense. Although the Registrar-General himself in this report has warned against the unrestricted use of these data as the coverage is not complete and quite a few events of deaths are missed.

However, it is a pertinent question as to what exact uses they could be put to. First, the PHCs, where this scheme is operative, are not at all the representative of the states. Then the coverage is doubted as all events are not netted. As for the quality of the data, the broad headings of the causes of death rule out specificity. The classification adopted then needs to be assessed as to what practical purpose it serves. The epidemiologists of public health administrators are not content with these scanty data with doubtful accuracy.

However, it is worthwhile to examine even then how the present classifications should suit the data accrued from the scheme. The appropriateness of statistical classification should be judged from the following considerations:

(*i*) The categories should be mutually exclusive and clearly defined;

(*ii*) The number of classes in the classification scheme should be kept to a minimum;

(*iii*) Description of every case should have a place in one of the classes;

(*iv*) Appreciable frequency should be there to justify existence as a separate entity; and

(*v*) Residual class for different conditions which cannot be put under more specific class should contain comparatively few descriptions.

While the first three criteria are met to some extent, the last two do not appear to fit well. As far as the 1971 data are concerned, the detailed list which covers sub groups under each main group contains some classes for which sufficient deaths were not available *e.g.* under main group 'cough' streptoccocal sore throat of tongue, 'under' swelling group and under 'fever' group 'diphtheria' and 'malaria'. The most important observation in this scheme of tabulation which makes the data dubious is the preponderance of the number of deaths in the residual category under each main heading. The percentage of reported deaths in the residual categories under various groups are reproduced in the table on the next page.

The scheme is virtually the post-mortem survey to establish the cause of death. The information is collected from households. Obviously the information can only provide a description as was apparent. This description is limited only to some symptoms and outward conditions.

In many such cases *it* is virtually impossible to come out with a

Cause of death	Percentage of deaths classified in the residual category under the cause of death mentioned in col. (*i*) 1971	1972
Violence or and injury	14.8	11.0
Child birth and complicated pregnancy	25.8	20.2
Diarrhoea	29.0	38.4
Cough		
(*i*) Broncho pneumonia, pneumonia, bronchitis, influenza, streptococcal sore throat, whooping cough	6.6	7.0
(*ii*) Tuberculosis of respiratory system	6.9	11.2
Swellings	17.5	19.3
Fevers		
(*i*) With skin eruptions	9.1	9.5
(*ii*) With headache and stiff neck	8.7	2.4
(*iii*) With repeated attacks:		
(*a*) Malaria	13.2	10.6
(*b*) Typhoid, diphtheria, septicaemia, pynemia etc., tuberculosis of other forms	27.5	32.8
Other infant deaths	23.5	28.1

definite diagnosis even if the investigator is a medical man. A similar scheme to collect lay reports of cause of death was carried out by Gordon *et al* in the early sixties in a few villages of Punjab. The study area is popularly known as Khanna study. Every death in the study area was probed into by physicians. The evidence as to the probable cause was gathered from as many sources as possible.

Many deceased had no medical attention of any kind. After investigation in the field, each death and the concerning evidence as to its cause were reviewed in clinical conference of two or more doctors to decide the most probable cause of death. Even with all this precaution, the decisions taken were recognized as of varying reliability sometimes because of the nature of the disease and sometimes because of incomplete information.

Such methodology of post-mortem diagnosis of cause of death by interviewing the relation of the deceased provides data of doubtful validity, significance of which should be adequately appreciated before making any attempt to interpret them.

It is worthwhile here to give the experiences the present author had in this regard in connection with a field surveillance carried out in Kashmere Gate area of Delhi under the auspices of National Institute of Communicable Diseases, Delhi. The surveillance programme was initiated in 1968 and continued well beyond 1974 but the author was associated with programme till 1973. The programme started with 2,112 families and later was extended to cover 4,545 families with 24,421 population. The primary purpose of this surveillance was to follow up each individual of the family to observe the different types of illnesses that come from time to time. In the course of this follow-up, deaths occurring to the families under surveillance were also recorded. These deaths were later ascertained if they were registered or not.

In course of this matching, some of the enthusiastic investigators noted down the causes of death as recorded in the death register. There are 32 non-hospitalized deaths for which cause of death as registered in the official register were known. For all these 32 deaths, the record of illnesses covered from one year to five years were also available. The diagnosis recorded in the death register were compared with surveillance record. They presented a very interesting picture.

Though nothing could be generalised from these scanty data, the indication that about 50% of deaths even in an urban set-up go misreported in regard to cause is well suggestive.

SUGGESTIONS

The foregoing discussion is not meant for deprecating the importance of the Registrar General's Model Registration scheme. In spite of its weakness, it is a deserving attempt to fill in this information gap to get as much information as possible on cause of death from rural areas of the country. What is needed to improve the quality of data is the continued evaluation of the scheme.

In the foreword of report entitled "Cause of Death—A Survey—1972" the Registrar General, India, however, has informed us of setting up of an evaluation team to suggest improvement. What renovation has been incorporated at the suggestion of the evaluation team and as a result how the data have improved are not yet known. The propensity observed in the Registrar General's report in making sweeping generalisation and inter-regional comparison over these data whose significance is not fully understood is wholly unwelcome. Attempt should be made to weigh the data for its relevance.

For example, take maternal deaths, what proportion of maternal deaths have been probably included in the group or sub-groups of conditions in denoting maternal deaths and how much have been left out or misclassified? Each group or sub-group in the list should have an estimate as to the degree of acceptability. At the same time rubrics of each group and sub-group may be extended, expanded and reshuffled to arrive at a list relatively best suited to this type of data.

Further, the data accrued from these two schemes of Registrar-General are divergent in as much as cause of death as determined from medical certificates is the underlying cause, whereas the lay reports obtained from rural areas may be any thing, not necessarily underlying cause. It is desirable to develop an acceptable method of collation of these two types of data to bring forth an overall picture of mortality even if it may be a crude one. Pattern of delivery of health services in this country is now being reoriented to introduce multipurpose workers scheme. The Registrar-General may very well take advantage of this new situation to generate more meaningful statistics of cause of death.

Morbidity and Cause of Death Statistics

ASOK MITRA*

When the first sample census of births and deaths was taken in 1952-53 under the auspices of the Registrar-General, an attempt was made to devise a table for each state on the cause of death. The state of the art at that time can be judged from the fact that the Director of Health was called upon to publish an analysis of the reported deaths under eight main causes—cholera, smallpox, plague, fevers, dysentery and diarrhoea, respiratory diseases, injuries and other causes. The residuary category "other causes" accounted every year even for a state like Bombay, for more than half the registered deaths. The result was "that no one could be sure of what the most important half dozen causes of deaths in Bombay state were."

Despite the recommendations of the Bhore Committee, it was realized that it is often difficult enough for doctors to say what the cause of death was. For lay police patels or chowkidars, it is generally impossible. It was suggested therefore that directors of public health should publish a brief pamphlet to help registration authorities to identify causes of death. That would be useful. The second stage should be to have home visits from vaccinators or other staff with some medical background. They could record the symptoms for subsequent evaluation by doctors. A sample inquiry of this type might prove useful. The pattern obtained by it could be compared with that obtained under normal registration.

However, improvement in the level of births and deaths reporting being considered more important than evaluation of the causes of death, the latter has always suffered in as much as the former claimed about all the attention it could. The point only needs to be stated to be realized that extension of medical facilities will be necessary before any real improvement in the reporting of causes of death can be expected.

Between the experimental census of 1952-53 and 1958-64 when the

*Professor, Jawaharlal Nehru University, New Delhi.

Registrar-General launched a variety of attempts to stimulate the state directorates of health services to pay greater attention to the international classification, the abbreviate Yves Biraud classification, and the still more abbreviated Registrar-General's list, much attention was paid on a small-scale to recording of cause of death in responsive states and under the auspices of the All-India Institute of Hygiene and Public Health in places like Singur in West Bengal.

By way of illustration of the kind of effort that went into these investigations may be mentioned the several excellent reports on the short general health survey conducted around 1954-56 of several of the first generation of community development blocks throughout India under the leadership of S.C. Seal, Professor of Epidemiology of AIIHPH, Calcutta. Unfortunately, already these reports, published between 1954 and 1957, have gone very rare and some are even unavailable. Morbidity varied from block to block. For example, guinea worm claimed the highest morbidity in Dungarpur block of Rajasthan while the same cause was quite low down the list in West Bengal (Saktigarh). But the staples were fairly regular: fevers, scabies and skin disease, asthma, bronchitis, diseases of the digestive system, diarrhoea and dysentery, malaria, diseases due to pregnancy and childbirth, anaemia, diseases of the respiratory and circulatory systems etc. As to causes of sickness and death according to morbidity the following table for Dungarpur block is typical.

TABLE 1: *The first eight numerically important causes of sickness and deaths according to morbidity per 1,00,000 population during 12 months prior to survey: Dungarpur Community Development Block Rajasthan, 1956*

	Morbidity rate per 1,00,000 population
Fevers, other	3,478
Guinea worm infection	2,932
Diarrhoea and dysentery	1,059
Other ill-defined causes	511
Bronchitis	443
Typhoid and paratyphoid fevers	307
Skin and other diseases	273
Pneumonia	239
Cataract	239

Source: Report published by AIIHPH, Calcutta, 1956, p. 52.

Table 2 relates to the distribution of population according to morbidity rates, mortality rates and duration of sickness for different periods of life.

TABLE 2: *Distribution of population according to morbidity rates, mortality rates and duration of sickness for different periods of life in Dungarpur block 1956*

	Sample population	*Morbidity*		*Mortality*		*Duration of sickness in days excluding death*	
		No. suffered	*Rate per mille*	*No. dead*	*Rate per mille*	*Per sick person*	*Per head of population*
Infant (year)	127	5	39.4	2	15.2	3.4	0.15
Pre-School (1-5 years)	357	21	58.4	—	—	16.3	0.95
School age (5-15 years)	824	84	101.9	—	—	16.4	1.7
Adult (15-55 years)	1,506	168	111.6	4	—	62.6	7.0
Old age (55+)	119	23	193.3	—	—	51.0	9.9
All age groups	2,933	301	102.6	6	2.0	44.8	4.6

Source: Table L XIII, p. 56 of report published by AIIHPH, Calcutta.

The actual morbidity rate was highest among old persons above 55 years of age—193.3 per 1,000 with an average duration of 9.0 days per head—but the loss of working efficiency due to morbidity in the working age 15-55 is even more appalling; for the duration of sickness per sick person was highest among persons of this working age, the average loss being 63 days. The duration of sickness in pre-school and school age is not inconsiderable either and is an explanation in a large measure of the high rate of wastages and dropouts at school.

Table 3 gives an idea of the average number of days per year during which persons were sick. This Table, too, throws light on the enormous loss of efficiency and interruptions that sickness inflicts on people of working age 15-55 as well on children of pre-school and school age.

TABLE 3: *The average duration of sickness per person per year according to different blocks surveyed, 1954-56*

(*Figures in days*)

Name of block	*Age*					*Average of all ages*
	Less than 1	*1 to 5*	*5 to 15*	*15 to 55*	*55+*	
Saktigarh	26.4	60.9	43.2	111.7	155.8	95.7
Dabra	56.4	44.4	24.9	16.5	133.5	67.0
Ekangarsarai	30.4	43.3	63.8	102.2	135.7	90.3
Dungarpur	3.4	16.3	16.4	62.6	51.0	44.8

Source: Table L XIII A, p. 57 of Report on Dungarpur Block, 1956.

The Central Bureau of Health Intelligence of the Director-General of Health Services having concentrated its efforts on a narrow core of epidemiology covering epidemics and infectious diseases, the wider examination of the cause of death statistics was assumed towards the end of the fifties by the Registrar-General of India, who began publishing his annual reports on vital statistics in a comprehensive form 1958 onwards. The report of 1960 laid special emphasis on cause of death.

Having regard to the aim of this paper, we shall pick out particularly those aspects which have greater bearing on public health or the preventive aspect than on medical or the curative aspect of cause of death statistics. When the systematic appraisal by the Registrar-General began in 1958, the 1959 report could rely only on the statistics of hospital deaths by causes certified in the international form by practitioners of modern medicine in Nagpur for 1957 and 1958; in Rajasthan for 1959; and for Bombay city for four years, 1956-59. The 1960 Report added statistics for Poona city for three financial years ending 1959-60.

Nagpur data related to deaths occurring in private and government hospitals, maternity homes, jails and railway hospitals. Rajasthan data covered deaths occurring in government public hospitals in rural and urban areas, the bulk of the data relating, however, to urban areas, since nearly 90 per cent of beds were in urban hospitals. Bombay data were not certified in the international form but carried certificates by medical practitioners who attended the deceased during his last illness. Poona data were a mixture of the international form and medical certificates admitted for cremations or burials. The 1960

Report published special reports for West Bengal and nine districts of Mysore.

The promotional work performed in the 1950s by Dr Enid Charles, then attached to WHO, Delhi, amply brought out the fact that there was no conflict between the interests of demography and public health in the field of vital statistics. In fact the interests were very complementary; demography being interested in potentials and trends and public health in current measures.

The caution that must be borne in mind in contemplating the statistics is that (*1*) since the cases are all hospitalized cases, they are over-represented by the more complicated and serious ones resulting in death; (*2*) hospitalization being far from universal, the availability of hospital services and their acceptance by the people being limited, these factors may have over-represented certain diseases and socio-economic groups in the population; (*3*) hospital facilities for treatment being usually superior to what are available to those that die outside hospitals, the mortality pattern of these tables reflect the serious types of illnesses calling for curative skill and under-represent the more general and widespread epidemiological illnesses; and (*4*) the precise social, economic and medical influence of selective forces of the illnesses registered is not properly known. Nonetheless, the statistics yield a broad picture of the state of public health and medical services available under, of course, severely restricted environs.

The emphasis here being deliberately restricted more to public health areas—although it must be immediately acknowledged that the line between public health and medical in this field is often very thin—we shall exclude statistics relating to ten of the 17 major groups of the international list of cause of death—(*I*) infective and parasitic diseases; (*II*) neoplasms; (*III*) allergic, endocrine system, metabolic and nutritional diseases; (*IV*) diseases of the blood and blood forming organs; (*V*) mental psycho-neurotio and personality disorders; (*VI*) diseases of the nervous system and sense organs; (*VII*) disease of the circulatory system; (*VIII*) diseases of the respiratory system; (*IX*) diseases of the digestive system; (*X*) diseases of the genito-urinary system; (*XI*) deliveries and complications of pregnancy, child birth and the puerperium; (*XII*) diseases of the skin and cellular tissue; (*XIII*) disease of the bones and organs of movement; (*XIV*) congenital malformations; (*XV*) certain diseases of early infancy; (*XVI*) symptoms, senility and ill-defined conditions; and (*XVII*) accidents, poisoning and violence. The emphasis will thus be mainly on the remaining seven major groups of the International list. Among these major groups again only a very few specific causes in each have been picked up for discussion.

The discussion may well open with a summary table of proportion of deaths in each of the seven selected groups to total deaths for the years 1957-62, wherever data are available.

Two first comments will be in order. First, that these seven major groups of diseases out of a total of 17 claim the majority of deaths even in the best of city municipal areas, where at least potable water and a minimum of certain public health, sanitation and medical care services and amenities are assured, and that these seven major groups are primarily a manifestation of the level or lack of them of these services and amenities. Second, that, although the four areas exhibit four distinct regional patterns of permutations and combinations of the seven major groups, reflecting in great measure, particularly in respect of groups I and IX, the state of the municipal sanitary and public health care services and amenities, the *inter se* proportions among the seven major groups in each of the four areas, however, exhibit a remarkable unity of pattern, each highlighting the problems of infections and parasitic diseases, diseases of the circulatory, respiratory and digestive systems and diseases peculiar to early infancy that waited to be tackled in all these four areas. What is more, all these groups were primarily the concern of public health care, or preventive medicine, authorities.

In Bombay and Poona, which have particularly good environmental and sanitary conditions, proportionate mortality due to infections and parasitic diseases and diseases of digestive system is distinctly lower than in Nagpur, West Bengal (for which figures are not given) and Rajathan. On the other hand, mortality from diseases of the respiratory system and of allergic, endocrine system, metabolic and nutritional diseases, the former group, including great killers like pneumonia and bronchopneumonia, was markedly higher in the city areas of Bombay and Poona than in Nagpur and Rajasthan. This picture agrees with the accepted notion that in communities with relatively poor health, sanitary condition and nutrition, infective and parasitic diseases are the most important killers, but, even as they are brought under control, diseases of the respiratory system and of metabolism and nutrition assume greater significance.

By far the big killers were, in descending order of numerical importance, infectious and parasitic diseases, certain diseases of early

TABLE 4: *Proportionate deaths under selected major groups of international list of cause of death, 1957-1961.*

Description *Major Group No.*	*Nagpur*				*Bombay*				*Poona*			*Rajasthan*		
	1957-59	*1960*	*1961*	*1962*	*1959-60*	*1959-61*	*1961*	*1962*	*1957-60*	*1959-61*	*1962*	*1959-61*	*1961*	*1962*
Total Deaths	8,689	3,260	3,753	3,661	1,51,830	92,041	32,506	39,551	27,453	20,134	7,239	13,402	4,576	5,915
I Infectious & parasitic diseases	28.5	28.2	29.8	27.0	13.7	14.6	14.2	12.3	14.5	14.2	15.1	22.7	22 0	21.8
III Allergic, Endocrine system, metabolic & nutritional diseases	2.2	1.5	1.5	1.5	5.6	4.4	4.6	4.7	1.5	4.1	6.5	1.5	1.0	1.4
VII Diseases of the circulatory system	5.7	5.7	5.6	5.6	7.0	7.8	3.0	10.1	5.2	6.3	6.6	6.3	6.6	8.1
VIII Diseases of the respiratory system	6.6	6.9	5.1	5.4	18.9	20.7	22.3	15.8	11.6	10.6	10.9	9.5	9.0	8.3
IX Diseases of the digestive system	10.8	10.5	10.1	11.4	7.6	6.4	2.9	7.4	7.5	9.4	10.6	13 7	12.7	12.2
XI Deliveries & complications of pregnancy, child-birth and the puerperium	3.5	2.0	2.1	2.6	0.2	0.4	0.4	0.3	0.4	0.4	0.4	4.3	5.0	3 1
XV Certain diseases of early infancy	16.2	14.4	18.0	15.9	11.4	11.6	11.3	13.7	17.0	14.4	11.4	10.3	12 6	11.7
Total of 7 major groups	73.5	69.2	72.2	69.4	64.4	65.9	58.7	64.3	57.7	59.4	61.5	68.3	68 9	66 6
Grand Total	100	100	100	100	100	100	100	100	100	100	100	100	100	100

Sources: Vital Statistics of India 1961, Table 36 A, p. LVIII, and Vital Statistics of India, 1962, Table 14. p xii.

infancy (they go together), diseases of the digestive system, diseases of the respiratory system, deseases of the circulatory system, deliveries and complications of pregnancy, childbirth and the puerperium and allergic, endocrine system, metabolic and nutritional diseases. Every one of these primarily depends on the state of excellence and availability of public health measures and preventive services.

Coming to some of the detailed causes within the seven major International groups, the Report for 1960 considered proportionat deaths per thousand of deaths in each major group. The following table is abstracted from Table 3 (p. xxxii—xxxiv) of the 1960 Report.

TABLE 5: *Proportionate deaths per thousand of deaths in each of the seven selected major groups of the international list of cause of death, 1959-60.*

Cause group with detailed list Nos.	*Nagpur (1959)*	*Rajasthan (1960)*	*West Bengal (1960)*	*Bombay (1960)*	*Poona (1960)*
1	*2*	*3*	*4*	*5*	*6*
Major Group I Infactive and Parasitic Diseases (001-138)					
1. Tuberculosis of respiratory system (010)	302	148	136	396	336
2. Tuberculosis of meninges & central nervous system (010)	126	39	67	114	86
7. Typhoid fever (040)	50	199	66	47	24
12. Diphtheria (055)	63	60	125	29	45
16. Tetanus (061)	217	202	41	59	88
18. Small pox (084)	1	17	2	169	35
19. Measles (085)	1	64	6	41	77
24. Malaria (110-117)	25	36	10	1	—
25. Diseases due to helminths (124,126-130)	21	11	17	7	12
26. All other diseases classified as infective and parasitic (Rest of Major Group I)	20	12	166	18	91
Major Group III (Allergic, endocrine system, metabolic& nutritional diseases)					

1	*2*	*3*	*4*	*5*	*6*
31. 1 Rickets (283-284)	43	70	5	280	N.A.
31. 2 A vitaminosis & other deficiency states (280-282) (285-286)	69	22	367	2	583
32. Anaemias (290-293)	35	76	38	11	83
Major Group VII Circulatory system (460-468)					
38. Rheumatic fever		17	22	9	4
Major Group VIII (Respiratory system (470-475))					
46. 2 Bronchopneumonia (491)	631	540	494	587	681
46. 3 Primary atypical, other & unspecified Pneumonia (492-493)	51	82	168	297	57
47. Bronchitis (500-502)	61	133	127	45	200
Major Group IX (Digestive system (530-587))					
53. Gastritis, duodenitis enteritis, & colitie except diarrhoea of the new born	505	468	391	650	738
Major Group XI (Deliveries & complications of pregnancy etc.)					
60. Sepsis of pregnancy, & child birth & puerperiam (640, 6 , 681, 682, 684)	137	150	53	182	79
61. Toxaemias of pregnancy & puerperium (642. 652, 685, 686)	266	218	356	—	184
62.1 Placenta praevia & anteparatium haemorrhage (643 & 670)	56	114	75	55	N.A.
62.2 Other haemorrhages of pregnancy and child birth (644, 671-672)	40	83	108	172	158
65.1 Anaemia of pregnancy (646)	194	130	112	N.A.	N.A.
65.2 Rest of major Group XI	282	243	241	500	500
Major Groups XV (Early Infancy)					

1	*2*	*3*	*4*	*5*	*6*
69. Postnatal asphyxia & atelactasis (762)	145	115	157	98	56
70. Pneumonia, diarrhoea & other infections of new born (765-768)	90	185	147	38	124
71.1 Rest of major group XV with mention of immaturity	630	432	386	449	706
71.2 Rest of major group XV without mention of immaturity	95	206	257	402	69

The Registrar-General's annual reports of vital statistics for 1960, 1961 and 1962 have given an interesting set of uniform tables of mortality of boy and girl infants from a few of the most important specific causes, which shows that mortality of male infants is distinctly higher than that of female infants. "The differences are marked and do not seem to be wholly accountable to the greater proportion of male births, which does not exceed by more than 106 per 100 female births." Rather they reflect on the greater biological vulnerability of male infants in the first year of life.

TABLE 6: *Cause-specific infant mortality (absolute numbers) by sex in three cities of India (1960-62)*

	1960 Infant Deaths			*1961* Infant Deaths			*1962* Infant Deaths	
	M	*F*		*M*	*F*		*M*	*F*
			A. Bombay					
Congenital malformation	982	862	Tuberculosis	46	49	Tuberculosis	82	83
Prematurity	854	626	Small pox	95	89	Small pox	4	5
Tuberculosis	47	34	Pneumonia	1,324	1,391	Pneumonia	1,140	1,114
Diphtheria	18	12	Congenital malformation	1,123	965	Congenital malformation	110	85
			Injury at birth	—	—	Injury at birth	290	188
			Premature birth	887	703	Premature birth	2,011	1,605

			B. Calcutta					
Congenital debility	79	46	All Bowel complaints	725	642	All Bowel complaints	576	550
Prematurity	1055	893	Respitatory diseases	1,064	946	Respiratory diseases	980	915
Respiratory diseases except TB	1049	936	Premature birth	1,076	800	Premature birth	994	751
Tetanus	90	49	Congenital debility	76	49	Congenital debility	36	40
			Tetanus	104	37	Tetanus	118	60
			C. Nagpur					
Anaemia	17	8	Convulsions	8	4	Convulsions	7	4
Convulsion	11	2	Tetanus	21	24	Tetanus	40	32
Respiratory Diseases	40	24	Rickets	3	1	Rickets	1	2
Tetanus	23	20	Broncho-pneumonia	41	23	Gastroente-ritis & Colitis	36	39
			Gastroen-terities & Colitis	27	28	Postnatal asphyxia & ateletasis	50	37
			Pneumonia new born	20	11	Tuberculosis	2	1
			Postnatal asphyxia & atelectasis	32	22			
			Tuberculosis	7	6			

Sourec: Registrar-General, India, Vital Statistics, 1960, 1961, 1962: Tables 28 (a), (b), (c), (d).

All that has so far been discussed, however, amounts to refinements of a situation whose lineaments are still so broad and coarse that they defy refinement. The basic fact of mortality in India must not be lost sight of—that the main causes of death on which returns from rural and urban areas of all states and union territories are compiled for meaningful, operational and classificatory significance, are still eight in the main, with three subsidiary ones. The eight causes are: cholera, smallpox, plague, dysentery and diarrhoea, respiratory diseases, fevers, accidents and injuries, and all other causes. The last cause includes three more: diphtheria, whooping cough and maternal deaths.

The only conclusion that is possible is that mortality in India is still overwhelmingly a public health and preventive problem which will have to be tackled for a long time yet.

Joining hands with the Registrar-General's effort, the Central Bureau of Health Intelligence brought out an important publication called *Geographical Pathology of India* which, with a few other publications of the same directorate, fills up the picture for the 1960's until we come to a better array of information again around 1970. Unfortunately, the volume was published only in mimeograph, and has become rare. It is important, therefore, to retrieve some of its material for the record.

First, the distribution of mortality by causes in India in 1962-64 was as follows:

TABLE 7: *Percentage distribution of deaths during 1962-64, in broad groups of causes (based on medical certification of cause of death)*

Description	*Bombay 1962-64*	*Nagpur 1962-64*	*Poona 1962-64*	*Rajasthan 1962-64*	*West Bengal 1962-54*
Infective and Parasitic Diseases	12.59	25.37	12.64	20.66	25.74
Neoplasm	4.61	3.83	3.38	2.80	3.65
Allergic, Endocrine System, Metabolic & Nutritional Diseases and Diseases of the Blood-Forming Organs	9.71	6.64	8.39	3.65	3.08
Mental, Psychoneurotic & Personality Disorders	0.06	0.21	0.14	0.28	N.A.
Diseases of the Nervous System and Sense Organs	4.42	7.70	4.13	4.81	5.56
Diseases of the Circulatory System	10.26	5.76	7.12	8.02	5.45
Diseases of the Respiratory System	15.78	5.73	9 20	8.16	3.87
Diseases of the Digestive System	8 10	11.54	11 31	12.45	10.51
Diseases of the Genito-Urinary System	0.87	1 45	1.19	2.06	1.04
Deliveries & Complications of Pregnancy, Childbirth and the Puerperium	0.33	2.17	0.46	3.72	4.55

Diseases of the Skin, Cellular Tissue Bones and Organs of Movement	0.30	0 52	0.09	0.63	N.A.
Congenital Malformations	0 57	1.36	0.87.	1.12	0 45
Certain Diseases of Early Infancy	13.23	15.88	13.07	12.64	9.24
Symptoms, Senility and ill-defined conditions	12.30	5.55	23.95	8.81	16 54
Accidents, Poisonings and Violence	6.87	6.29	4.06	10.19	10 37
TOTAL	100.00	100.00	100.00	100.00	100.00

Source: S.K. Sengupta & P.N. Kapoor: Principal Causes of Deaths in India, 1970; Table II, pp. 47-48.

CHOLERA

TABLE 8: *Incidence and distribution of cholera in India, 1954-64*

	Attack rate (no. of persons per 100,000 of population)	*Case fatality rate (per cent of attacks)*	*Death Rate per 100,000 of population*
Andhra Pradesh	10.01 – 15.00	41.87	6.16
Assam	> 5.00	50.15	1.41
Bihar	15.01 – 20.00	36.38	6.01
Gujarat	> 5.00	17.90	0.33
Karnataka	10.01 – 15.00	39.32	4.40
Kerala	> 5.00	52.85	0.06
Madhya Pradesh	5.01 – 10.00	44.17	2.60
Maharashtra	10.01 – 15.00	31.59	3.81
Orissa	10.01 – 15.00	46.99	6.97
Punjab (including Haryana)	> 5.00	24.77	0.05
Rajasthan	> 5.00	33.83	0 04
Tamil Nadu	10.01 – 15.00	43.01	5.14
Uttar Pradesh	> 5.00	34.36	0.62
West Bengal	20.01 – 25.00	39.40	9.52
Delhi		8.70	0.19
Himachal Pradesh	> 5 00	40.00	0.08
Manipur	> 5.00	34.38	0.54
Pondicherry	25.01 & above	32.56	10.00
Tripura	5 01 – 10.00	43.22	2.88

A more detailed geographical picture is available in *Statistical Review of Cholera Problem in India* by K.C. Patnaik and P.N. Kapoor (1967). This book says that during 1961-65 India alone was responsible for 73.9 per cent of total world cases and 84.9 per cent of total world deaths. This in spite of the fact that the mean annual death rate which was as high as 1.58 (deaths per 1,000 population) during 1900-24 dropped to 0.74 during 1925-47 and still further to 0.17 during 1948-63. "There is not a single week when cholera is not reported from some part or the other of the country," although the incidence varies with the seasons, rainfall, humidity and temperature.

Some of the important factors which favour persistence of cholera in India, singly or jointly, are (*1*) close proximity between the frankly endemic and the potentially epidemic areas—both within the state and the neighbouring states; (*2*) delayed and defective notification: (*3*) poor and primitive environmental conditions including water supply and sewage disposal system; (*4*) lack of facilities for epidemiological investigations and statistical intelligence; (*5*) supporting laboratory and ambulance services; and (*6*) lack of facilities of isolation and treatment centres. Rail, river, road traffic and particularly fairs and festivals play a pre-eminent role in the spread and persistence of cholera. The bastions of cholera are Pondicherry, West Bengal, Orissa, Andhra Pradesh, Bihar, Tamil Nadu, Karnataka and Maharashtra. Together they accounted for about 90 per cent of total deaths reported in India during 1956-66. Of these again, Bihar's contribution was 20.84 per cent, West Bengal's 18.57 per cent, Andhra Pradesh's 13.52 per cent, Maharashtra's 12.09 per cent, Tamil Nadu's 10.70 per cent, Orissa's 6.07 per cent and Karanataka's 5.93 per cent.

As for rural urban distribution, Andhra Pradesh, Bihar, Madhya Pradesh and Maharashtra reported higher attack rates in rural areas for both 1963 and 1964 whereas only West Bengal consistently reported higher rates for urban areas than rural.

As for death rates, as distinct from attack rates, Bihar, Maharashtra, Karnataka and Orissa consistently reported higher death rates in rural areas whereas Bengal reported higher death rates from urban areas. Out of 314 districts classified for endemicity, 43 were in the hyperendemic category, 126 in the intermediate-endemicity category, and 145 were in the low-endemicity (including non-endemic) category. Out of 43 hyperendemic districts, 10 belonged to Andhra Pradesh, 7 to Bihar, 7 to Maharashtra, 6 to Karnataka, 5 to West Bengal, 4 to Tamil Nadu, 3 to Orissa and 1 to Assam. Of these again, 12 districts

—East Godavari (A.P.), Gaya, Monghyr, Patna, Shahabad (Bihar), South Arcot, Tanjore (Tamil Nadu), Cuttack (Orissa), Calcutta, Howrah, Midnapur and 24 Parganas (W. Bengal) were responsible for 38 per cent of the total cases recorded in India during 1954-64.

It is interesting that some of the areas are identical with those classified by Satya Swaroop as far back as 1951 on the basis of three tests: "(*a*) cholera mean mortality rate for ten years recording the lowest incidence of the disease during the period 1901-45 on five-yearly moving averages of death rates; (*b*) mean duration in months for which a district remained free from cholera deaths during the last 30 years; and (*c*) average number of weekly periods free from cholera cases during last ten years."

Both K.C. Patnaik and P.N. Kapoor (1967), and S.K. Sengupta and P.N. Kapoor (February 1972), applied the following tests for low, intermediate and high endemicity of cholera. They accepted two criteria: (*a*) persistence level (PL) and (*b*) minimum monthly incidence rate (MMIR), PL and MMIR being defined as follows:

$$PL = \frac{\text{Number of weeks reporting incidence of one or more cholera cases}}{\text{Total number of weeks during period}} \times 100$$

$$MMIR = \frac{\text{Arithmetic mean of three lowest monthly figures of cases for each year of the total period considered}}{\text{Population of area considered in lakhs}}$$

The limits were defined as follows:

(1) Low endemicity	: $PL < 10 + MMIR < 0.1$
(2) Intermediate endemicity	: All districts not included in categories of non, low and hyper-endemicity
(3) Hyper endemicity	: $PL \geqslant 20 + MMIR \geqslant 0.1$ or PL 10 to $20 + MMIR \geqslant 0.2$
(4) Non-endemic	: Districts reporting nil incidence

On the basis of these tests the changes in the incidence of cholera between 1954 and 1970 have been abstracted in the following table:

TABLE 9: *Changes in level of endemicity of cholera of states & districts, 1954-64 to 1965-70*

	Low (L)		*Interme-diate*		*High (H)*		*Non Endemic*		*Not Available*		*Top Hyper-endemic but included in*	
	1954-64	*1965-70*	*1954-65*	*1965-70*	*1954-64*	*1965-70*	*1954-64*	*1965-70*	*1954-64*	*1965-70*	*1954-64*	*1965-70*
Andhra Pradesh	—	4	10	15	10	1	—	—	—	—	4	—
Assam	5	3	5	7	1	—	1	—	—	—	—	—
Bihar	3	5	7	10	7	1	—	1	—	—	1	—
Gujarat	10	5	4	10	—	1	3	2	1	—	—	—
Haryana	4	4	1	1	—	—	1	2	1	—	—	—
Kerala	3	4	—	5	—	—	6	—	—	—	—	—
Madhya Pradesh	13	7	27	4	—	—	3	32	—	—	—	—
Tamil Nadu	1	1	9	9	4	2	—	1	—	1	2	2
Maharashtra	4	11	15	12	7	12	—	1	4	—	1	—
Mysore	4	2	8	14	6	1	1	2	—	—	3	—
Orissa	—	6	10	6	3	–	—	1	—	—	2	—
Punjab	4	5	1	—	—	—	5	5	—	—	—	—
Rajasthan	6	15	4	1	—	—	16	10	—	—	—	—
Uttar Pradesh	32	27	15	21	—	1	7	5	—	—	—	—
West Bengal	3	8	8	6	5	1	—	1	—	—	4	—

Source: Statistical Review of Cholera Problem in India by K.C. Patnaik and P.N. Kapoor, 1967 (printed)

Changing pattern of Cholera Endemicity in India by S.K. Sengupta and P.N. Kapoor, Fabruary 1972 (Mimeograph).

The table presents a mixed picture. In Andhra Pradesh, although the districts of high endemicity (H) decreased from 10 to 1 (Cuddapah), clearly the decrease distributed itself promptly in two groups: 5 to the intermediate (I) and 4 to the low (L) category. The intermediate category swelled and the low category boasted of new accretion. In Assam, Kamrup of high endemicity in 1954-64 disappeared from that group but appeared in I category in 1965-70. The I category increased in number although the low category decreased. In Bihar, the number of H districts decreased from 7 to 1 but there were increases in both L and I. In Gujarat, there were retrograde increase in M and I marked by decrease in L. In Haryana, the position held unchanged but Kerala distinctly deteriorated in the second period, while Madhya Pradesh improved considerably. Tamil Nadu slightly improved its position only in H while in Maharashtra there was overall and rather marked deterioration. Karnataka (Mysore) improved in H and L but deteriorated in I. Punjab showed an overall improvement but Rajasthan saw a steep, more than three-fold, rise in L. In Uttar Pradesh, the situation deteriorated in so far as I and H were concerned. The situation in West Bengal distinctly improved in H and I but deteriorated in L.

No similar exhaustive analysis is available subsequent to 1970, but the information indicates that although the virulence of cholera seems to have diminished, the geographical extent of endemicity has not shrunk. In other words, it cannot be conclusively asserted that the non-endemic districts have definitely increased in number since 1970, nor that the areas declared non-endemic are absolutely invulnerable.

SMALLPOX

Since it has been observed that in general high or low peaks of cholera and smallpox follow each other or run concurrently, we shall look into smallpox in our country next.

Geographical Patholagy of India yields the following table on smallpox 1958-64.

TABLE 10: *Incidence and distribution of smallpox in India, 1958-64*

	Attack rate (No. of persons per 100,000 population	*Case fatality rate (per cent of attacks)*	*Death rate (per 100,000 of population*
Andhra Pradesh	10.1 to 20	24.9	3.6
Assam	0 to 10	26.8	1.0
Bihar	0 to 10	29 1	2 3
Gujarat	0 to 10	30.1	2.8
Jammu & Kashmir	10.1 to 20	25.0	3.2
Karnataka	10.1 to 20	23.1	2.8
Kerala	0 to 10	35.0	2.5

Maharashtra	20.1 to 30	24.1	5 7
Madhya Pradesh	10.1 to 20	18.4	3.4
Orissa	30.1 to 40	24.2	8.1
Punjab (incl Haryana)	0 to 10	17.2	1.2
Rajasthan	10 1 to 20	23.0	3.8
Uttar Pradesh	10.1 to 20	33.8	4.2
West Bengal	20.1 to 30	42.2	9.0
Himachal Pradesh	0 to 10	24.2	1.3
Delhi	30.1 to 40	23.1	4.3
Manipur	0 to 10	24.3	0.5
Tripura	0 to 10	18 2	0.6
Pondicharry	40.1 to 55	55.8	44.1

In an earlier (1966) volume, *Statistical Review of Smallpox Problem in India,* K.C. Patnaik and P.N. Kapoor observed that during 1959-63 India contributed 62.7 per cent of all smallpox cases in the world, Africa contributing 22.6 per cent, other countries of Asia contributing 11.4 per cent, the Americans contributing 3.2 per cent and Europe 0.1 per cent.

The decline of smallpox has occurred in three phases in the current century:

(1) 1900-20 : Death rate varied from 0.19 to 0.80 with mean annual death rate of 0.37 per 1,000 population.

(2) 1921-46 : Death rate varied from 0.09 to 0.70 with mean annual death rate of 0.29 per 1,000 population.

(3) 1947-67 : Death rate varied from 0.02 to 0.44 with mean annual death rate of 0.15 per 1,000 population.

There was a reduction of nearly 20 per cent in 1921-46 as compared to 1900-29, and of nearly 56.2 per cent in 1947-64, as compared to 1921-46. This by itself may not appear as a revolutionary improvement in the periodicity waves of smallpox and their duration. Thus relatively high incidence has been recorded during the years 1902-03, 1906-09, 1913-15, 1918-20, 1925-28, 1933-36, 1940, 1943-45, 1950-51 and 1957-58. While epidemic waves in the past had longer durations generally, the duration has shortened in recent decades.

As can be surmised from Table 10 above, Uttar Pradesh 13.8 per cent, Maharashtra 13.4 per cent, Tamil Nadu 12.1 per cent, West Bengal 11.2 per cent, Madhya Pradesh 8.9 per cent, Orissa 8.7 per cent, Andhra Pradesh 7.7 per cent, Bihar 5.6 per cent, Rajasthan 5.1 per cent accounted for 86.5 per cent of the total incidence and 86.9 per cent of the total deaths from smallpox. The reasons for these will be found in (*a*) indifferent notification of cases and deaths from smallpox; (*b*) higher virulence of the disease; (*c*) relatively slower action on the part of local Public Health Authorities in prompt notification and subsequent adequate isolation and treatment and hospitalization facilities; (*d*) incomplete coverage under vaccination and revaccination programmes; and (*e*) endemicity and epidemicity of the disease.

One of the facts that should cause concern is that "there was no significant difference between attack rates in rural and urban areas in 1964." Case fatality rates were the highest (43.5 per cent in 1963) in the age group 0-4, patently betraying widespread lack of primary vaccination in infancy and lack of enforcement of the compulsory statutory provision. The next higher case fatality rates occurred in the age group 5-14 (21 per cent), also betraying lack of primary vaccination and revaccination.

The nature of the contagious disease is demonstrated by the positive association between density of population and other factors like level of emdemicity, degree of endemicity and case fatality rates.

S.K. Sengupta and P.N. Kapoor producing their report on *Changing Pattern of Smallpox Endemicity in India* in February 1972 (mimeograph) applied the same test of K.C. Patnaik and P.N. Kapoor of low, intermediate and high endemicity as follows: Their definitions of low, intermediate and high endemicity were as follows:

A is persistence level defined as

$$PL = \frac{\textit{No. of weeks reporting incidence of one or more cases of smallpox}}{\textit{Total number of weeks during period}} \times 100$$

B is minimum monthly incidence rate (MMIR) defined as

$$MMIR = \frac{\textit{Arithmetic mean of the three lowest monthly figures of cases for each of the years under review}}{\textit{Population in 100,000's of the districts}}$$

1. Non-endemic : Districts reporting nil incidence
2. Low endemicity : A < 20% + B < 0.2
3. Intermediate endemicity : All districts not included in the categories of non-low and hyper endemicity.

4. Hyper endemicity : A ⩾ 50%
+ B ⩾ 0.2
OR A = Between 20 and 50%
+ B ⩾ 0.5

On the uniform application of these tests between 1958-64 and 1965-70, with the National Smallpox Eradication Programme operating continuously from 1962-63, the results were as follows:

TABLE 11: *Changes in level of endemicity of smallpox of state and districts, 1958-64 to 1965-70*

	Low		*Inter-mediate*		*High (H)*		*Non-endemic*		*Not Available*		*Top Hyper-endemic but included in column (H)*	
	1958-64	*1965-70*	*1958-64*	*1965-70*	*1958-64*	*1965-70*	*1958-64*	*1965-70*	*1958-64*	*1965-70*	*1958-64*	*1965-70*
Andhra Pradesh	7	7	6	9	—	4	—	—	—	—	1	1
Assam	8	6	2	4	—	—	1	1	—	—	—	—
Bihar	7	7	10	10	—	—	—	—	—	—	—	—
Gujarat	11	12	6	6	—	—	—	—	1	—	—	—
Haryana	1	—	5	5	—	—	—	—	1	2	—	—
Jammu & Kashmir	—	3	—	—	—	—	—	6	9	—	—	—
Kerala	1	—	7	2	1	—	—	—	—	—	1	—
Madhya Pradesh	13	24	24	18	3	—	3	1	—	—	—	—
Tamil Nadu	—	7	4	5	9	—	—	2	1	—	7	—
Maharashtra	8	9	15	16	3	1	—	—	—	—	—	—
Mysore	2	12	15	7	2	—	—	—	—	—	—	—
Orissa	—	10	7	3	6	—	—	—	—	—	—	—
Punjab	5	6	5	2	—	—	—	—	—	2	—	—
Rajasthan	4	10	21	16	1	—	—	—	—	—	—	—
Uttar Pradesh	6	36	47	18	1	—	—	—	—	—	—	—
West Bengal	3	8	10	8	3	—	—	—	—	—	—	—

Sources: K.C. Patnaik & P.N. Kapoor: Statistical Review of Smallpox Problem in India, 1966.

S.K. Sengupta & P.N. Kapoor: Changing Pattern of Smallpox Endemicity in India, February 1972 (Mimeograph).

Several facts immediately strike the eye. As in cholera, no major state was free from smallpox as late as 1970. On the other hand, as late as 1954-64 as many as 10 major states had varying numbers of high endemic districts. The number H states dwindled to 2 in 1965-70 bearing testimony to the results that a determined national programme of eradication can achieve. But that this programme achieved not much more than demonstration effect is proved by the persistence of large numbers of I and L districts even in 1965-70 in all major states except Jammu and Kashmir. The heaping in I districts bears a tell-tale character. At the other end, the number of non-endemic districts is small and they are located mostly wide apart except in Jammu and Kashmir.

What happened after 1970 in the field of smallpox in India is a tribute to what determined effort is capable of in a short time. According to the Central Bureau of Health Intelligence, 83,943 cases were reported in 1961 in India resulting in 26,225 deaths. In 1971 these figures declined to 16,166 and 2,706 respectively. But there was a progressive rise from 1972 to 1974 which is explained by the vigorous surveillance that was mounted around 1970, the tempo of which accelerated in the next few years and brought out many usually undetected cases into the open, followed by a sudden collapse resulting in claimed extinction by 5 July 1975. The all-India figures are as follows:

	1971		*1972*		*1973*		*1974*		*1975*	
	Cases	*Deaths*	*Cases*	*Deaths*	*Cases*	*Deaths*	*Cases*	*Deaths*	*Cases*	*Deaths*
All-India	16,166	2,706	27,047	5,457	88,110	15,434	186,003	31,262	1,436	176

The authorities defined a new outbreak as a geographical area from which one or more cases were reported, and an active area as one where there was a case within the last six weeks of a previous case. In 1972, 1973, 1974 and 1975, the total number of districts reporting smallpox were 157, 211, 215 and 59 respectively out of a total of 386 in all India. The CBHI report observes that in 1973, 94 per cent of the cases were reported from Uttar Pradesh, Bihar, West Bengal and Madhya Pradesh. These four states were classified as endemic states, while Andhra Pradesh, Assam, Haryana, Jammu and Kashmir, Maharashtra, Meghalaya, Orissa, Punjab, Rajasthan and Delhi were classified as low incidence states. The other states and

Union territories were considered to be smallpox free as most of the outbreaks reported were documented to be imported. The government announced a reward of Rs 1,000 for any reported smallpox case proving correct. This helped intensify active search. Nonetheless, the unevenness of supervision and vigilance is reflected in the following fluctuating figures for 1972-75 documented by CBHI.

The following table has been constructed from Appendix L of the same mimeographed report.

TABLE 12: *Last case of smallpox outbreak reported in India, 1974-75*

State	*Date of onset of first case*	*Date of onset of last case*	*Date of Notification*
Andhra Pradesh	10.8.74	16.8.74	16 8.74
Assam	24.5.75	24.5 75	26.5.75
Bihar	5.3.75	17.5.75	8.5.75
Gujarat	2.5.75	2.5.75	11.5.75
Haryana	15.7.74	6.8.74	23.7.74
Himachal Pradesh	10.5.75	10.5.74	28.5.74
Jammu & Kashmir	27.9.74	27.9.74	5.10.74
Karnataka	6.5.74	6.5.74	9.5.74
Kerala	5.5.74	5 5.74	11.5.74
Madhya Pradesh	27.10.74	23.12.74	—
Maharashtra	12.8.74	12.8.74	17.8.74
Manipur	15.6.74	10.9.74	23.9.74
Meghalaya	20.4.75	20.4.75	22.4.75
Nagaland	13.7.74	13.7.74	22.7.74
Orissa	6.1.75	6.1.75	7.1.75
Punjab	28.8.74	28.8.74	14.9.74
Rajasthan	18.4.74	9.9.74	4.9.74
Sikkim	9.3.73	16.5.73	24.4.73
Tamil Nadu	4.7.74	4.7.74	7.7.74
Tripura	30.4.75	19.5.75	22.5.75
Uttar Pradesh	12.2.75	8.3.75	12.3.75
West Bengal	26.4.75	15.5.75	3.5.75
Arunachal Pradesh	22.4.74	22.4.74	28.4.74
Chandigarh	16.5.70	16.5.70	19.5.70
Delhi	15.9.74	15.9.74	28.9.74
Goa, Daman & Diu	6.8.70	6.8.70	9.8.70
Mizoram	26.4.73	26.4.73	1.5.73

Against such a background, as recent as 1974, the claim, just established by the Ministry of Health and Family Planning that since

5 July 1975 the country has not seen a single case of smallpox proper bears testimony to what can be achieved by a determined national eradication campaign such as the National Smallpox Eradication Campaign, started as late as 1962-63.

Smallpox differs from cholera or malaria in the sense that it is a direct person to person communication disease, while cholera is mainly water and food borne and malaria has the ubiquitously breeding mosquito as its vehicle. It is comparatively easy to break the smallpox chain and prevent its extension. Nonetheless, the spectacular and total disappearance of smallpox for no less than nine months is a feat of no mean order.

Of course, disappearance of such duration cannot be claimed as total eradication and at least two whole years must elapse of an entirely smallpox-free continuum before we can reasonably compliment ourselves, particularly so because the eradication organisation needs an all embracing and enduring network of very rigorous surveillance backed up by vaccination and revaccination machinery and segregation, quarantine and hospitalization support to isolate and take care of stray cases and incidences of containable magnitude. For, most impressive as the record of the last five years has been, the level of smallpox incidence as late as 1974 demands that the utmost vigilance and follow-up must be exercised for several years to secure the gains of recent years. For premature complacency, as we shall presently see happened in the case of malaria, can undo much good national effort.

Although the production of freeze-dried smallpox vaccine in the four production centres of India is claimed to be ample, the field staff of paramedical assistants, supervisors at the rate of one for every four vaccinators in rural areas and vaccinators at the rate of three to four for every primary health centre (for urban areas, one vaccinator for every 25,000 urban population and one supervisor for every four vaccinators) may not be adequate for the optimum rate of revaccination on top of primary vaccination, particularly if this field staff is expected to perform other kinds of duties, including helping in the family planning programme. A great deal depends on touring and peripatetic supervision for which adequate travelling facilities must be ensured.

PLAGUE

In Chart No. 7 of his Geographical Pathology of India, K.C. Patnaik gave the following figures for plague:

TABLE 13: *Average annual attack rate, case fertiliiy rate and death rate from plague, per 100,000 of population, 1960-64*

State/ District	*Average annual attack rate per 100,000 population*	*Case fatality rate*	*Death rate per lakh of population*
Andhra Pradesh			
Chittor	0.26 to 1.50	17.97	0.24
Tamil Nadu			
Salem	0.26 to 1.50	20.78	0.25
Karnataka			
Bijapur	0.00 to 0.10	Not certain	Not certain
Bangalore	0.00 to 0.10	33.33	0.02
Mysore	0.11 to 0.25	14 23	0.01
Kolar	1.51 and above	11.97	2.01

Source: Geographical Pathology of India, Chart 7.

Plague persisted in a small pocket of districts consisting of Mysore, Bangalore, Kolar, Chittor and Salem centred on the trijunction of the three states—Andhra Pradesh, Karnataka and Tamil Nadu – with the exception of Bijapur in the northern extremity of Karnataka. But in 1950, the number of cases was as large as 42,555 in all India and the deaths 7,823 with an attack rate and death rate respectively of 11.91 and 2.19 per lakh of population which dwindled to 11 attacks and 8 deaths in 1966. In 1966, there were two cases of plague reported from Mahasu (Himachal Pradesh) of which one resulted in death. In 1970 CBHI reported nil attacks and nil deaths since 1967. But until the geographical focus described above continuously reports no incidence for several years and until the collateral effort of the recrudescence of malaria, kala-azar and plague is observed to be inconsequential, there will still be the unfortunate possibility of plague continuing to be dormant as distinct from its total eradication.

GUINEA WORM

This is so far as the infections that occupy the most fearful place in the public mind are concerned. But the perniciously debilitating diseases are still dysentery and diarrhoea, respiratory diseases and malaria. The compass of this paper will not warrant any detailed mention of leprosy, trachoma, goitre or venereal diseases which are quite widespread but take lesser tolls of human lives, but as an example of its widespread, almost ubiquitous prevalence, on account of poor state of water supply, sewage and zoonosis (animals sharing the same housing space as man), the incidence of guinea worm will also be briefly noticed.

The only available authoritative information is perhaps contained in K.C. Patnaik and P.N. Kapoor's *Incidence and Endemicity of Guinea Worm in India* (Indian Journal of Medical Research, Vol. 55, No. 11, January 1967). This paper covers guinea worm alone, but the other equally pernicious helminths like hookworm, roundworm, ringworm, tapeworm, etc. have not been adequately surveyed.

There are still other diseases caused by the living together of human beings and animals like the camel, horse, cattle, buffalo, sheep, goat and poultry not only in the same building but very often in the same room, by which helminths, spores and other infections are constantly transmitted to humans. There are helminths which are transmitted to human beings through standing and even running water in ponds, streams and rivers. The association between helminthic diseases, intestinal diseases and malnutrition is very close, for intestinal and other parasites eat up much of what nutrition a person takes through food and drink, leaving the host greatly destituted.

It becomes difficult in certain situations to pronounce authoritatively which should be the first priority: to rid a particular population first of helminthic infestation or to rid it of intestinal diseases or to correct its nutritional status. But whichever programme is first begun it becomes quite clear shortly that unless these invisible or visible parasites are got rid of, some time or other they are capable of robbing the human body silently and devastatingly.

How extensive the prevalence of guinea worm was and still is can be judged from the following table of endemicity abstracted from Patnaik and Kapoor. Of a total of 342 districts considered no information was available on 29 districts (including all of Andhra Pradesh for which sketchy information was available only in 1963). Of the remaining 313 districts, only 100 were considered free from endemicity, 42 were considered subject to low endemicity, 82 to intermediate endemicity and as many as 91 to hyperendemicity. Hyperendemicity prevailed in a small part of Gujarat, considerable portions of Madhya Pradesh, the bulk of Maharashtra, Orissa, Rajasthan and Uttar Pradesh, and a substantial part of Tamil Nadu.

Intermediate endemicity prevailed in part in Gujarat, Himachal Pradesh, Maharashtra, Orissa, Rajasthan and West Bengal but in considerable portions of Madhya Pradesh, Mysore, Tamil Nadu, Uttar Pradesh and West Bengal. Low endemicity prevailed in considerable portions of Gujarat, Madhya Pradesh, Mysore and West Bengal but in small areas of Haryana, Orissa, Punjab and Uttar Pradesh. Assam, Bihar, Jammu and Kashmir, Kerala and all the Union Territories were free from endemicity, while no district of Maharashtra, Mysore, Orissa and Rajasthan was free from endemicity. The other States enjoyed varying extents of freedom from endemicity.

TABLE 14: *Endemicity of guinea worm, 1950-1964*

	Free from Endemicity	*Low Endemicity*	*Intermediate Endemicity*	*High Endemicity*	*Not Available*
Andhra Pradesh	—	—	—	—	20
Assam	11	—	—	—	—
Bihar	17	—	—	—	—
Gujarat	5	8	3	1	—
Himachal Pradesh	6	—	1	—	1
Jammu & Kashmir	9	—	—	—	—
Kerala	9	—	—	—	—
Madhya Pradesh	4	7	22	10	—
Maharashtra	—	—	5	21	—
Manipur	5	—	—	—	—
Meghalaya	2	—	—	—	—
Mysore	—	9	10	—	—
Nagaland	3	—	—	—	—
Orissa	—	2	3	8	—
Punjab	12	2	—	—	5
Rajasthan	—	—	4	22	—
Tamil Nadu	3	—	5	5	—
Tripura	3	—	—	—	—
Uttar Pradesh	2	4	24	24	—

West Bengal (incl. Sikkim)	1	10	5	—	—
Goa, Daman & Diu	3	—	—	—	—
Delhi	1	—	—	—	—
Lakshadweep	1	—	—	—	—
Mizoram	1	—	—	—	—
A & N Islands	1	—	—	—	—
Arunachal Pradesh	—	—	—	—	1
Chandigarh	1	—	—	—	—
Pondicherry	—	—	—	—	—
Total	100	42	82	91	27

Source: K.C. Patnaik and P.N. Kapoor: Incidence and Endemicity of Guinea Worm, India (1967); Table II, pp. 6-10.

DYSENTERY AND DIARRHOEA

It is difficult to arrive at any realistic assessment of dysentery and diarrhoea obtaining in the country which includes the entire range from simple diarrhoea to food poisoning, cholera, dysentery and all forms of gastroenteritis. Then again, CBHI and Registrar-General, India, have confined themselves to reports obtained from those hospitals which they have been able to enlist for reporting. The following table constructed from K.C. Patnaik and P.N. Kapoor's *Geographical Pathology of India*, Registrar-General, India's Report on Survey of Cause of Death 1966-67, Causes of Death 1971 and Vital Statistics of India 1970 must therefore be interpreted with much caution. It does not give the true picture by any means but represents the best that we have by way of statistics.

TABLE 15: *Deaths due io dysentery and diarrhoea 1960-63, 1966-67 and 1971*

	Average annual death rate per 1000 population	*State's share (Per cent) to total deaths from dysentery and diarrhoea in the country*			
	1960-63	*1960-63*	*1966*	*1967*	*1971*
Andhra Pradesh	0.26 to 0.50	5.00 to 9.99	11.9	8.4	3.63
Assam	0.26 to 0.50	1.00 to 4.99	21.3	19.3	9.85
Bihar	0.01 to 0.25	1.00 to 4.99	8.5	11.8	1.29
Gujarat	0.26 to 0.50	1.00 to 4.99	6.6	6.2	1.97

Arunachal Pradesh	0.51 to 1.00	0.01 to 0.99	—	—	14.58
Jammu & Kashmir	1.01 to 1.50	1.00 to 4.99	—	4.0	2.65
Kerala	0.26 to 0 50	1.00 to 4.99	12.2	4.5	2.31
Karnataka	0.51 to 1.00	5.00 to 9.99	—	13.5	11.83
Madhya Pradesh	0.26 to 0.50	5.00 to 9.99	—	11.8	5.71
Maharashtra	0.51 to 1.00	10.00 to 15.00+	—	10.8	4.55
Orissa	0.51 to 1.00	5.00 to 9.00	23.7	18.6	7.04
Punjab (incl. Haryana)	0.26 to 0.50	1.00 to 4.99	8.1	8.1*	1.40
Rajasthan	0.26 to 0.50	0.01 to 0.99	9.7	N.A.	7.93
Tamil Nadu	0.51 to 1.50	10.00 to 15.00+	10.0	8.4	6.48
Uttar Pradesh	0.51 to 1.00	10.00 to 15.00+	—	6.6	3.86
West Bengal	0.26 to 0.50	5.00 to 9.99	18.8	14.2	6.89
Delhi	1.51 to 2.00+	0.01 to 0.99	—	—	2.52
Pondicherry	1.51 to 2.00+	0.01 to 0.99	—	—	7.47

*Excluding Haryana.
N.A.—Not available.

Since dysentery and diarrhoea are mainly public health problems, we may conclude this section by examining the distribution of deaths reported by field agents (see explanation in the section on Respiratory Diseases) from diarrhoea (which includes food poisoning, cholera, dysentery and all forms of gastroenteritis) such as is available by sex among the principal age groups from the Registrar General's Report on Survey of Causes of Death 1966-67 (published 1969).

Respiratory Diseases

The incidence of repiratory diseases for the early years of the 1960's is furnished in K.C. Patnaik, and P.N. Kapoor's *Geographical Pathology of India* as follows. This supplements information already commented upon.

Table 16 is a testimony to the number of beds available for treatment of respiratory diseases than of the share of this cause of deaths among all causes. The Registrar-General's surveys of causes of death undertaken in 1966 and 1967 and again in 1971 were however undertaken as field surveys. About 660 primary health centre villages were selected throughout the country roughly on the basis of one PHC village per million of population.

The 1966 analysis was based on the experience of 544 PHC villages, the 1967 analysis on 714 PHC villages and the 1971 analysis on 770

TABLE 16: *Average annual reported death rates, percentage share of each state of reported deaths due to respiratory diseases to total deaths, 1960-63*

	Average annual death rates per mille	Percentage share of each State of Reported Deaths due to Respiratory Diseases to Total Deaths	
		1960	1963
Andhra Pradesh	0.51-1.00	5.01-10.00	N.A.
Assam	0.11-0.50	0.01- 5.00	0.01- 0.99
Bihar	0.01-0.10	0.01- 5.00	0.01- 0.99
Gujarat	1.01-2.00	5.01-10 00	15.00 above
Himachal Pradesh	0.11-0.50	0.01- 5.00	0.01- 0.99
Jammu & Kashmir	1.01-2.00	0.01- 5.00	0.01- 0.99
Kerala	0.51-1.00	0.01- 5.00	1.00- 4.99
Karnataka	1.01-2.00	5.01-10.00	10.00-14.99
Madhya Pradesh	0.11-0.50	5.01-10.00	5.00- 9.99
Maharashtra	1.01-2.00	20.01-25.00	15.00 above
Orissa	0.11-0.50	0.01- 5.00	0.01- 0.99
Punjab (incl. Haryana)	1.01-2.00	5.01-10.00	1.00- 4.99
Rajasthan	0.51-1.00	0.01- 5.00	0.01- 0.99
Tamil Nadu	1.01-2.00	10.01-15.00	5.00- 9.99
Uttar Pradesh	0.51-1.00	15.01-20.00	10.00-14.99
West Bengal	N.A.	N,A.	5.00- 9.99
Delhi	1.01-2.00	N.A.	N.A.
Pondicherry	1.01-2.00	N.A.	N.A.

PHC villages. The information was collected by a field agent who was either a vaccinator, a social health worker, a sanitary inspector or a compounder, whose particular qualification would be no more than that he should be familiar with the locally prevailing diseases in his area and possess an elementary understanding of the cause and symptomatology of certain common diseases The field agent, usually a local resident, would depend upon his own awareness of the occurrence of a death and upon the clues supplied by an informant. An informant was usually a public functionary, such as midwife, chowkidar, watchman, the village headman or an official of the village panchayat or an institutional functionary like the village barber or the community priest presiding over funeral rites.

The emphasis was on collection of information in respect of a village and not in respect of an individual or household: the place of

TABLE 17: *Percentage share by sex and selected age groups of deaths from cough to total surveyed deaths from 9 main causes of death in selected states of India, 1966, 1967 and 1971*

		Age Group											
		Less than one		1-4		5-14		15-34		35-54		55 Plus	
		M	F	M	F	M	F	M	F	M	F	M	F
1	2	3	4	5	6	7	8	9	10	11	12	13	14
Andhra Pradesh	1966	5.7	6.6	14.4	12.7	9.2	13.0	23.1	11.5	26.9	21.0	11.4	10.0
	1967	5.6	5.3	7.5	10.1	14.5	9.3	17.5	15.6	24.9	15.7	13.2	7.2
	1971	2.1	1.9	8.2	10.7	15.2	9.8	17.1	9.9	29.3	18.7	10.1	9.3
Assam	1966	20.0	31.2	42.9	25.0	33.3	12.5	50.0	—	37.5	27.3	18.2	41.7
	1967	15.6	16.7	33.3	31.8	28.6	13.0	20.0	10.0	55.6	28.1	28.9	12.5
	1971	—	19.4	30.0	12.5	—	8.3	57.1	13.6	27.6	45.0	25.4	42.4
Bihar	1966	34.5	32.0	34.3	24.1	23.8	29.3	37.7	25.0	38.0	34.3	33.3	21.1
	1967	28.6	20.6	21.3	32.9	18.4	13.3	29.3	21.2	35.1	18.1	18.4	13.4
	1971	22.0	26.7	24.5	30.2	18.8	21.9	21.4	20.0	22.7	15.6	12.9	15.6
Gujarat	1966	18.3	21.1	40.0	25.9	26.1	28.1	27.3	29.0	54.0	46.0	31.4	37.5
	1967	18.9	17.1	21.9	24.5	27.1	24.0	38.5	19.5	38.5	29.0	27.7	20.3
	1971	12.9	12.8	13.6	10.5	10.7	17.9	32.0	33.3	44.9	32.4	40.5	29.8
Haryana	1966	—	—	—	—	—	—	—	—	—	—	—	—
	1967	26.8	23.6	27.0	32.5	25.7	20.0	25.9	28.2	36.4	41.0	45.8	37.9
	1971	23.1	33.3	30.0	25.0	22.2	20.0	16.7	15.4	54.2	21.7	47.9	58.5
Jammu &	1966	—	—	—	—	—	—	—	—	—	—	—	—
Kashmir	1967	46.1	37.5	44.5	75.0	20.0	33.3	—	—	30.8	20.0	27.3	30.0
	1971	60.0	50.0	80.0	69.2	33.3	67.7	—	20.0	14.3	14.3	20.7	29.2
Kerala	1966	9.6	20.7	26.9	22.2	31.6	11.1	50.0	12.5	19.1	22.2	12.0	5.7
	1967	16.7	33.3	42.8	10.0	16.7	—	30.0	25.0	36.4	—	9.6	8.2
	1971	—	6.3	25.0	14.3	33.4	50.0	16.7	15.4	35.3	23.1	19.1	11.9

1	2	3	4	5	6	7	8	9	10	11	12	13	14
Madhya Pradesh	1966	—	—	—	—	—	—	—	—	—	—	—	—
	1967	28.0	25.3	35.2	30.9	21.3	11.0	24.4	18.9	36.6	28.5	26.9	13.2
	1971	30.1	32.0	39.0	34.9	15.4	16.3	25.6	23.6	32.2	27.5	22.8	18.4
Maharashtra	1966	—	—	—	—	—	—	—	—	—	—	—	—
	1967	11.3	9.4	16.2	13.3	14.0	12.2	30.4	15.0	20.2	21.5	31.8	24.9
	1971	15.2	16.1	29.7	26.9	15.7	10.9	29.4	23.7	36.3	36.5	37.9	30.3
Mysore	1966	—	—	—	—	—	—	—	—	—	—	—	—
	1967	12.9	—	6.7	—	14.2	20.0	20.0	42.9	18.8	16.7	21.2	17.4
	1971	4.6	12.5	18.4	17.1	—	13.3	8.3	10.7	32.5	26.5	30.2	17.5
Orissa	1966	14.5	10.2	11.3	17.3	19.4	17.9	6.1	5.6	12.5	9.3	8.5	5.4
	1967	5.9	7.5	7.6	6.8	3.4	6.3	10.3	6.7	13.3	25.5	3.4	5.9
	1971	10.0	13.5	11.1	31.6	15.8	35.7	21.0	9.5	16.7	13.6	8.4	3.6
Punjab	1966	31.4	31.6	29.4	39.5	24.0	25.7	30.1	29.1	38.1	37.9	40.4	37.8
	1967	26.4	22.3	29.4	33.0	20.4	15.5	27.3	19.7	36.8	28.8	35.4	31.7
	1971	29.9	34.4	25.0	37.9	15.4	15.6	17.5	19.4	27.5	31.1	28.4	27.7
Rajasthan	1966	35.1	27.9	38.3	31.6	22.4	21.4	29.5	19.7	45.6	39.7	41.9	29.0
	1967	32.9	32.1	39.1	32.9	15.4	20.0	24.3	18.7	42.3	32.3	41.4	29.3
	1971	—	—	—	—	—	—	—	—	—	—	—	—
Tamil Nadu	1966	5.1	12.9	21.6	23.5	10.3	11.1	30.0	20.5	23.2	12.5	10.0	5.0
	1967	14.1	21.5	19.4	26.5	9.5	21.0	6.9	23.5	16.2	25.5	9.3	3.9
	1971	8.6	10.9	17.6	21.6	15.2	20.6	20.7	13.9	23.1	20.8	9.1	7.7
Uttar Pradesh	1966	—	—	—	—	—	—	—	—	—	—	—	—
	1967	22.5	27.3	30.4	37.5	—	—	61.5	10.0	35.7	53.9	36.8	25.0
	1971	30.0	26.2	28.9	37.3	34.2	24.5	21.3	32.8	40.0	33.3	42.2	35.6

1	*2*	*3*	*4*	*5*	*6*	*7*	*8*	*9*	*10*	*11*	*12*	*13*	*14*
West Bengal	1966	24.3	19.9	17.7	26.5	22.2	6.5	20.7	22.7	35.9	23.2	25.5	22.2
	1967	23.3	19.4	11.5	19.7	7.4	15.1	30.0	22.7	25.3	25.0	29.8	26.1
	1971	3.6	17.7	26.7	11.1	8.3	33.3	22.2	27.3	15.8	10.0	25.3	18.6
All-India	1966	25.5	23.6	29.0	27.7	20.4	19.5	27.8	19.6	35.5	30.2	29.9	23.1
	1967	22.0	20.5	26.9	26.3	17.6	15.4	24.9	18.5	32.7	26.1	27.9	20.0
	1971	17.2	18.3	24.0	25.9	15.5	16.4	20.9	18.8	31.2	26.2	25.3	21.0

Note: The figures in this table indicate deaths due to 'cough' in a particular sex and age group expressed as percentage of deaths from all causes in that sex-age group.

Source: Report on Survey of Cause of Death 1966 & 1967 and Causes of Death 1971 Survey, Registrar-General, India.

occurrence was the important thing. The field agent was provided with (*a*) a copy of Yves Biraud's "A Method for Recording of Crude Causes of Death by Laymen in Underdeveloped Areas" (submitted at the African Conference on Vital & Health Statistics—Brazzaville, November 1956), which formed the mainstay of the Registrar General's effort since 1958; and (*b*) a synoptic key of this primer drawn up by D.K. Viswanathan and T.B. Patel to assist a paramedical investigator in fixing the cause of death.

In this scheme a set of nine major diseases is provided—(1) violence or injury, (2) childbirth or complicated pregnancy, (3) diarrhoea, (4) cough, (5) swellings, (6) fevers, (7) other infant deaths, (8) other clear symptoms, (9) others—(*a*) extreme old age without any known cause, (*b*) the rest. Each major disease is subdivided into several diseases again, based mainly on symptoms.

Thus the major group, cough, was provided with symptoms which could lead to further classification into (*a*) bronchopneumonia, (*b*) pneumonia, (*c*) bronchitis, (*d*) influenza, (*e*) streptococcal sore throat, (*f*) whooping cough, (*g*) tuberculosis of the respiratory system, and (*h*) others. Two sets of tables are quoted from each of the reports for 1966, 1967 and 1971. The first gives the place of cough in the setting of the nine major causes. The second gives the distribution of the eight main subgroups of diseases under cough. Each set gives the distribution of death by main age groups.

The picture taken as a whole brings out rather forcefully the persisting effects of exposure, lack of adequate clothing and housing, congestion and bad ventilation, and certainly of underlying malnutrition on Indian mortalily particularly in states which undergo marked seasonal variation in temperature and humidity.

Mortality Statistics in India

R.B. LAL*

INTRODUCTION

The history of mortality statistics in the country dates back to the middle of the nineteenth century. Deaths began to be registered with a view to assessing the health conditions of the people. The quality of statistics collected, however, was not satisfactory, being highly deficient in quality and completeness. As a step towards improvement, the government directed the Sanitary Commissioner in 1868 to prepare a series of forms for the collection of vital statistics in respect of the general population.

In 1873 the Bengal Births and Deaths Registration Act was passed, and was subsequently extended to neighbouring Bihar and Orissa. In 1886 the government placed on the statute book a measure called Births, Deaths and Marriages Registration Act to provide for voluntary registration of births, deaths and marriages throughout the country. The Act had a very limited application and remained a dead letter as far as the general population was concerned. Registration was carried out in urban areas under municipal bye-laws, and in rural areas on the basis of executive orders and instructions to the village officials under the revenue codes and police manuals.

By 1903, about 80 per cent of the population came under the registration system. This system was deficient in regard to coverage and content. It could not give cause of death correctly. Several experimental enquiries were conducted to ascertain the cause of death statistics in Bengal, Uttar Pradesh and Madras.

In 1919 the Sanitary Commissioner introduced the supplementary annual form of tabular statements. Detailed classification of infant

*Deputy Registrar-General, India.

deaths according to age at death was also introduced. The importance of mortality statistics in the study of manpower and health conditions prevailing among different groups of population was highlighted by the Royal Commission on Agriculture (1924) and the Royal Commission on Labour (1938). These commissions recommended the appointment of medical registrars in larger towns and industrial areas for proper classification of the causes of death.

The Health Survey and Development Committee (popularly known as the Bhore Committee) which made an extensive survey of the problem of public health in India made several useful recommendations in 1946 for improving vital statistics. The committee recommended the setting up of registration offices in each primary health unit and the public health nurses and midwives being made registrars of births and deaths. In areas where there were no primary health centres, the deployment of non-medical personnel having elementary training was recommended.

A conference of the state representatives concerned with the collection of vital statistics was convened by the Registrar-General in April 1961. This conference made several useful recommendations for improving the collection of birth and death data. In pursuance of these recommendations a central legislation for registration of births and deaths was enacted in 1969.

The establishment of an efficient registration system is a long and slow process. To measure the growth of population, the office of the Registrar-General initiated a scheme of sample registration of births and deaths with the main objective of providing reliable estimates of vital rates for the state and the country pending establishment of an efficient birth and death registration system. Most of the deaths that occur are domiciliary in nature, and are not attended by qualified doctors. Medical certification of causes of deaths in such cases is not feasible.

Attempts are, therefore, to be made to fix cause of death by post-mortem verification through lay reporting. Model registration—a survey of cause of death—was introduced by the office of the Registrar-General in a number of primary health centres through para-medical personnel. The scheme provides the mortality pattern by broad groups of diseases.

Need for Mortality Statistics

In recent times there has been an increasing demand for the collection of mortality statistics for health planning. Information on number of deaths in a year by geographical divisions helps to identify areas which require greater medical and health facilities. Cause of death statistics are the base for taking preventive and curative measures against communicable and other diseases and to improve health conditions of the people. Mortality statistics by age, sex and socio-economic variables enable us to identify specific vulnerable sections of population and to provide necessary medical and health facilities to them. The data available at present are scanty and cannot be utilised for assessing the requirement for medical and health facilities at the micro level.

Sources of Data

The three main sources of collection of mortality data are: (*i*) registration statistics; (*ii*) sample surveys; and (*iii*) population censuses. These are described in the following paragraphs.

Civil Registration

The potential source of information on mortality data is the civil registration system which is the conventional method of obtaining vital events whereby events reported and recorded shortly after their occurence. Events reported and recorded as and when they occur are likely to be more complete and the accuracy of the information is greater than if reporting depends on a later visit through an interviewer or recall of facts by the respondent. The collection of death statistics through the civil registration system entails the cooperation and coordination of the staff engaged in the different departments in the collection of data and to a greater extent, on the awareness among the general public about the need for registering vital events.

In India, the problem of collection of vital data by the traditional method is handicapped by the low level of literacy, the overwhelmingly illiterate rural population scattered throughout the length and breadth of the country with insufficient means of transport and communication and the inadequacy of the registration machinery.

The information collected from civil registration includes age, sex, nationatity, religion, place of death of the deceased, cause of death, whether medically certified or not and type of medical attention received at the time of death. Information on still birth is also collected separately. The data on mortality are tabulated broadly by (*1*) death by age and sex, (*2*) death by month of occurrence, (*3*) deaths by causes, age and sex, (*4*) infant deaths by age and sex, and (*5*) material deaths by age at death.

The quality of death statistics collected from civil registration is unsatisfactory in regard to coverage and completeness. The deaths are often not reported especially the infant deaths. The extent of under-registration is over 50 per cent. The degree of under-registration differs from state to state depending upon the level of efficiency of the civil registration machinery. Some of the measures of mortality as obtained from civil registration are given in the following tables.

All these mortality indices suffer from a high degree of under-registration.

TABLE 1

	Area	*Death rate*	*Still birth rate*	*Per cent infant deaths to total deaths*
1968	R	7.4	4.3	16.3
	U	8.4	22.3	16.2
	T	7.6	9.6	16.3
1969	R	7.2	6.3	17.1
	U	8.8	22.9	18.7
	T	7.5	11.4	18.0
1970	R	7.3	6.4	16.5
	U	7.8	23.1	16.9
	T	7.5	11.7	16.8
1971	R	7.4	5.8	16.0
	U	7.6	22.2	18.0
	T	7.4	12.3	16.5
1972	R	7.8	—	14.4
	U	8.2	—	17.7
	T	7.9	12.1	15.3

Table 1 shows that the death rate for rural areas is lower than the urban death rate, indicating greater under-registration in the rural areas. The sex-wise composition of the mortality indices presented in

Table 2 reveals that quite a large proportion of female deaths escaped registration. The infant death rate is appreciably low both in the rural and urban areas.

TABLE 2

	Infant mortality rate			*Neo-natal mortality*			*Post-natal mortality*			*Perinatal mortality*
	M	*F*	*T*	*M*	*F*	*T*	*M*	*F*	*T*	
1968	61.7	58.0	60.0	30.0	30.2	30.1	31.7	27.8	29.9	28.3
1969	62.4	58.7	60.6	30.5	26.6	28.6	31.9	32.1	32.0	28.2
1970	62.8	58.9	61.0	32.6	28.0	30.4	30.2	31.9	30.6	29.8
1971	57.7	55.0	56.4	30.5	26.6	28.6	27.2	28.9	27.8	29.1
1972	60.5	57.9	59.2	30.5	26.6	28.6	30.0	31.3	30.6	26.3

Sample Surveys

In the absence of dependable data on vital events from civil registration for providing estimates of vital rates on a current and continuous basis, alternative methods for gathering population data have been devised through the application of sampling techniques. Such methods include both single and multiple round retrospective surveys and dual record systems. In single round retrospective surveys, information is collected on vital events which occurred to members of the households during the interval specified in the enquiry. The reference period of this type of enquiry is a fixed period preferably twelve months preceding the enquiry.

The multi-round survey consists of making periodic observations on the same set of sampled areas by repeated interview. Experience in censuses and surveys has shown that it is extremely difficult to obtain reliable information about vital events occurring during a given reference period by enquiring about such events in a single round retrospective survey. The dual record system makes use of two independent records of vital events such as continuous enumeration and retrospective household surveys. The two records are matched event by event and the doubtful cases are re-verified in the field to get an unduplicated count of correct vital events.

Most of the studies on mortality in the past were fragmentary in nature and were restricted to local areas and so did not provide firm estimates at the state or national level. The sample census conducted by the office of the Registrar-General during 1960, 1964 and 1965-67 also collected information on deaths. The data obtained from the surveys were not found to be reliable due to response bias. Surveys conducted by the NSS since 1958 have attempted to provide comprehensive data on all aspects of population. NSS surveys were single round retrospective surveys. Information was collected on vital events which occurred to members of the sampled households during the twelve months proceding the enquiry. A comprehensive survey on population, fertility, family planning and mortality was introduced in the 28th round (1973-74) of the National Sample Survey (NSS). The estimates obtained from such surveys are subject to large recall lapse and do not seem to have added much to the meagre availability of mortality data.

The sample registration system is a dual reporting and recording system which in effect consists of continuous enumeration of births and deaths by an enumerator who is by profession mainly a school teacher and an independent survey every six months by a whole time field investigator. The data obtained through these two records are matched. The partially mached and unmatched events are verified to obtain an unduplicated count of correct vital events in the sample area. A base-line survey of the sample unit is also carried out in order to provide population base for working out vital rates. At the end of each six month period the population figure is updated. The system has thus the advantages of a longitudnal enumeration as well as a retrospective six monthly survey.

The information collected in SRS includes age, sex of the deceased, type of medical attention received at the time of death and still births. Similar data was also collected in the NSS. This type of data provides estimates of death rate, age and sex specific death rates, deaths by type of medical attention, infant mortality rate and its components, still birth rate and peri-natal mortality. In the accompanying table the results showing death rate and infant mortality rate obtained from the NSS and SRS are presented.

Mortality during the first year of life can be broken up into two main components, each with a distinctive etiology namely, neo-natal mortality occurring within the first four weeks and post-natal mortality occurring within the remainder of the first year after birth. Neonatal mortality serves as an approximate index of that component which is attributable to edogenous factors, while the postnatal mortality indicator serves as an index of exogenous factors responsible for infant mortality. Post-natal mortality is therefore amenable to control by environmental and medical measures unlike neo-natal mortality. The endogenous causes responsible for the neo-natal deaths include genetic factors inherent in the cellular growth of the organism, birth injuries and conditions arising from the hazards of delivery while exogenous causes relate to infections and parasitic diseases, arising from unhealthy feeding and environmental factors. It is therefore necessary to provide separate estimates of components of infant mortality.

As pointed out earlier, civil registration does not provide dependable figures on infant mortality and its components. The National Sample Survey had collected data on infant deaths by age and sex. The important source from where this type of information is obtained covering the entire country on a yearly basis is the sample registration system. Infant mortality rate as revealed by the NSS is lower than the SRS rate. A comparison of the figures from NSS and SRS is shown in Table 3.

TABLE 3

Source	*Period*	*Infant mortality rate*				
		Below 7 days	*7-28 days*	*29 days to 6 months*	*7 months to one year*	*Total*
SRS	1968 (rural)	43	31	39	24	137
	1969 (rural)	43	32	43	22	140
	1970 (rural)	48	32	37	20	137
	1971 (rural)	50	32	34	17	133
	1972* (rural)	49	31	45	25	150
	1970 (urban)	32	17	27	14	90
	1971 (urban)	31	15	23	11	80
	1972 (urban)	32	14	26	13	85
NSS 19th round (rural)		*0-3 weeks*		*3-51 weeks*		*Total*
	July '64-June '65	63		51		114

*Provisional.

Information on still births is necessary to compute a measure of the pregnancy wastage indicated by still birth rate. The bulk of the birth in the rural areas is domiciliary in nature. There is no medical attention of any description in a large proportion of cases. There is thus every likelihood of misclassification of still-birth and under-reporting of infant deaths. The pei-natal mortality which takes into account infant deaths below one week and still births may be a better indicator.

A knowledge of the differential pattern of mortality for the various sections of the population in the different stages of life is useful for health planners. The only dependable source of information on deaths by age and sex is the sample registration system. In the accompanying Table 4 the age specific death rates by age groups and sex are shown :

TABLE 4

Age Group	*Rural*			*Urban*		
	1970	*1971*	*1972*	*1970*	*1971*	*1972*
0-4	58 1	56.7	62 4	32 3	31.6	33.4
5-9	5.2	5.2	5.9	3.2	2.7	2 8
10-14	2.3	2.2	2.5	1.6	1 4	1.2
15-19	3 2	2.7	3.4	2.1	1.6	1.7
20-24	4.1	4.0	4 7	2.3	2.4	2.3
25-29	4.4	4.1	4 7	2.7	2.5	2.6
30-34	4.8	5.0	5.4	3.4	3.4	4.2
35-39	5.4	6.1	6.0	4 0	4.3	4.1
40-44	7.8	6.9	8.6	5.5	5.9	6.3
45-49	11.2	9.8	11.6	8.1	7.7	9.8
50-54	16 8	17.5	17.8	13.1	14.6	18.1
55-59	23.5	21.0	26.2	17 4	18 8	21.3
60-64	39 3	36.3	42.7	34.1	38.8	32.4
65-69	50.9	47.8	63.0	41 4	41.3	48.1
70+	115.8	113.8	132.8	97 1	94.2	109.7

Source: Sample Registration System.

In India mortality among females in the reproductive age group is found to be higher than among males. It is due to the high incidence of maternal mortality. It has also contributed to the continuing decline in the sex ratio of the population since the beginning of the century. The collection of maternal mortality data is essential for MCH planners.

Civil registration provides data on maternal deaths. The maternal mortality derived from civil registration is an under estimate and is not reliable. Model registration—a survey of cause of death has collected information on maternal deaths in the rural areas. Table 5 gives the maternal mortality rates (per 10,000 live births) as obtained from civil registration and model registration in the rural areas.

TABLE 5

	Civil Registration	*Model Registration*
1970	23.2	389
1971	20.5	376
1972	16 5	418
1973	—	393

Causes of death statistics. As mentioned earlier, the majority of deaths in India are domiciliary in nature. Medical services are inadequate, particularly in the rural areas. Medical certification of cause of death therefore is not feasible.

Pune and Bombay provide medical certification of cause of death. The available medical facilities for specialized treatment attract a large number of patients from outside the city. Thus the statistics obtained from these sources do not give a correct pattern of mortality by causes.

Model registration—a survey of cause of death initiated by the office of the Registrar General—is an experimental study in the collection of reliable death statistics by causes in the primary hea centres through the para-medical personnel. The scheme is based o ascertaining broad symptoms and conditions, anatomical site and duration of complaint by personal enquiries from the family of the deceased by the para-medical personnel. The modus operandi is that the field agent visits the concerned household and obtains the necessary information about the symptoms, anatomical site and duration of illness to assign the probable cause of death. A manual of instructions has been prescribed for this purpose. To achieve greater reliability, all the events observed by the field agent in a month are checked for consistency at the primary health centre. This is further scrutinised in regard to causes of death by the medical officer attached to the primary health centre. The scheme has yielded reliable pattern of mortality by broad groups of diseases. The results obtained from model registration are presented in Table 6.

TABLE 6

Cause and/or prominent symptoms	*Per cent deaths*			
	1970	*1971*	*1972*	*1973*
Accidents & injuries	4.0	4.2	4.0	4.0
Child-birth & Pregnancy	1.1	1.2	1.3	1.2
Fevers	14.9	15.0	14.3	14.5
Digestive disorders	8.7	7.9	7.9	9.6
Coughs (disorders of respiratory system)	24.0	22.1	23.1	22.0
Disorders of central nervous system	1.2	0.7	0.6	2.3
Disorders of circulatory system	2.8	3.2	3.7	5.6
Other clear symptoms	10.7	11.2	9.1	8.6
Causes peculiar to infancy	11.5	10.9	11 6	11.8
Senility (old age)	12.1	12.8	14.4	13.9
Others	9.0	10.8	10.0	6.5
All causes:	100.0	100.0	100.0	100.0

(iii) Population Censuses

Another source of mortality data is the population census. If two consecutive censuses give an accurate account of population by age and sex, it is possible to make reasonably accurate estimates of death rate for the inter-censal period using reverse survival method. The census age returns have been subject to extensive misreporting of ages. Problems with age misstatements and age-heaping can be partly solved by smoothening with the aid of polynomials. Thus the reliability of the results mainly depends on the soundness of the underlying assumptions. Other techniques based upon census data are the application of stable and quasi-stable population techniques. While these techniques are found useful in many of the developing countries, their assumption of constant fertility is to be seriously considered.

Since mortality rates in developing countries are high especially for infants and children, it is necessary to have better techniques of estimating infant and child mortality. Two indirect procedures have been developed by Brass for measuring infant and child mortality.

The Brass technique requires tabulation on mean number of children ever born and mean number of surviving women of the child-bearing age group. In the absence of adequate vital statistics data, this is likely to be the best source of information on infant and child mortality. Brass has recently developed a second indirect technique for estimating adult mortality called the orphanhood method. Reliable estimates of mortality may be obtained for age groups commencing with the earliest age of child-bearing.

Comparison with other Countries

The table below gives the crude death rate and infant mortality for developing and developed countries :

TABLE 7

Country	*Year*	*DR*	*IDR*
Sri Lanka	1972	7.7	45.1
Thailand	1972	10.4	27.0
Philippines	1965-70	12.0	67.9
India	1975	15.8	136.4 (1972)
Japan	1973	6.6	11.3
Sweden	1974	10.6	9.2
U.K.	1974	12.1	17.2
U.S.A.	1974	9.1	16.5

In India, infant mortality continues to be high mainly on account of persistence of exogenous causes arising from environmental and nutritional factors. Much of the success in reducing infant mortality to a level consistent with that of advanced countries depends on creating proper conditions, institutionalisation of births, additional trained doctors and nurses through an integrated health, maternal and child welfare programme.

Deaths by Ages

The pattern of mortality in the different age groups as measured by the proportion of deaths in the various countries is shown in Table 8. In India over 50 per cent of deaths occur in the age group (0-4) while in Japan one in twenty deaths belong to this age group. Child mortality in India is considerably high. In the older age group, the proportion of deaths increases faster than the proportion in India.

Reduction in mortality is possible by reducing infant and child mortality for which there is need for setting up an integrated programme for maternal and child care and making available the services of more hospitals, doctors and nurses in the rural areas.

TABLE 8

Age group	*Japan (1967)*		*Sri Lanka (1967)*		*India (1969)*	
	M	*F*	*M*	*F*	*M*	*F*
0-4	5.7	5.0	29.9	32.1	50.5	55.0
5-9	0.7	0.5	2.9	3.6	4.6	5.2
10-14	0.5	0.4	1.6	1.8	2.1	1.6
15-19	1.4	0.8	1.8	1.9	1.0	1.8
20-24	1.7	1.1	2.1	2.3	1.5	2.2
25-29	1.8	1.3	1.9	2.4	1.4	2.0
30-34	2.1	1.5	1.7	2.1	1.5	2.3
35-39	2.7	1.9	2.6	2.8	2.1	1.8
40-44	3.0	2.4	2.6	2.0	2.5	2.0
45-49	3.2	3.0	3.8	2.5	3.1	1.9
50-54	4.9	4.2	3.9	2.8	4.1	3.1
55-59	7.6	5.7	5.0	3.4	3.9	2.4
60-64	10.2	7.3	5.6	4.2	6.2	5.1
65-69	13.4	10.2	7.3	5.9	4.4	3.4
70+	41.1	54.5	28.3	30.2	11.1	10.3

CONCLUSION

As will be clear from the preceding account of the state of mortality data in India there are several deficiencies of coverage, quality and timeliness. Serious attempts are being made to strengthen the civil registration system to obtain complete and timely information on the various aspects of mortality. This is the only system which provides mortality statistics at the lowest level for purposes of local socio-economic planning. Civil registration being a vast administrative and organisational task, involving the cooperation of several state agencies, it will take a long time to reach a satisfactory level of efficiency. While vigorous attempts are being made to strengthen the system, as an alternative the S.P.S. have proved its utility in providing reliable estimates of mortality at the state and national level.

Malaria Statistics in India

S. PATTANAYAK and V.P. PATHAK*

The occurrence of malarial fevers in India is known since ancient time. Some of the earlier references to this fever are available in the *Athara Veda* which is believed to have been composed about 1500 B.C. From the numerous references it would appear that it was the commonest fever.

Modern history of research in malaria dates from 1845, when the British Army Commission was appointed to investigate the causation of malaria following the opening of the Western Jamuna Canal. The determination of the spleen rate as a malaria-metric index was employed for the first time by Dr T.E. Dempster who was a member of this commission. This index (spleen rate) was a most valuable measure of estimating the incidence of malaria. But spleen rate by itself is crude though simple. Therefore, a method for measuring every enlarged spleen was developed by Hackett in 1944. By this method average enlarged spleen (A.E.S.) could be worked out.

Before and During the National Malaria Control Programme

Malaria-metric surveys, which included spleen rate, determination of average enlarged spleen, child parasite rate and infant parasite rate were carried out in different areas to estimate the incidence of malaria and malaria endemicity. These were the sample surveys. The results obtained were applied to whole tracts to estimate the figures. Another source of data was the vital statistics published by the Public Health Commissioner. For example, in 1981, 60 per cent of the total mortality in the country was ascribed to fevers, of which one-third or one-fourth were attributed to malaria. Still another im-

*Directorate of National Malaria Eradication Programme, Delhi.

portant source was the dispensary and hospital statistics. The proportion of malaria cases to the total cases attending the hospitals and dispensaries and expressed as percentage is the proportional case rate. The proportional case rate for different years can be compared to assess the rise or decline of incidence of malaria.

Agencies Collecting the Data and the Types of Data Collected

During the National Malaria Control Programme, which was launched in 1953 and later converted to an eradication programme in 1958, insecticidal spray in the dwelling houses and cattle sheds etc. was carried out throughout the length and breadth of the country with the objective of interruption of malaria transmission. After some years of insecticidal protective coverage, the incidence of malaria fell drastically with the result that traditional malaria-metric indices, vital statistics and even the hospital and dispensary statistics (which recorded cases of clinical malaria only) became insensitive.

A total coverage of the population under a surveillance mechanism was aimed at. Under this mechanism where all the fever cases are screened by both active and passive agencies, the blood of the fever cases is examined microscopically and the cases are administered presumptive and radical treatment as the case may be. The objectives of surveillance are both operational to wipe out the residual infections and epidemiological intelligence by data collection. The following agencies are concerned with the collection, tabulation and furnishing the data.

(*i*) National Malaria Eradication Programme units and district health authorities collect surveillance/vigilance data and spray data.

(*ii*) Entomological organisations of the states and the regional coordinating organisations collect entomological data mainly about the vector density and their susceptibility status.

(*iii*) Hospitals and dispensaries collect data regarding the total cases, fever cases and microscopically, positive malaria cases attending these institutions.

It may be pointed out here that routine reports asked for from the periphery which are not very complicated, special investigations are sometimes necessary either to verify the field data or to gather additional information (*e.g.* sociological or economic aspects). Often a multidisciplinary approach is needed for the latter. Problem areas also need in-depth study which cannot be taken up by the staff engaged in routine work. The type of data obtained is as under.

(*a*) *Through active surveillance/vigilance and passive surveillance/vigilance*

(*i*) Basic data regarding the number of districts/units, primary health centres/sub-units, number of sectors, sections and villages. The number of houses in each village. The number of inmates of each house, population of each village etc. This data is updated in the beginning of each year.

(*ii*) The number of fever cases, or cases with a recent history of fever encountered at the time of the visit of surveillance worker/basic health worker.

(*iii*) The number of blood slides taken from the fever cases from each village during the fortnight/month depending on the periodicity of the visit and the annual blood examination rates in different areas.

(*iv*) The number of cases found microscopically positive. The species of malaria parasite responsible for the infection.

(*v*) The age and sex distribution of the population suffering from fever/malaria.

(*vi*) The number of fever cases given presumptive treatment with chloroquine and radical treatment with primaquine.

(*vii*) The number of positive cases followed up every month for one year and their result. The number of mass blood surveys carried out around positive cases and their result.

(*viii*) The number of malaria foci.

(*ix*) Covered with focal spray.

(*x*) Epidemiological classification of the positive cases.

(*xi*) The number of blood smears in backlog for examination.

(*xii*) Time interval between collection of blood smear and the communication of result by the laboratory.

(*xiii*) The result of cross-checking of blood smears both at the state cross-checking laboratories and regional coordinating organization cross-checking laboratories.

(*xiv*) Total cases attending hospitals and dispensaries, the number of blood smears collected and found positive for malaria.

(*b*) *Data regarding spray coverage*

(*i*) Delimitation of malarious areas extent and attitude.

(*ii*) Timing of spray operations in relation to transmission season.

(*iii*) The type of insecticide used and the number of spray rounds planned and actually carried out.

(*iv*) The number of units/sub-units, districts/PHCs, sections and villages covered with insecticidal spray.

(*v*) The number of houses sprayed, refused, locked and missed and percentage coverage of houses.

(*vi*) The number of houses covered partially. Room coverage percentage.

(*vii*) The number of serviceable spray pumps available and the spray teams employed.

(*c*) *Data regarding logistics*

(*i*) Availability or transport in the units/districts. Road worthy or off road.

(*ii*) Availability of insecticides.

(*iii*) Spray equipments and spare parts for spray equipment.

(*iv*) Antimalarial drugs.

(*v*) Microslides.

(*vi*) Microscopes—in working order, repairable or unserviceable.

(*d*) *Entomological data*

(*i*) Vector densities during different parts of the year. The densities of other anopheline mosquitoes.

(*ii*) The susceptibility status of the vector in relation to different insecticides used when adequate number of mosquitoes are available.

Gaps in data from the point of view of Social and Economic Planning

Some of the important gaps in the available data are outlined below:

(*a*) *Epidemiological data*

(*i*) In the areas where the incidence has gone up abnormally after the resurgence or malaria, the data obtained through the usual surveillance agencies has become inadequate and insensitive. This is because the usual surveillance machinery is geared only to be effective when the case load in the community is below a certain level. Beyond this level, this machinery is unable to detect cases, because of the staff and laboratory inadequacies.

(*ii*) The data is inadequate regarding major and minor industrial or constructional projects which attract labour from malarious or non-malarious areas, so also regarding the major or minor irrigation projects which are conducive to water-logging and creation of mosquito-genic conditions.

(*iii*) Data is deficient on vulnerability and receptivity of different areas.

(*iv*) Data regarding the problem areas and their delimitation is sometime inadequate.

(*v*) Population structure—tribal, non-tribal and religion of the population is not covered under surveillance data.

(*vi*) Out-door occupations—nomadism and different routes and timings of migration from one place to another.

(*b*) *Data is inadequate regarding habits and attitudes of the people*

(*i*) Attitude to spraying.

(*ii*) Refusals to accept spray and reasons for the same.

—Religious grounds.

—Silk-worm rearing.

—Spoiling of furniture or distempered walls.

—Bed-bugs.

—Loss of collateral benefits like resistance by other insects.

—Inconvenience of cleaning the floors and other household articles after spray.

—Local custom of not allowing others to enter kitchen and the temple room.

—Storage of foodgrains and fodder etc.

(*iii*) Habit of mud-plastering. Extent of its presence and its role in loss of insecticidal protection.

(*iv*) Out-door sleeping—use of mosquito-nets. Occupations which require staying out-doors at night.

(*v*) Level of health education and educational inputs.

(*vi*) Population movements. How often and their pattern.

(*c*) *Entomological data*

(*i*) Data regarding the physiological resistance in vectors should be collected vigorously from more areas where no entomological studies have been done so far with WHO standard kit.

(*ii*) Estimated man-biting densities per person per night inside sprayed rooms and outside.

(*iii*) Proportion of parous females in samples caught biting or freshly-fed.

(*iv*) 25-hour outlet trap survival rate in captures from sprayed structures.

(*v*) Data regarding behavioural changes in the vectors like out-door biting and out-door resting.

(*vi*) Role of secondary vectors.

(*d*) *Data about cost benefit of National Malaria Eradication Programme*

(*i*) Inputs of the anti-malaria programme and the out-puts of the programme in the form of reduced morbidity and mortality and its role in economic development.

(*ii*) Cost effectiveness of alternative strategies.

(*e*) *Data regarding staff of the Malaria Organisations in the States*

(*i*) Training status of different categories.

(*ii*) Morale of the staff.

(*iii*) Rate of turn-over of staff.

WHAT NEW ITEMS OF DATA COLLECTION ARE SUGGESTED

Enidemiological data. In the areas where the incidence of malaria is very high say above 10 per 1000 in a few representative sections, total coverage should be achieved in respect of surveillance by deploying more staff for a smaller population depending on the case load. All the blood smears collected from these sections could be given top priority. The data from these sections (index sections) will be more valuable in indicating the trends of incidence and the impact of remedial measures than the data collected by routine surveillance.

The actual transmission season varies in different areas depending on the climatic and other factors. The data regarding this is absolutely necessary for proper timing of the spray operations. In certain areas the actual transmission may be starting early before the spray coverage is given. This will reduce the impact of insecticidal spray on this transmission.

The data regarding major and industrial, agricultural, forest irrigational or constructional projects available with the malaria organizations is not always complete. These projects attract labour from distant areas. More often than not this labour comes from malarious areas and harbours malaria parasites in their blood. They are responsible for many focal outbreaks in the group as well as in the local communities. The labourers live in temporary shelters which are difficult to treat with insecticidal application. These projects being the focal points from where malaria disseminates have to be provided special attention. Therefore, fairly satisfactory system of data collection about them has to be evolved and implemented.

Certain areas are more vulnerable and susceptible to malaria transmission than others. Complete data about them should be collected and appropriate measures to prevent reestablishment of malaria endemicity applied.

There are problem areas where the eradication measures do not prove to be as fruitful as in others. To make any appreciable impact in such areas special methods may have to be applied. Therefore, such areas should be delimited and complete data about them should be collected.

In a few small pockets in Assam and Meghalaya, studies have revealed that plasmodium falciparum has developed tolerance or resistance to chloroquine. These studies should be expanded to know the extent of this phenomenon. The areas should be delimited so that alternative drugs may be used in such areas.

India is a vast country with a variety of terrain and different levels of development of means of communications. The quantum of staff required for spray and surveillance and also supervision will be more in areas with difficult terrain even if the population to be served is less. Complete data regarding these areas specially with reference to the population or the area which a worker can cover without undue difficulty. A realistic pattern of staff should be worked out in the light of such data.

The nomadic groups are responsible for spread of malaria. They have set patterns of movement. The usual anti-malaria methods like spray and surveillance are difficult to apply in their case. Special methods are needed to protect them from malaria. Complete data regarding their numbers, patterns of their movement and other social and cultural habits may be useful to apply appropriate anti-malaria measures in their case.

Data regarding spray coverage. Data regarding types and sprayable surface per house is necessary for planning the frequency of application of insecticides, and the quantity of insecticides to be supplied in different areas. The sprayable surface per house can be worked out on sample basis in representative villages and then applied to the whole district.

The rate of turnover of the houses is also very important. The construction of new houses, additions and extensions in the existing houses, replastering of walls or alterations in the ceilings etc. are the important factors which have an effect on the efficacy of the spray operations. Temporary shelters are difficult to treat with insecticides and require more frequent applications.

The spray coverage should be worked out as percentage of the total sprayable surface which should have been treated with the insecticide. This data will give the real picture to assess the impact of spray operations. In most of the areas the locked and closed houses are not taken into account while working out coverage which gives a false idea. The rooms in the closed and locked houses can be estimated by the average number of rooms per house in the village.

The strength of the spray-squads should be worked out in the light of local terrain and means of communications. So complete data about the terrain etc. must be collected.

Data regarding refusals to accept spray must be collected according to the reasons for such refusals, as described in the earlier paragraphs so that appropriate corrective measures could be applied.

The habit of mud-plastering specially in some tribal areas is an important factor which negatives the effect of insecticidal spray. The data regarding the extent of this habit and its effect on malaria transmission should be collected.

Data regarding out-door sleeping during transmission months and the percentage of people who may be using mosquito-nets has a bearing on malaria transmission.

The level of health education and the inputs being made in this area will influence the future course of events by influencing people's cooperation in spray operations and other anti-malarial activities.

Entomological data. Under the modified plan of operations which is being implemented next year, the entomological component has been provided at the zonal level. There are 72 such zones in the country. Therefore, the entomological work has to be intensified manifold. The data on the lines indicated in the earlier paragraphs should be collected so that the anti-malaria operations could be carried out on more scientific lines depending on the information provided by the entomological parameters. More elaborate studies are required in the problem areas.

Cost-benefit data. The data about the cost benefit of National Malaria Eradication Programme is scanty at present. More detailed studies are necessary to bring out the economic benefits brought about by the malaria eradication programme vis-a-vis the investments made. The cost effectiveness of the alternative strategies also needs scientific study.

Data regarding staff. It is the staff in the states who are responsible for the efficient implementation and adequate supervision in the states. Therefore, a complete data about the training status, morale and the rate of turnover is very essential for future planning of the programme in different states.

Leprosy Statistics in India

S.K. NOORDEEN*

Data base for health in general and for chronic diseases like leprosy in particular is generally unsatisfactory. Even while collecting information on communicable diseases in general leprosy is often left out. This is because for a long time leprosy has been considered as something different from other diseases, largely due to the social overtones connected with it.

The very term "leprosy" carried different meanings to different people depending upon their own areas of interest. To the medical worker a leprosy patient is anyone who has certain clinical signs and symptoms characteristic of the disease, irrespective of the stage or type of disease and irrespective of the fact whether or not he is going to be a problem otherwise. To the public health-worker only leprosy patients who are capable of communicating the disease to others are of serious concern. To the social-worker leprosy is a problem only when patients are recognized as such by the community leading to ostracism and social handicap. To the health economist the disease is of interest mainly because it causes physical disability in an otherwise wage-earning group leading to economic loss. The understanding of the disease from different points of view generally does not cause any problem, except when data on leprosy collected from one point of view is attempted to be utilized for another.

Till about thirty years back information on leprosy from any point of view was very scanty, and even those available were not reliable for any scientific planning. Attempts to collect information on leprosy through official census enumerators were made in the decennial census operations beginning from 1872, but the information that came out turned out to be quite unreliable. On the other hand, in

*Deputy Director, Central Leprosy Teaching and Research Institute, Tamilnadu.

early days collection of accurate information on any large scale through any organized attempt was not considered possible.

Even so, the then Indian branch of the British Empire Leprosy Relief Association did carry out total population surveys in few areas in the country where leprosy was considered a serious problem. However, the first official estimate on leprosy for the country was essentially based on data collected by census enumerators after applying certain corrections for which the data from the limited surveys carried out by the early workers appear to have been utilized.

Although data from the early surveys provided information on total leprosy, information on certain vital aspects such as disability etc. were not available. In fact till recently information on several aspects of leprosy came from data collected from patients admitted to institutions. The institutions variously known as sanatoria, colony, etc., attracted only patients with certain characteristics and the institutionalised patients in general did not represent the true situation of the leprosy patients in the community.

With the development of the National Leprosy Control Programme as part of plan schemes the situation on data collection in leprosy improved. An important constituent of the programme was active case finding through various methods including total population surveys. These total population surveys, when properly carried out, gave good information on leprosy in the community studied.

However, collection of information through such surveys takes a very long time due to various reasons and constraints. In the last 25 years, since organized leprosy control work started, it has been possible to obtain such information at least in part in about one-half of the country to which the programme has been extended. Even then estimates made from such surveys are subject to certain errors, which might in certain situations be quite serious. For instance, most of the estimates are based on one time surveys where the field worker fails, due to technical reasons, to distinguish between active cases of leprosy and inactive cases of leprosy, and as a result the total numbers of patients mentioned include a proportion of leprosy patients which should not have been included.

Another important source of error in these surveys is the poor coverage for examination. The leprosy situation in the unexamined population has often been known to be different from that in the examined population, as a number of leprosy patients particularly escape examination due to social stigma attached to the disease, and remain in the unexamined population. Apart from all these the limited training of the field worker, and the unsatisfactory examination of the female population due to employment of male field workers, themselves contribute to certain types of errors.

Lastly, for estimating leprosy prevalence in large geographic areas such as districts or States the data utilized are from restricted areas where surveys have been carried out in those districts or states. In general such surveys are carried out in areas which are known to be highly endemic, and estimates made from such areas may not reflect the true situation.

Although the total population survey component of the National Leprosy Control Programme admirably combines the case finding purpose as well as data collection, the emphasis on data collection has increased very much in recent years. In fact the tendency to collect more and more data at the field level has led to a situation when the field worker is loaded with forms, registers and reports to fill in leading to dilution of other control activities. It is felt that data collection is often ill planned, unnecessarily copious, and not directed towards any specific purpose.

Apart from government agencies in recent years several voluntary agencies in leprosy have extended their services to field programmes, and many of the voluntary agencies are collecting useful and reliable information in leprosy particularly in certain areas.

From the point of view of social and economic planning the data available at present is far from adequate. We have only a very rough idea about the proportion of leprosy patients who are disabled. A leprosy patient may suffer from physical disability, social disability or both. We have practically no data on social disability in leprosy. With regard to physical disability in leprosy we have no information on its relative importance with reference to other disabling conditions in the community such as blindness, orthopaedic handicap, etc.

Lastly we have no information on the effect of physical or social disability on the economic life of individuals and the community under varying conditions.

In order to improve the data base in leprosy it is very necessary to take into consideration certain factors. Firstly the primary responsibility to collect basic information on leprosy should be that of the health services responsible for control of the disease. Although at present leprosy control activities are carried out as a specialized vertical programme it is expected that in course of time it will be part of general health services, in which case data collection for leprosy will be part and parcel of data collection for other communicable diseases. The major emphasis in data collection at the basic level should be to develop a simple system which will provide accurate information through simple forms.

In large geographic areas where leprosy service is yet to be provided it may be necessary to collect basic information through sample surveys. This might require specially trained personnel. Even in areas where reliable information is thought to be available it may be useful to check such information through sample surveys. In fact periodic sample surveys could provide very useful additional information not only on the disease situation but also on other related matters. Further such periodic data collection could be very useful in studying time trends.

The collection of information required for social and economic planning should be integrated with collection of such information for other health programmes. The items of information could include not only data on physical and social disability in leprosy but also the degree of economic dislocation caused by the disease. In such situations it is often difficult to study leprosy in isolation. The interaction between one or more health situation and the social and economic setting in the community can be quite complex.

One problem that often attracts the attention of social workers is the problem of beggars with leprosy. The problem of beggars as a public health menace has often been overstated, and there is a need to study the problem objectively, and deal with it as part of a general problem of beggars.

It is concluded that there is a vast scope for improvement of data base in leprosy, and all future planning should take into consideration not only collection of information on basic disease situation in leprosy but also on the impact of the disease on the social and economic setting. The need to look at leprosy as part of total health problem affecting the community should also not be lost sight of.

Statistics on Communicable Diseases

B.B. GAITONDE and
D.M. RENAPURKAR*

India has still to overcome the challenge of communicable diseases as in other developing countries. However, since independence there has been a considerable progress in increasing efficiency of health delivery system and widening its horizon. We have succeeded in reaching the target of "zero" incidence of smallpox. No case of plague has been reported during the last 10 years and cholera incidence has shown a definite decline.

Yet we have other communicable diseases persisting or staging a comeback. Malaria, which was on the point of eradication, is returning in full swing. In 1966, "The picture has altered so radically that we are finding it difficult to obtain material for imparting adequate knowledge about this disease to our undergraduates." In 1972, the incidence of malaria reached 1.2 million, in 1973 it soared to 1.5 million and in 1976, the incidence is seen continuing its further upward trend.

Filariasis, another mosquito-borne communicable disease, is spreading in enormous proportions. In 1953, about 25 million population was estimated to be exposed to the risk of filariasis. In 1960, it was shown that 64 million people were exposed to the risk of filariasis of which 5.4 million people were microfilaria carriers. In 1971, 136 million people were shown to live in filariasis endemic areas with 12 million people as microfilaria carriers (Sharma, 1976).

Leprosy continues to be a major problem in India. The estimates show three million leprosy cases to be there of which about 20-25 per cent are infectious. The incidence of tuberculosis is on an increase. In 1955-58, the number of active and probably active cases of tuberculosis varied between 13 and 25 per 1000 population. Tuber-

*Hoffkins Institute, Bombay.

culosis accounted for 6.96 per cent of total institutional deaths reported during 1962-64.

The north-western states of India have high prevalence rates of trachoma. Trachoma and keratomalacia due to Vitamin A deficiency are responsible for much of the blindness in the country. There are believed to be five million blind persons in India.

The incidence of cholera is falling steadily; the mean annual death rate which was 1.58 per 1,000 in 1900-24, had come down to 0.016 by 1964-69. There has also been a substantial reduction in the attack rate for cholera.

Venereal diseases are showing an upward trend as in the other parts of the world. There is, however, no accurate data to assess the gravity of the problem. The incidence of tetanus, diphtheria and pertussis needs accurate evaluation. Magnitude of problems of diarrhoeal diseases and several viral infections has yet to be assessed. There is no country-wide data on poliomyelitis. Virus Research Centre, Poona, has shown the presence in varying degree of intensity, of many of the virus diseases, some already known to us and some discovered in recent years, and others introduced only recently from other regions. There is no information about their distribution and density in different parts of the country.

Infective and parasitic diseases constituted the leading group among medically certified deaths in 1962-4 in some parts of India, contributing 14.42 per cent to total mortality (*see* Table 1 on p. 182). The next groups in order of importance were diseases of the respiratory system, disorders of early infancy, diseases of circulatory and digestive system, and metabolic and nutritional disorders. Tetanus constituted a leading individual cause of death with a contribution of 7.08 per cent to total mortality; next in order was gastroenteritis and colitis (5.0 per cent), pulmonary tuberculosis (4.11 per cent) and anaemias (4.01 per cent).

Other important diseases figuring among the first twenty causes of mortality were dysentery of all types, malnutrition, typhoid fever, disorders of the heart, cholera, and cirrhosis of the liver. From the information accumulated on institutional morbidity under the Sample Registration System in nine states of India it would appear that, the 'infectious and parasitic' diseases constituted the major cause of disease accounting for 18.1 per cent of the total morbidity.

PRESENT STATUS OF STATISTICAL DATA ON SOME MAJOR COMMUNICABLE DISEASES

Malaria. No other communicable disease is as satisfactorily recorded as malaria thanks to fairly orderly surveillance system. However, many things went wrong and incidence of malaria seems to be on increase. This may be due to several factors such as inadequate case detection and reporting, complacency in laboratory diagnosis, want of effective vector control measures, non-involvement of people in the programme, and last but not the least casual attitude to data collection and analysis etc.

Classification of different areas with regard to malaria endemicity on the basis of splenic index used for the first time in India by Dempster in 1848 was a suitable method in the pre-DDT era. Today the data on malaria incidence in different parts of country is indeed available. In fact, entry of different areas from one phase to the other as a part of operational design for eradication of the disease—from attack phase to surveillance phase—has been worked on the basis of this index.

On pragmatic considerations, it is apparent that strategy of malaria eradication to that of its effective control seems to be the need of the hour. Epidemiologically, therefore areas with regard to disease endemicity, receptivity and transmission potential are to be precisely and clearly demarcated, so that control measures are tailored to the specific purpose. To achieve this end the available data on disease incidence from different areas in the country should be made use of.

Studies are urgently required to be undertaken to demonstrate the social and economic gains following malaria control and eradication. Methods and techniques are to be developed for the quantification of cost benefit and cost effectiveness aspects of the programme in economic terms. This is necessary for getting the support of administrators and planners for such programme. Such an investigation should be entrusted to a multidisciplinary team consisting of malariologist, health administrator, biostatistician, social scientist and management consultants.

Filariasis. Filariasis has not been paid the attention it deserves. It was estimated in 1953, that about 25 million population was exposed to the risk of bancroftian filariasis. This estimate was based on limited data available then. Large scale filariasis surveys undertaken during 1955-1960 revealed that about 64 million people were living in filarious areas of which 5.4 million people were microfilaria carriers and 4.4 million were suffering from various types of disease manifestations.

In 1971 it was revealed that about 136 million people lived in areas endemic for W. bancrofti of which 12 million people suffered from disease manifestations. The apparent increase in morbidity is due to detection of infection in new areas, public awareness of the disease and increase of population (Sharma, 1976).

The problem of filariasis in most of the states has not been completely delineated. Still 130 districts out of 289 districts in endemic states are to be surveyed. Status of disease in non-endemic areas has not been evaluated. The disease is now reported to be spreading to non-endemic areas. Surveys carried out so far in non-endemic states of north western region of India such as Rajasthan, Punjab, Himachal Pradesh and Jammu and Kashmir showed the presence of microfilaria carriers who either migrated from the endemic areas or lived in those areas for a considerable period of time. There is no data on the infection in mosquito Vector population a facet vital for the total containment/eradication of the disease.

In short inspite of the fact that filariasis has been a national public health problem and a lot of work has been done in regard to its epidemiology, case detection etc., enough statistical data is not available on the basis of which a strategy can be evolved for control/eradication of the disease from different parts of the country.

Cholera. Since 1900 the incidence as well as frequency of epidemics due to cholera have declined particularly following the institution of National Water Supply and Sanitation Programme in 1951. The case fatality rate has also shown a considerable decline in the recent years due to better methods and improved facilities of treatment being available (*see* Table 2 on p. 183).

Though cholera incidence has been keeping low since 1966, a wider area of the country has been affected every year. As against six to ten different states reporting cholera in the past, the disease has been reported every year since 1966 from 16 or more states, some of which had been free from cholera for a long period (Kerala, Gujarat, Haryana, Punjab, Rajasthan) or had never known the disease (Andaman and Nicobar Islands).

On the average, annually 26,483 cases and 6,253 deaths have been reported in the country during 1964-73 as against the average of 36,606 cases and 10,596 deaths during the previous decade (1954-63). The case fatality rate has also declined during the recent decade (1964-73) to about 24 per cent as compared to about 40 per cent during the previous decade (1954-63).

The main bottleneck in cholera surveillance is delay in reporting of outbreak of the disease which in the initial stages is often reported as cases of gastroenteritis. In addition to delay in reporting and misreporting of cases, there is a lot of underreporting particularly in rural areas inspite of legal provisions in this regard. Stray cases are seldom reported and there is a tendency to report cases only when the epidemic is fully established and a large number of cases have occurred with same deaths. Another factor is the inadequate facilities for laboratory diagnosis. Statistical data on environmental conditions are wanting. Data on socio-economic status of population, environment climatic conditions, water supply position, contributing to the epidemiology of the disease are faulty and inadequate.

Smallpox. Statistics on smallpox also suffered from inadequate reporting and this was the major problem faced by those engaged in smallpox eradication campaign. This lacuna was removed with the introduction of intensified campaign against smallpox and India succeeded in achieving smallpox free status. Urgent instructions were issued for launching operation smallpox "Target Zero" in January 1975. The results of this emergency programme were very fruitful and the number of outbreaks began to decline and continued to do so, until 24 May 1975, the data of the last case reported in India (*see* Table 3 on p. 184).

Although India has now recorded a zero incidence for the first time in its history, active surveillance activities must be continued for a further few years so as to confirm that not a single case of smallpox, either indigenous or imported, remains undetected. The work during the next few years must be carried out with the same determination and passion, if smallpox is to be officially declared eradicated in India. If each worker who has been involved in this miracle, the human miracle, wishes to ensure that never again shall an Indian child die, be blinded or be disfigured by smallpox. Factors conducive for virus to be latently growing are present. They need to be identified and programme for their containment or eradication must be planned.

Leprosy. Leprosy is prevalent in our country since time immemorial as evidenced by reference about the disease in *Shushrut Samhita* and *Manusmriti*. In the absence of a preventive vaccination the only method available for controlling leprosy is to treat all infectious cases.

Case detection is the major factor in the treatment and control of leprosy. At the time of launching the leprosy control programme in 1954-55 it was contemplated that the result in the form of reduction in prevalence and incidence would be apparent in about 10-15 years. However, barring in a few study centres these expectations have not been fulfilled.

The last two decades have witnessed considerable expansion in the governmental programmes for leprosy control. The programme is now in operation in 25 states, Union and Territories covering nearly all areas of high and moderate endemicity. There are 278 leprosy control units and 2,243 survey education and treatment centres. Besides these several national and international agencies are also participating in the National Leprosy Control Programme.

Despite all efforts made for the control of leprosy the disease continues to be a major public health problem in our country with all its social ramifications.

It is estimated that out of more than twelve million leprosy cases in the world about 3.2 million are in India as shown below.

Endemic population	372	million
No. of cases in India	3.2	million
infectious cases	8	lakhs
deformed cases	8	lakhs
beggar patients	6	lakhs
children leprosy cases	10	lakhs
new cases detected every year	0.64	lakhs
Population covered upto date	132.9	million

Out of the total population of 547 million in India, 372 million live in the endemic belt; only 166.2 million of this population have so far been covered by the programme. Also out of the estimated total number of 3.2 million cases of leprosy only 1.25 million cases have been detected and only about one million patients are taking treatment regularly (1976).

The National Leprosy Control Programme today has three objectives: (1) to detect the early cases by survey; (2) to carry on intensive health education, and (3) treatment of index cases. The work so far has not resulted in the detection of adequate number of cases. Statistical data are inadequate. We have still to detect more than two million patients out of the total expected 3.2 million cases in India. Surveys of school children, industrial establishments, slum areas and closed communities are very few. These are essential for leprosy control programme as these will play a major role in early detection and treatment of cases and prevention of deformities. As such these data particularly in relation to school children are very important.

As one is aware, leprosy is a disease with a long incubation period. Early detection of the disease particularly in children has a major role to play in the control and treatment of the disease and prevention of disability. However, there are no statistical data to show the status of disease in children. Intensive and extensive epidemiological studies are needed to show the susceptibility of children to leprosy in the interest of evolving a strategy for the future. Similarly, population based epidemiological studies on leprosy are very few. Since the inception of sulphide treatment and leprosy control programmes, there are, however, many records available of case finding surveys some of which allow for prevalence rate calculations.

The interval between two successive surveys being often five years or longer and because of poor recording, these data are unsuitable for incidence rate calculation and in turn for planning suitable measures, Longitudinal surveys of defined population at short intervals to define epidemiological variables like age and sex and other environmental factors are badly needed. Apart from this statistical information on factors such as mass movement of population due to floods or natural calamities from areas of high endemicity to low endemicity, effect of industrialization of an area resulting in the immigration of labour is wanting.

One of the biggest lacuna that exists in statistics on leprosy is inadequate data on contacts. We do not know about the type of contact which transmits leprosy. We have many reports to indicate aggregation of leprosy in certain families. We have no data to answer questions like, "In what way does a family contact differ from other type of contacts." The old theory of close and prolonged contacts does not provide the reply, because it is agreed that doctors and nurses working in close contact with leprosy do not have a higher incidence as compared to general population.

In addition to the physical proximity, the familial aggregation has some aggregation of genetic factors as well. It is very difficult to say whether this clustering of cases in families with history of disease in previous generation is due to genetic factor or due to continuance of the same socioeconomic environment favourable for the transmission of leprosy.

Lastly, all efforts at the control of leprosy are doomed to failure unless the significance of stigma and the associated social and economic factors are not given due consideration. It must be appreciated that the achievement of necessary psychological changes in a disease like leprosy, is a much more subtle and formidable task than the technical problems of treatment. Need or consideration of socioeconomic factors while planning leprosy control programme is imminent. There is also dire need to investigate the "drop-outs" discontinuing the treatment programmes and evaluate the extent of these drop-outs. The problem of DDS resistance also needs statistical appraisal. Statistical evaluation of these problems is necessary for future planning of leprosy control measures.

Tuberculosis. Tuberculosis is the foremost public health problem in India. There are at present at least six million cases of active tuberculosis, of which more than two million are excreting tubercle bacilli in their sputum and are thus responsible for the spread of the disease in the community. The estimated economic loss to the nation resulting from the death of patients and disablement of patients is of the order of Rs 2,000 crores. From the economic and public health points of view there is a great need for combating tuberculosis on a priority basis by undertaking efficient and energetic control measures on a country-wide scale.

The first major attempt to determine the size and extent of the tuberculosis problem in India was a National Sample Survey carried out under the auspices of the Indian Council of Medical Research in 1955-58. The survey covered six cities, 30 towns and 151 villages; the population covered was approximately 3,00,000 all aged 5 years or above. The survey revealed that the prevalence rate for active and probably active tuberculosis varied from 13 to 25 per 1,000 population in cities, towns and villages, average being 18 per thousand. The prevalence rate for bacteriologically positive cases varied from 2-8 per 1,00,000 population, the average being four per 1,000. The prevalence rates were found to be broadly similar in cities, towns and villages and in general the prevalence rate showed a continuous increase with age.

Based on these findings, the total number of active and probably active cases of tuberculosis is estimated to be about eight million including about two million sputum positive cases.

To tackle the tuberculosis problem, the Centre launched the National Tuberculosis Programme. This is a permanent country-wide programme based on the epidemiological and socio-economic conditions in the country and is integrated into the general health and medical facilities at both the rural and urban levels. The district tuberculosis programme is the basic organisational unit of the NRP.

The activities of the DTP can be broadly classified into three categories as case finding treatment and prevention. The district TB centre is responsible for not only to provide diagnosis and treatment to those reporting to these centres but also to organize case finding and treatment in all the existing peripheral health and medical institutions in the district as an integral part of the general health services in the district. 270 districts have been covered to date with a district TB centre in each (*see* Table 4 on p. 185).

The programme has been in operation for quite some time. The question often asked now is that whether the prevalence rate of tuberculosis has remained the same or decreased or increased. The situation is not known. With the increase in population, better diagnostic facilities, more public awareness more number of cases are being detected. This may create a false impression that the prevalence rate of tuberculosis is on the increase. Fresh surveys are required to be undertaken to determine the prevalence and impact of our control programme on the problem of tuberculosis.

In this connection it is very important to evaluate the change in the infection and prevalence among children as this is a very sensitive index to indicate the way in which wind is blowing. The ecology is changing everywhere. Rapid industrialization, movement of rural population to urban centres, crowding of population in slums, prevalent malnutrition in certain communities, socio-economic status of community are some of the factors that need to be measured for working out tuberculosis indices for different localities to exercise effective control programme. Unfortunately, these factors have not been paid proper attention.

There is no doubt that for our country BCG vaccination is the most effective preventive measure. So far, nearly 125 million persons have been BCG vaccinated by 230 BCG teams working in the country. The cost benefit analysis studies show that investment in BCG vaccination programme is the most economic way of combating tuberculosis and therefore BCG vaccination must be give topmost priority. Everywhere one often hears about drug resistance.

There are frequent reports of drug default. However, no such indices exist for treatment schedules followed for tuberculosis. It is necessary to obtain statistical indices on the problem of drug resistance and its impact on control programme. The problem of drug default and irregularity in treatment has affected NEP control programme seriously at many centres. There is an imminent need to obtain data on this problem and underlying causes behind this phenomenon.

The success of the National Tuberculosis Programme depends upon (*i*) the service provided, and (*ii*) the opinion of the community about ability and capacity of these services to meet their demands which lead to community participation in utilisation of services. Hence, research on the overall health care delivery system of the general health services is essential for providing scientific data to (*a*) modify or evolve the NTP to suit the changing community needs and demands with respect to tuberculosis and (*b*) take corrective actions to improve the National Tuberculosis Programme. Epidemiological, sociological and operational studies which could lead to the formulation of health care programmes that the large proportion of population suffering from tuberculosis could demandare long over due.

Venereal Diseases. Venereal diseases pose a serious threat to country's health. There is no doubt that they are on an increase. There are no exact statistical indices to evaluate the extent of infection. As in other parts of the world the menace is growing as is seen from periodically published reports. At present there are 262 V.D. clinics working throughout the country and 50 more clinics are proposed to be opened shortly. Intensive anti-V.D. programme is also operating in the border areas of U.P. Facilities for training in the modern treatment and control are available at the Training and Demonstration Centre, New Delhi and the Institute of Venereology, Madras (*see* Table 5 on p. 186).

There is a great need for more reliable statistics at state level. In the first place these could establish trends and perhaps later give an indication of incidence.

Other Communicable Diseases. The situation on statistical information on other communicable diseases is worse. There are no reliable data on typhoid, diarrhoeal disease, poliomyelitis and virus infections obtained from different parts of country. We have to rely on data based on hospital or clinical statistics and periodically published survey reports for obtaining data. All statistical indices available relating to these diseases do not provide any assessment of extent and severity of these infections in the Indian community.

AGENCIES RESPONSIBLE FOR COLLECTION OF DATA ON COMMUNICABLE DISEASES

At Rural Level. The responsibility of collecting vital statistics in rural areas has not yet been finally fixed. It has been shifted from person to person *e.g.*, village headman, chowkidar, police sanitary inspector and auxillary health personnel working in the field as supplementary agencies. The end result of these changes is that the collection of vital statistics has still remained defective and unreliable.

Now with the introduction of the village panchayat as the agency for rural administration the work of registration of vital events has been entrusted to the secretary of the village panchayat. The health centre has also been provided with adequate machinery for compilation of vital and health statistics for onward transmission to the Bureau of Health Intelligence at Director General of Health Services Office, New Delhi.

After the establishment of panchayat raj, registration is done by the secretary of the village panchayat who is known as the Registrar of Births and Deaths. Panchayats register births, still births and deaths and their causes. They send copies of the registered events to the taluka development officer at the taluka panchayat office who consolidates the reports village-wise and sends them to the State Bureau of Health and copies to the district health officer and statistical officer at the district panchayat. In borough municipalities and corporations, the chief officer or executive officer is the registrar, and he sends the monthly report directly to the state directorate. The registration of births is compulsory in all states, but it is not strictly enforced.

Notification of epidemic diseases such as cholera, smallpox and plague is compulsory for village panchayat officers such as secretaries of village panchayats. They inform the taluka office who conveys the same by telegram to the collector, district health officer and director of health services, for immediate action. In borough municipalities and corporations it is compulsory on the part of physician to notify attending the case of notifiable disease. It is also compulsory for the head of the family or landlord, who must inform the local health authority. There are prescribed rules and procedures for this. The data obtained through such agencies are usually incomplete and often unreliable for want of correct diagnosis of the disease. Registration and collection is done at the state level from where reports go to the World Health Organisation.

In 1951, the WHO selected six diseases termed as "quarantinable" in any part of the world and decided that they should be reported by the national health authority. These six diseases are smallpox, plague, cholera, typhus fever, yellow fever and replapsing fever. Apart from the obligation to report these six diseases, every country was obliged to include a few other diseases for reporting according to local importance.

The consolidated weekly reports of the six quarantinable diseases in various districts of India are received from every state through telegrams in the Central Bureau of Health Intelligence, New Delhi, within five or six days after the end of the week. The weekly report giving revised figures of incidence are received within about three weeks. Weekly reports showing incidence of quarantinable diseases in different local areas namely districts or sea or airport or cities are prepared in the Central Bureau of Health Intelligence and sent every week to the WHO office, Geneva, within about 10-12 days of the end of the week. These reports are also published in the supplement to the Government of India Gazette for wider circulation.

The weekly epidemiological disease report in every major airport and seaport in the country is, however, sent to the WHO within four or five days. The health authorities in each local area are required to intimate the fresh outbreak of any quarantinable disease in their area to CBHI as soon as fresh outbreak is reported to them and they are also required to report freedom from the disease when the prescribed period of freedom from the infection has elapsed.

Data from Institutional Records. These records include returns from hospitals, health centres, dispensaries and maternity homes. The institutions record all indoor and outdoor cases that come for treatment with diagnosis and result. Monthly returns are filed to Director of Health Services. The data cannot be used to measure morbidity as they do not cover any specified area or population, though they can give a gross picture of disease prevalent in the catchment area of the institution.

Data from Reports of Surveys. Well documented and comprehensive surveys provide many useful data about the health status of the community, status of communicable diseases and the progress made in measures adopted. Epidemiological surveys about malaria incidence, combined with entomological surveys about the vector, breeding places etc. before and after DDT spray give useful data on the epidemiology of malaria. Comprehensive surveys are carried out for the assessment of tuberculosis, filariasis, leprosy and cancer prevalence.

Data from Miscellaneous Sources. Data on causes of death recorded by insurance companies may be useful. Morbidity and mortality data recorded by some of the industrial managements with well developed factory health departments are very useful for assessment of health of worker and occupational hazards.

Other Sources (Published material). Other sources of statistical information are mentioned below. These are published from routine recording such as (*i*) vital statistics, (*ii*) meteorological data (*iii*) sociological and economic data from the Government gazettes and reports of Central Statistical Organisation, National Sample Survey, Bhore Committee, Indian Census, Director Health Services of various states, Director-General of Health Services, Indian Council of Medical Research Reports and Health and Morbidity Surveys.

METHODS OF DATA COLLECTION EMPLOYED IN INDIA

1. Personal interviews for sample surveys or house to house investigations.
2. Data collection through agents and organisations.
3. Data through mailed cards or through questionnaire.
4. Data collection in a well designed programme, the exact nature of which will depend upon the requirements and size of the enquiry and the methods used for laboratories and analysis.
5. Special house to house investigations.

Gaps in data from the point of view of social and economic planning

Defects in notification system. Although a system of notification of communicable diseases has many uses, its main purposes are (*a*) to permit immediate action by the health authorities, (*b*) provide a permanent record and (*c*) plan strategy for control/eradication.

WHO Expert Committee (1968) recommended following improvements in the notification system.

Sampling methods based on particular areas, periods of time, or physicians to provide notification data of better quality than might be obtainable by large scale procedures.

The use of trained paramedical personnel for notification.

Specification of the diagnostic criteria used in deciding whether to report a given case, so that such criteria could be included in statistical reports.

The use of special procedures in defined areas so as to identify the cause of incomplete notification and to develop improved systems of reporting.

Regional studies of comparability, possibly by means of establishing minimum common list of notifiable diseases.

Notification implies the mandatory reporting of certain prescribed diseases whenever they are encountered. Although the primary purpose of notification is not statistical, health statistical agencies have made use of it as a source data. Furthermore, it may be argued that the detection of significant changes in the occurrence of disease is a statistical problem.

Although, notification may be a valuable source of data, the extent to which it can be used as such is limited by a number of inherent disadvantages, the most important of which is the restricted number of diseases that can be made notifiable. There is no agreement between different states about the notifiability of different diseases and as such list of notifiable diseases varies from state to state.

Apart from this notification data are often incomplete and their representativeness is variable and often unknown, for many purposes, this consideration makes notification data unsuitable.

However, despite these disadvantages, it seems clear that for many years notification has successfully fulfilled its primary purpose, in that fluctuations in the level of notification have provided useful indications in the imminence of disease outbreak. For some disease at least, it has provided valid long term data on trends in occurrence. Particularly in India, we have been solely relying on our notification system, however faulty it may be. It has served us well despite its pitfalls. All major outbreaks of communicable diseases have been documented because of our notification.

In combating and assessing trends of incidence of cholera, smallpox and plague our notification system has proved very useful. This has also helped us in demarcating areas of high endemicity for important communicable diseases like cholera, smallpox, plague, poliomyelitis etc.

Unfortunately as mentioned before our notification system is full of many imperfections and many of the reasons for the imperfection are well known. The diagnosis is often open to question, especially, when owing to shortage of doctors, notification is made by non-medical persons and that too by a chowkidar at the village level. The notification procedure may aggravate the inaccuracy of diagnosis, by calling for urgent notification on suspicion of disease so that control measures can be put into the operation. Another factor affecting the accuracy of diagnosis is the availability of facilities for bacteriological, virological or, serological examinations. In many parts of the country, well equipped laboratory facilities are wanting.

The factors making for inaccuracy in notification data may be divided in two main groups (WHO 1965):

Those depending upon the social and environmental conditions of the locality for which prospects for improvement lie in economic and educational developments, and

Those inherent in the notification system which are susceptible of improvement by administrative action within the health services.

The existence of adequate bacteriological and virological facilities in a country can affect notifications in two ways. First by increasing the general level of accuracy of diagnosis and secondly by affecting the numbers of cases of certain diseases brought to light since with some infectious diseases the symptoms are non-specific and the true nature of the disease can be discovered only in the laboratory.

In this respect, it would be worthwhile to recall an attempt that is being made by Maharashtra to set up a network of laboratory services in the state. The pattern proposed is accounted here. There will be a field laboratory attached to the primary health centres. These laboratories will have basic facilities for diagnosis of major tropical diseases and are expected to serve as tributaries of more advance laboratory facility situated at the district level for carrying out important investigations and providing guidelines to the field laboratories.

All district laboratories will be connected to zone – which in turn will be connected to state laboratory or national laboratories like Haffkins Institute, National Institute of Communicable Diseases, Central Drug Research Institute etc. The laboratories at zonal level, apart from participating in research investigations will collaborate with national laboratories in major epidemiological investigations.

A laboratory system of this nature is badly needed today for our country, particularly when country is facing the population explosion and socio economic upheavals. This is particularly so since we are planning up to improve our health care delivery system. Establishment of efficient laboratory system of this nature will not only help to improve documentation of our statistical data on communicable diseases by providing reliable statistics, it will also serve to control communicable diseases and prevent its spread in time.

Other defects in our notification system are as follows: When notification of infectious diseases is compared with deaths from these diseases, many anomalies are found: these are partly from the fact that whereas death registration may be complete or incomplete, notification of infectious diseases is grossly defective. Confusions may also arise from the fact that some diseases for example, tuberculosis, tend to run a protracted course, and that many years may elapse between the time of diagnosis (and notification) and the time of death. The figures for deaths and notifications in any year are likely to refer to different persons.

Regularity of Data

An important factor in the compilation of complete statistics is the regularity of submission of data. In the statistics of infectious diseases periods of high incidence may alternate with long periods during which no cases occur. Such fluctuations have been shown to occur particularly in many communicable diseases like plague, cholera, polyomyelitis. As one glances through the history of plague, one will often notice that periods of pandemics are often interrupted by periods of quiescence.

India has no reported case of plague since 1967. Still this is no matter for complacence. Plague has been shown to remain dormant for years and reappear again even after 30 years or even more. Similar phenomenon has been shown to occur in the case of cholera. Apart from this, in sporadic outbreaks of communicable diseases in non-endemic areas and remote places reporting is irregular. In these areas, no regular data is maintained after the outbreak subsides and no returns are filed.

To be sure that no outbreaks are occurring it is essential to file "nil" reports for local authorities during the periods in which no cases occur. This will help in building up statistics and ensure the control authority that no cases are occurring and help in future planning in the long run.

Epidemic Evaluation: Epidemic is the occurrence of an illness in a community clearly in excess of natural expectation. Frequencies and fluctuations in occurrence of various epidemics of communicable diseases do occur and collection of information of occurrence of epidemics helps in forecasting future outbreaks.

Among the principles of evaluation of epidemics constant vigilance (surveillance) carries extreme significance. Prompt and proper reporting, dissemination of information and collection of information requires sound machinery at all levels of health and connected organisations both at the national and international level. It is only by throwing effective feelers allround that the change in the environment and smouldering of epidemic can be sensed or perceived.

Since it is not possible to arm oneself with accurate morbidity and mortality data for each disease for the whole country, sampling techniques could be employed for investigating outbreaks. Health and morbidity surveys of statistically chosen sections of the population and controlled studies would provide valuable information applicable to the entire community. Long term prospective epidemiology is a useful tool in forecasting epidemic occurrences. Statistician, sociologist, epidemiologist, pathologist, sanitarian and geographist have a large part to play in a successful epidemic evaluation study. Epidemic evaluation study is the need of the day. Unless this is done future strategy will suffer for want of improvement.

Adequate number of health statisticians: Acute shortage of adequate number of trained health statisticians is one of the major causes of gaps in the statistical system employed for communicable diseases. In advanced countries health statistician: doctor ratio has been shown to be 1:400. On the other hand the ratio in India is observed to be 1:1381. Unless the situation improves, it is very difficult to build up a sound statistical base.

To sum up, statistics on communicable diseases suffers from serious inadequacies. Reporting system for communicable diseases is faulty. There is no correlation between various statistical indices. *i.e.* mortality rate, morbidity rate. Various statistical indices with respect to communicable diseases need to be evaluated in relation to growing population, environmental changes, socio-economic infrastructure and meteorological conditions. Data retrieval system is very poor. Processing of statistical data at the central level involves considerable delays. On many occasions publications of reports are delayed to such an extent that they lose their significance.

The position on statistics on communicable diseases will improve only when the responsibility at the village level is entrusted to basic health worker. Today, we have projects for controlling several communicable diseases. The one employed for the control and eradication of malaria would offer the ideal system for obtaining statistical data on malaria, other communicable diseases, and for obtaining all statistical data. Integration of various schemes like National Malaria Eradication Programme, National Filaria Control Programme National Tuberculosis Control Programme, National Leprosy Control Programme, would serve to make us more basic health workers available. It would also help to allot one basic worker to the population of 5,000-10,000.

At this stage, it would be worthwhile to project the concept of Multi-purpose Health Workers tailored to suit the needs of Indian Society. The worker in question should be provided adequate training to meet basic health needs of rural community. Further, he should be provided adequate education in collecting and processing statistical data relating to health problems.

The basic worker should be entrusted to prepare folders on every family in his jurisdiction and collect data by paying a visit once in two weeks. He should register all statistical information including vital statistics for the population covered by him. The basic health worker should be answerable to the medical officer, primary health centre. Further it should be made compulsory for all medical practitioners, paramedics, village officers and head of the family to report notifiable diseases to the medical officer incharge primary health centre or to panchayat officer.

The medical officer-in-charge, primary health centre should be responsible for receiving and compiling all morbidity data on notifiable diseases, and he should prepare returns simply with other illness for regular submission to the bureau. His staff should be authorised to verify correctness.

Every effort should be made to expedite the data to centralised agency and proper feed-back of the processed data should be ensured for timely evaluation of the progress.

The new questions that health administrators have been asking are not just concerned with the quantity and population distribution of disease, the determinants and therefore preventability of diseases and curative services, or even the costs of health services; these matters have been of interest to those responsible for health planning. The health administrators were concerned with relevance of information to forward planning; with the comparison in terms of cost effectiveness of optional strategies to combat predicted pressures in the future, and with the relationship between health services planning and other sectors of social and economic planning especially with other aspects of social policy.

More specifically, for the statistician the problem is that of predicting the trend of health indicators in the future in such a way that they can be translated into demand for action; and of predicting the cost and benefits of action. Within the information system to meet these problems there are a number of syb-systems.

Health indicators embrace not only more comprehensive measure of morbidity or of anthropometric and physiological characteristics of the population but also measure of those social and economic characteristics that are the determinants of levels of morbidity (WHO 1974). Much more needs to be known, too of the activity surrounding patients in health service facilities. Activity analysis, the measurement of reasources, utilisation in relation to prophylactic procedures, provides a whole new field of statistical units of activity.

On the economic side, there is a need to study the satisfaction or dissatisfaction and indeed the motivation of those who use health services and those who do not use them.

There would have to be a determined move towards a statistical system that would meet modern needs. Such a system would have to conform to a logical design, however gradually approached. It must be planned. This design would have to be related to the objectives of health services. Components of a health information system should include:

Indicators of state of the population (morbidity or mortality data, psychological or physiological parameters, the outcome of specific preventive or treatment measures);

Measures of the utilisation of services of various kinds;

Statistics of resources available to support this utilisation, especially manpower;

Financial statistics (costs, expenditure related to particular objectives);

Demographic, social and environmental data.

With the training and motivation of basic health worker and involvement of the population to whom the benefit will accrue it will be possible for us to obtain sound data of this nature. Needless to say that only extensive data of this nature, specified above would prove valuable from the point of view of social and economic planning.

References

BASU, R.N., (1976) Evolution of smallpox eradication programme in India, Ind. Jour. Pub. Health 20:51, 1976.

CENTRAL BUREAU OF HEALTH INTELLIGENCE. Pocket Book of Health Statistics, Central Bureau of Health Intelligence, Director General of Health Services, Government of India, New Delhi, 1973.

GOVT. OF INDIA, Report of the Health Survey and Development Committee (Bhore Committee, 1946) Planning Commission, New Delhi, 1946.

GOVT. OF INDIA, Report of the Health Survey and Planning Committee (Mudaliar Committee, 1961) Planning, Commission, New Delhi, 1952.

GOVT. OF INDIA, National Leprosy Control Programme of the Government of India—Report for the period from April to December 1974, Leprosy in India 48:183, 1976.

MAITRA, S.S., Workshop on promotion of leprosy, work in India. Leprosy in India 48:61, 1976.

MITTAL, M.C., Vaidya, N.K., and Joshi, R.V., Defaults in Collection of Vital Statistics in a Rural area in Indore, Ind. Jour. Pub. Hlth. 11:58, 1967.

PANDIT, C.G., Assessment of the National Filaria Control Programme, India 1961-1970, Indian Council of Med. Res. Tech. Rep. Ser. 10, 1971.

RAO, N.S.N. AND MARWAH, S.M., A Health Statistical Unit for a Township with. Illustrations from Benaras Hindu University Campus, Ind. Jour. Pub. Hlth. 15:77.

SEN, M., Editorial:Health Statistics, Ind. Jour. Pub. Hlth. 10:113, 1966.

SENGUPTA, S.K. AND KAPUR P.N., Principal causes of Death in India, Jour. Com-Dis: 4:40, 1972.

SHARMA, M.I.D., Problem of Filarasis, Jour. Com. Dis. 8:95, 1976.

WORLD HEALTH ORGANIZATION, Trends in the study of Morbidity and Mortality, Pub. Hlth Papers 27:9, 1965.

——Morbidity Statistics, Twelfth Report of the WHO Expert Committee on Health Statistics, Wld. Hlth. Org. Tech. Rep. Ser. 389, 1968.

——New Approaches in Health Statistics, Report of the Second International Conference of National Committees on Vital and Health Statistics, Wld. Hlth. Org. Tech. Rep. Ser., 1974.

APPENDIX

TABLE 1—*Percentage contribution to total mortality/morbidity by major groups of causes (according to WHO International Classification of Diseases, 1955)*

Major group	*Mortality*		*Morbidity*	
	Institutional deaths	*Medically certified deaths*	*Inpatients*	*CD* block surveyed*
Class	(*1961-4*)	(*1962-4*)	(*1962-4*)	(*1955-8*)
Infective and parasitic diseases	27.81	14.42	18.10	20.88
Neoplasms	2.96	4.20	1.54	0.21
Allergic, endocrine, metabolic, and nutritional diseases and diseases of blood-forming organs	7.84	8.65	6.99	3.37
Mental, psychoneurotic and personality disorders	0.41	0.11	0.59	0.17
Diseases of the nervous system and sense organs	3.73	4.67	7.37	6.69
Diseases of circulatory system	7.20	9.27	2.43	0.77
Diseases of respiratory system	6.58	13.27	8.95	36.07
Diseases of digestive system	12.91	9.24	10.05	8.60
Diseases of genitourinary system	2.98	1.08	6.73	0.60
Deliveries and complications of pregnancy, childbirth, and the puerperium	4.56	0.85	16.44	0.59
Diseases of skin, cellular tissue, bones and organs of movement	1.25	0.83	4.46	8.44
Congenital malformations	0.65	0.73	0.43	0.02
Certain diseases of early infancy	6.63	13.84	8.42	0.24
Sympotoms, senility, and ill-defined conditions	2.76	12.91	1.96	22.18
Accidents, poisoning, and violence	11.73	6.83	10.54	1.17
All diseases	100.00	100.00	100.00	100.00

*CD=community development.

TABLE 2—*Notified Cholera Cases and Deaths (1969-1972)*

	1969		*1970*		*1971*		*1972*	
	C	*D*	*C*	*D*	*C*	*D*	*C*	*D*
1	*2*	*3*	*4*	*5*	*6*	*7*	*8*	*9*
Andhra Pradesh	640	151	527	38	581	47	821	109
Assam	486	217	348	69	250	66	—	—
Bihar	4,416	1,296	3,973	1,191	10,086	2,585	4,723	1,289
Gujarat	151	28	326	29	468	44	424	19
Haryana	58	18	—	—	8	—	78	4
Himachal Pradesh	—	—	—	—	—	—	—	—
Jammu & Kashmir	—	—	—	—	—	—	—	—
Kerala	186	26	37	6	—	—	—	1
Madhya Pradesh	67	6	2,341	507	320	82	5,834	627
Maharashtra	4,689	750	2,759	267	1,093	192	2,545	201
Mysore	693	170	601	125	305	45	414	58
Meghalaya	—	—	—	—	—	—	—	—
Manipur	—	—	—	—	—	—	—	—
Nagaland	—	—	—	—	—	—	—	—
Orissa	238	80	1,170	291	16	4	361	42
Punjab	4	—	11	4	4	—	—	—
Rajasthan	42	7	—	—	1	—	337	18
Tamil Nadu	5,460	634	1,414	377	2,469	173	3,674	205
Tripura	—	—	3	—	—	—	—	—
Uttar Pradesh	676	201	1,430	482	420	90	383	110
West Bengal	1,153	164	2,257	514	927	259	1,414	208
UNION TERRITORIES								
A. & N. Islands	—	—	—	—	—	—	—	—
Arunachal Pradesh	—	—	—	—	—	—	—	—
Chandigarh	—	—	—	—	—	—	—	—
D. & N. Haveli	—	—	—	—	—	—	—	—
Delhi	314	9	63	1	192	8	315	16
Goa, Daman and Diu	—	—	—	—	—	—	1	1
L. M. & A. Islands	—	—	—	—	—	—	—	—

1	2	3	4	5	6	7	8	9
Mizoram	—	—	—	—	—	—	—	—
Pondicherry	7	—	8	—	—	—	11	—
INDIA (Total)	19,280	3,757	17,268	3,801	17,140	3,595	21,331	2,908

C=Cases
D=Deaths
—=Nil

TABLE 3—*Attacks and Deaths due to Smallpox in India since 1950*

		Cases	*Deaths*
Pre N.S.E.P.	1950	157,487	41,201
	1951	253,332	54,580
	1952	74,836	17,116
	1953	37,311	9,072
	1954	46,619	11,375
	1955	41,887	8,598
	1956	45,109	10,931
	1957	78,666	23,150
	1958	168,216	45,848
	1959	47,693	12,183
	1960	31,091	7,903
	1961	45,380	12,480
N.S.E.P.	1962	55,595	15,084
	1963	83,423	26,360
	1964	40,256	11,831
	1965	33,402	9,058
	1966	32,616	8,482
National Assessment	1967	83,943	26,225
	1968	30,295	7,266
	1969	19,139	4,156
	1970	12,341	2,240
	1971	16,166	2,706
	1972	27,407	5,457
Intensive Campaign	1973	88,110	15,404
	1974	188,003	31,262
	1975	1,436	176

TABLE 4—*National T.B. Control Programme as on 12.1.1973*

	No. of T.B. De-monsteration Centres	*No. of T.B. Clinics*	*No. of Distt. VBCs under-taking Distt. VB Pro-gramme*	*No. of Beds available*	*No. of Persons Tuberculin-tested*	*No. of B.C.G. Vaccinated*
1	*2*	*3*	*4*	*5*	*6*	*7*
Andhra Pradesh	1	40	20	3281	12260	769423
Assam	1	15	8	1021	—	189210
Bihar	2	33	7	1173	3616	426378
Gujarat	1	24	17	2124	16284	632247
Haryana	—	8	7	211	179	370687
Himachal Pradesh	—	8	6	1174	—	89516
Jammu & Kashmir	1	13	9	600	5161	135964
Kerala	1	21	10	1936	29286	720479
Madhya Pradesh	1	42	28	1506	7144	827619
Maharashtra	1	32	20	5805	—	673551
Meghalya	—	—	—	—	+	+
Mysore	1	24	17	2558	5605	950783
Nagaland	—	2	—	125	—	29561
Orissa	1	15	12	691	17939	332857
Punjab	1	12	9	979	17373	176735
Rajasthan	1	25	26	1615	—	337088
Tamil Nadu	1	40	14	3358	69825	562794
Tripura	—	1	1	50	—	22294
Uttar Pradesh	1	77	40	2380	75298	1360348
West Bengal	1	98	15	5179	26469	1041285
UNION TERRITORIES						
A. & N. Islands	—	—	—	65	—	768
Arunachal Pradesh	—	—	—	—	—	6508
Chandigarh	—	1	—	—	+	+
Delhi	1	10	1	1462	75548	82906
Goa, Daman & Diu	—	1	1	251	—	42402
Mizoram	+	+	+	+	+	+
Pondicherry	—	1	1	120	10105	335592
D. & N. Haveli	+	+	+	+	—	284
Total	17	547*	270	37754	372092	9836515

*Includes 270 District TB Centres.

TABLE 5—*Number of V.D. cases seen and treated in the V.D. Clinics during 1960-1971*

	1968	*1969*	*1970*	*1971*
Andhra Pradesh	1,82,543	56,592	47,382	1,40,031
Bihar	3,612	4,702	11,215	17,346
Gujarat	1,607	679	347	252
Jammu & Kashmir	3,144	2,323	2,315	1,606
Kerala	14,102	16,409	10,094	7,483
Madhya Pradesh	5,042	5,505	1,037	10,333
Maharashtra	42,818	36,857	23,804	12,593
Mysore	3,111	4,733	4,008	2,923
Orissa	8,609	8,263	10,428	9,571
Himachal Pradesh	2,991	2,955	1,862	2,427
Tamil Nadu	19,958	25,761	9,976	9,169
Uttar Pradesh	8,721	3,423	2,408	8,113
West Bengal	25,151	32,143	34,593	28,624
UNION TERRITORIES				
A. & N. Islands	101	158	658	670
Delhi	24,584	21,781	18,771	20,871
Goa, Daman & Diu	1,481	1,591	1,105	1,287
Manipur	4,108	4,697	4,359	3,695
Pondicherry	—	6,295	7,767	10,267
Arunachal Pradesh (NEFA)	194	105	1,120	672
Tripura	8,291	7,561	10,686	5,235
Association for Moral and Social Hygiene	34,545	34,429	14,617	24,918
Total	3,94,683	2,76,962	2,18,552	3,17,986

Mental Health Statistics in India

R. L. KAPUR*

It is appropriate that till recently health planners in India have devoted their attention to combating killing diseases. Now, however, when we are in the process of gaining victory over these major scourges, it is time that resources are deployed against illnesses which may not kill but which, by crippling the human potential, disrupt and inhibit the social and economic growth of the country. Foremost among these is, perhaps, mental disorder. No one needs to be made aware of the severe anguish which mental disorder produces in the individual suffering from it and among his family. It is often forgotten, however, that by disrupting the social milieu, mental disorder prevents the whole community to which the patient belongs, from contributing its optimum to the society.

There is sufficient evidence that the nation is now preparing itself to meet the challenge of mental disorder. Ever since the All-India Institute of Mental Health came into being in 1954, a number of medical institutions have started offering higher qualifications to the medical graduates in the discipline of psychiatry. There has been a corresponding growth in the allied disciplines of clinical psychology, psychiatric social work and psychiatric nursing, though perhaps not as fast. More and more medical institutions and general hospitals have started attaining psychiatric beds and recruiting psychiatric teams to their staff. There is greater consciousness amongst the public at large that mental disorders are treatable and some of them even preventable. It would not however be wrong to say that most of this growth and awareness has been on ad-hoc rather than planned basis.

It is axiomatic that for proper planning against any disease those concerned with it should have the following information at their disposal:

*National Institute of Mental Health and Neuro-Sciences, Bangalore.

1. Its prevalence in the population.
2. Its incidence *i.e.* the rate of fresh cases occurring in a given period.
3. Information about the risk promoting factors and the high-risk groups.
4. Information on whether the incidence of disease is increasing or decreasing with passage of time as well as the reasons for this increase or decrease.
5. The "degree" of personal, social and economic morbidity caused by the illness in comparison with other illnesses which also require attention.
6. The degree of need (for help) experienced by the individual and those around him.
7. Agencies and facilities already available in the community for providing help.
8. Various methods of treatment and prevention.
9. The cost of the various treatment and prevention manoeuvres in relation to the benefits which could be derived from them.
10. The available resources for deployment against the illness.

Very little reliable and valid information is available regarding what has been mentioned above. This is not to say that statistics are not being collected; attempts are being made to assemble information regarding at least some of the items enumerated above. The fact however is that there are a variety of methodological obstacles which detract greatly from the quality of information obtained.

Methodological Problems of Mental Health Statistics

The foremost methodological problem is that of an absence of any absolute standard criteria for defining a psychiatric 'case'. There is no germ which can be demonstrated under a microscope nor are there any precise laboratory investigations which would distinguish a person suffering from mental disorder from one who is not. Definition of mental disorder is basically a question of value judgement; a psychiatric symptom being simply a mental state which is perceived as odd, distressful or harmful by the person suffering from it, or by those around him, or both. It is from these value judgements that the clinician derives his criteria of assessment and so crude is this method that different experts frequently differ about their decisions. Not only do the differences exist in defining a person normal or abnormal but once the decision about abnormality has been taken, clinicians differ about the diagnostic category to which the patient might belong. The diagnostic categories are based not on aetiology (which is usually multi-factorial) but on symptomatology, there being a substantial overlap, in the symptom content of various psychiatric syndromes.

A few examples will illustrate the points made above. Different surveys of prevalence of mental disorder using clinical assessment as the criterion for diagnosing a case, carried out in very similar populations produced case rates of mental disorder varying from 16.7 to 333 per 1,000 (Lin and Stanlley, 1962).

Kreitman *et al* (1961) showed that a pair of psychiatrists reached agreement on diagnostic category in only 65 per cent of cases.

In a study where 538 female patients were admitted to three different wards of the same hospital at random, the diagnosis of schizophrenia was given to 68 per cent, 29 per cent and 22 per cent of the patients admitted to the three wards respectively (Pasamanick, 1959).

One easy way out would be to operationally define as a psychiatric 'case' any one who has attended the facility of a psychiatric hospital (outpatient or inpatient). Hospital statistics, however, do not reflect the real case rate because they depend on the facilities available and the willingness of the people to make use of them. This is especially true of hospital statistics of mental disorder in the Indian setting, since hospital facilities are severely inadequate compared to the need. Even where facilities are available, people, conditioned by their beliefs about the causation of mental abnormality, often consult astrologers, mandarines or priest rather than go to a hospital. Some needy patients are deterred from going to a mental hospital because of the stigma attached to the latter or because of the distance or the expenses involved.

It is apparent, therefore, that if the true prevalence data are to be obtained they must be got through a population survey. The question of course is how to construct criteria which would make a population survey both reliable and valid.

Disappointed by the pitfalls of the clinical assessment approach, some workers have employed standard questionnaires and trained the investigators to use them similarly. A questionnaire, however, has several shortcomings. Its range of inquiry is limited by the number of questions. It is rigid and prevents the informal cross-examination which might be necessary to evaluate the subject's response. The answers are often dependent on the subject's response set. These shortcomings often make a questionnaire lose in validity what it gains in reliability.

A compromise between a clinical approach and a questionnaire approach is the structured interview schedule. This is similar to a questionnaire in providing a standard check list of symptoms and of questions designed to elicit these symptoms, but differs from the latter in that a cross-examination is permitted to clarify doubts and in that the decision about the prevalence or absence of psycho-pathology is made by the investigator, guided by a standard definition for various symptoms. The structured interview schedules retain the flexibility of a clinical approach but is more reliable because of the use of standard questions and definitions.

It must be realized that both a questionnaire and a structured interview schedule, reliable as they are, do nothing more than ascertain the presence or absence of psychiatric symptoms, and symptoms on their own do not make a person a psychiatric case if by 'case' we mean someone who needs help and treatment. Surveys designed to ascertain the prevalence of symptoms have often shown more than half the population to be manifesting some sort of psychological disturbance. It is difficult to accept, however, that more than half the population is in need of psychiatric help. To determine this need it is necessary to measure certain other parameters besides the presence of psychiatric symptoms.

'Need for help' is not a unitary concept. It may be felt by the individual, his family, his neighbours or by the society at large. The person himself, those around him and the society may agree or disagree about the presence and degree of need. Healers, priests and law enforcers in a given community may view the need differently from each other and from those who complain.

Need is related to, but not the same thing as, demand. The demand for psychiatric help may be suppressed because of fear, shame, ignorance or a sense of hopelessness. On the other hand there may be an over-demand because of propaganda or fashion, as one suspects has been the case in certain strata of society in the U.S.A.

Need is related to, but not the same thing as, morbidity if by the latter term we mean a clinically recognizable pathology. A clinical abnormality may not require help if it is not sufficiently distressful or does not interfere with day-to-day functioning. On the other hand, a person may be extremely distressed even though his condition does not fall into any of the diagnostic categories recognised in current clinical jargon.

In the medical model this problem of the subjective element in recognition of need is side-stepped through the use of the concept of a "clinically defined need" which is assumed to be present wherever a clinically recognizable "disease entity" is identified. Inherent in this assumption is the belief that the person who has the disease needs help and that if he does not himself experience this need now, he will do so in future. These diseases are entities recognized by standard signs and symptoms and often confirmed through laboratory tests.

Unfortunately the disease concept can be applied to only a few of the conditions considered to be in the realm of a psychiatrist. Most psychiatric symptoms fail to coalesce into indisputable syndromes with a predictable progress. Under these circumstances one has to fall back on the first order value judgements concerning the person's need for treatment, about which there may or may not be agreement between the individual, his family, the doctor, the priest, the law enforcer and the society at large. Whose value judgement should be accepted? What criterion is the most appropriate for measuring psychiatric need?

A number of prevalence surveys have been carried out in India but because of the difference in criteria the disparity is so much that the results of these costly surveys can do nothing but confound the health planners. The disparity will be obvious from the figures given in Table I.

TABLE 1—*Psychiatric 'case' rates in different Indian Population Surveys*

	Place	*rate/1000*
Surya *et al* (1964)	Pondicherry	9.5
Dube K.C. (1970)	Agra	18.0
Elnagar *et al* (1971)	Bengal	27.0
Sethi *et al* (1972)	Lucknow	72.7
Nandi *et al* (1975)	Bengal	102.8

What is the answer to this dilemma? Should we forego prevalence studies and resort to ad-hocism? Certainly not. Attempts are being made in India and internationally to develop techniques for studying mental morbidity in a standardised manner. In the Indian setting Carstairs and Kapur (1976) carried out a population survey using a structured interview schedule developed in India. Indian Psychiatric Survey Schedule (Kapur *et al*, 1974) had also made attempts to assess the degree of need in a standardised manner. The authors do not claim that their criteria are unique but only that they are explicit.

ICMR has now launched a project to first of all translate and standardise Indian psychiatric survey schedule in different Indian languages and then carry out a mental morbidity survey on similar lines in four centres: Bangalore, Delhi, Ranchi and Goa. The study will also endeavour to examine the question of risk factors, risk groups, degree of personal, social and economic morbidity caused by the psychiatric illness. One hopes that this attempt at standardising the techniques of measurement will provide the necessary information to the health planners.

The Problem of Classification

A problem closely related to that of case definition is the one of classification. As mentioned earlier the classification of psychiatric illness is based on symptoms and the boundaries of syndromes are not very clear. In fact, the boundaries become more and more hazy as one moves away from the cultures in which these syndromes were formulated. I have already alluded to the studies of Kreitman and Pasamanick who found such disparity in diagnosing a syndrome in the same setting. The differences are likely to be huge when patients from two different cultures are compared (Cooper, *et al* 1972).

We are still far from understanding the aetiology of mental illness and shall for a long time depend on 'symptoms' for classification. WHO is now doing a heroic job by clarifying the concepts underlying the different diagnostic categories. In the international classification of disease, Vol. 8, the psychiatric section gives an exhaustive glossary. Recently WHO has completed an international pilot project on Schizophrenia with the aim of clarifying the core concept of this illness across different cultures. They are now doing a similar project on the other inpatient psychiatric syndrome of Depression. These are commendable efforts.

From another direction workers are utilising techniques of cluster analysis and numerical taxonomy to permit an "objective" classification (Meguire, 1973). These methods must be pursued vigorously as they permit delineation of syndromes which may not yet exist in the current terminology.

THE IMPORTANCE OF INCIDENCE STUDIES

No incidence study has yet been carried out in India. We have no idea of the number of fresh cases which comes up in a given time. The frequently asked question whether the growth of industrialisation and urbanisation is leading to increase in mental stress and hence mental disorder, cannot be answered unless incidence studies are launched. Even the questions of risk factors and risk groups can best be answered by undertaking incidence studies and not through prevalence studies. One hopes that with the standardisation of techniques for determining cases in the population, incidence studies will soon follow .

STUDIES OF EXISTING FACILITIES AND EVALUATION OF SERVICES OFFERED

The Directorates of Health Services in various states and the Directorate-General of Health Services in Delhi do collect some information on the hospitals and clinics offering services to the mentally ill, but they can reach only a fraction of agencies providing care for the mentally disturbed in the country. Many mentally ill go to general practitioners presenting somatic symptoms or to social welfare agencies presenting social problems. A large majority utilises the help of traditional healers. It is commonly stated that there are no psychiatric facilities in the rural parts of India.

This should not be interpreted to mean that the mental patients in rural India do not get any help at all. In a recent study (Kapur, 1975) it was discovered that more than half of the patients who had been found to have psychiatric symptoms in an exhaustive population survey, had already visited one or other of the local agencies for help (Mantrawadi, Ayurvedic healer, temple priest, etc.) and all those with severe psychiatric disturbance had attended one of these traditional healers.

It is true that we have not evaluated the benefit the patients derived from these agencies but then for that matter we are still not clear about the benefits derived from the methods of treatment in modern psychiatry. As mentioned earlier the health planners will require information on agencies offering mental health care as well as the cost-benefit analysis of the help given. This lacuna has yet to be filled up.

Hospital Statistics

In earlier sections, I have criticised the relevance of hospital statistics to understand the prevalence of psychiatric disorder and psychiatric need in the country. This does not mean that hospital statistics are not useful. Kramer (1969) has written a splendid monograph on the method of collecting hospital statistics and their advantages. It is not possible to better his monograph and I shall only try to summarise some of the salient points.

Each inpatient facility should maintain separate records foı first admissions, conduct at least once a year census on the resident population and also keep a record on the movement of patients. The diagnosis should be based on the latest ICD manual (the 8th version of which has been referred to earlier). The method of collecting information should be standardised for all the facilities in the country.

Information required on the inpatient records

1. Identification number of patient within the facility
2. Patient's name (for married women, also maiden name)
3. Patient's address
4. Date of birth
5. Sex
6. Date of admission
7. Legal category of admission
8. Referral source
9. Education
10. Occupation
11. Marital status
12. Admission diagnosis
13. Places and dates of prior psychiatric treatment.

    Other items, usually recorded at the time of separation, are:

14. Date of separation
15. Whether patient was alive or dead
16. Final psychiatric diagnosis
17. Recommendations for further care

The first admission data can be compared over the years to examine the trend of admissions. For example, in the western countries, the old age group is increasing forming a higher population of the total admissions. This has led the health planner to provide for more geriatric homes. Another use of the first admission data is to illustrate situations where primary prevention has failed. Admission of persons with meningoencephalic syphylis, poisons, drugs, dietary deficiencies and brain trauma are cases of mental disorder which could have been prevented.

Another benefit of first admission data, which has not been clearly tackled by Kramer but which is very important in the Indian context, is the study (through comparison with population prevalence figures) of the socio-cultural indices which favour admission. With a similar clinical condition what are the socio-economic and cultural characteristics who get admitted. This will give us information about groups who need special education regarding the need for hospital treatment where indicated.

The analysis of resident patients gives an idea of long term disability and serves as a starting point for measures to prevent chronicity. It is evident in India that there is a wide variation in the relative proportion of long duration patients in the various hospitals. Changes in chronicity figures will show the advances a particular hospital is making.

It is being increasingly noticed that some hospitals, anxious to reduce chronicity, are discharging patients before they are ready for discharge. This leads to repeat admission soon afterwards and what has now come to be called the "revolving door" policy. Data derived from cohort studies (movement data) of patients admitted to hospitals can provide baseline information regarding the impact of programmes designed to increase the rate of return of patients to community and to maintain them in community.

Kramer recommends the maintenance of outpatient records which should include information on number of interviews carried out with the patients and relatives. Below is the list of items information on which must be collected by all agencies.

Information required in outpatient records

1. Age
2. Sex
3. Marital status
4. Source of referral
5. Residence
6. Type of admissions to the clinic (new, readmission)
7. Type of service rendered
   (*a*) Diagnostic study only

(*b*) Diagnostic study and treatment
(*c*) Psychological testing only, etc.

8. Number of interviews with patient, relations, guardian, etc.
9. Presenting problem
10. Admission diagnosis
11. Discharge diagnosis
12. Dates of admission to and discharge from the clinic
13. Follow-up services recommended

Comparative data on outpatients and inpatients can be useful in detecting imbalances that may exist in the provision of services. OPD record can be used to study trends of admission to outpatients specific for age, sex, diagnosis etc. Cohorts of admission can also be utilised to determine the probability of not receiving final interview within defined period following admission. Outpatient data can be very useful for follow-up studies (natural history of illness).

Psychiatric case register: The new community health programmes emphasise the need to integrate and co-ordinate inpatient, outpatient and intermediate services. Such programmes would necessitate integrated data on different facilities, their relative usage and pattern of patient flow from one facility to another. Psychiatric case registers which link up the records of a patient on the moves from one facility to another are being employed in some countries.

While the case register concept is excellent it will be soon time before it can be used in our country. The facilities are few and it is difficult as yet to guarantee the degree of communication between different facilities.

Kramer recommends a central agency which should collect the information from various outpatient and inpatient services, analyse it and feed it back to the agencies. The automatic feedback is essential because it is for the use of these agencies.

In India at present the D.G.H.S. collects all such information from various agencies. The information is, however, likely to be faulty for the following reasons:

*Poor keeping of inpatient and outpatient records because of lack of adequate staff and facilities.
*Non-utilization of ICD codes.
*Lack of clear cut instructions about how to collect data.
*Lack of feedback.

Much more organization input is needed before such information as collected by D.G.H.S. can be useful.

Summary and Recommendations

In the preceding pages I have highlighted the necessity as well as difficulties of maintaining useful mental health statistics. Some recommendations are outlined below:

1. There should be a central agency for collecting mental health statistics. The special problems of collecting the mental health statistics have been outlined above. These problems necessitate that the persons manning the agency should have special orientation in mental health problems. For this reason it would be ideal if the agency for collecting mental health statistics should be separate from that collecting information about other illnesses. It may still be housed in the D.G.H.S. It may be housed in a research oriented institution like the National Institute of Mental Health and Neuro-Sciences, Bangalore.

2. The central agency should make a survey of all facilities available for psychiatric help in the country. There should be a central directory of these facilities.

3. Inpatient and outpatient records on the given model should be maintained at all facilities. The central agency by sending manuals of instructions or even their officers to these facilities, should teach the facilities about how to maintain these records.

4. As far as possible, at least in bigger institutions there should be a separate psychiatric records office.

5. The analysis carried out by the central agency should be fed back automatically to the various facilities. A return on their endeavour will inspire them to take interest in their work.

6. Attempts should continue to be made on improvements in case definition, classification and tools for collecting information should continue.

7. Prevalence and incidence surveys using similar methodology and with specific issues in mind (e.g. impact of social change, economic dysfunction caused by mental illness etc.) should be carried out.

8. Cost-benefit analysis on various treatment and preventive manoeuvres should be conducted. This research will depend a lot on good statistical information.

References

LIN, T.Y. and STANDLEY, C.C., "The Scope of Epidemiology in Psychiatry", WHO public health paper: 16 November, 1962.

KREITMAN, N., SAINSBURY, P., MORRISSEY, J., TOWERS, J., and SCRIVENER, J., "The Reliability of Psychiatric Assessment: an Analysis," *J. Ment. Sci.*, p 107, 887, 1961.

PASAMANICK, B., DINITZ, S., and LEFTON, M., "Psychiatric Orientation and its Relation to Diagnosis and Treatment in a Mental Hospital," *Amer. J. Psychiat.*, p. 116, 127-132, 1959.

ELNAGAR, M.M., MAITRA, P., and RAO, M.M., "Mental Health in Indian Rural Community," *Brit. J. Psych.*, p. 118, 499-503, 1971.

DUBE, K.C., "A Study of Prevalence and Bio-social Variables in Mental Illness in a Rural and an Urban Community of Uttar Pradesh, India. *Acta. Psy. Scand.*, p. 46, 327, 1970.

NANDI, D.N., AGMANY, S., GANGULY, H., BANNERJEE, G., BORAL, G.C., GHOSH, A., and SARKAR, S., *Ind. J. Psych.*, p. 17, 87, 1975.

SETHI, B.B., GUPTA, S.C., Rajkumar, Promilla Kumari, "A Psychiatric Survey of 500 Rural families," *Ind. J. Psych.* p. 14, 183, 1972.

SURYA, N.C., DATTA, S.P., GOPALKRISHNA, R., SUNDERAM, D., and KUTTY, J., *Transactions of All India Institute of Mental Health*, p 50, 1964.

CARSTAIRS, G.M., and KAPUR, R.L., *The Great Universe of Kota*: Stress, Change and Mental Disorder in an Indian Village, London. Hogarth, 1976.

KAPUR, R.L., KAPUR, M., and CARSTAIRS, G.M., Indian Psychiatric Survey Schedule (IPSS), *Second Psychiatry*, p 9, 71-76, 1974.

COOPER, J.E., KENDALL, R.E., GURLAND, B.J., SHARPE, L., COPELAND, J.R.M. and SIMON, R., *Psychiatric Diagnosis in New York and London*, London, Oxford University Press, Maudsley Monograph No. 20, 1972.

MEGUIRE, R., Classification and the problem of diagnosis, *Handbook of Abnormal Psychology*, edited by H.J. Eysenck, Pitman Medical and Sons, Ltd., pp. 3-33, 1973.

KAPUR, R.L., "Mental Health Care in Rural India: A Study of Existing Patterns and Their Implications for Future Policy," *Brit. J. Psychiat.*, pp. 127, 286-93, 1975.

Community Health Survey

B.C. DAS*

The purpose of surveys is to forecast and allocate meagre resource in a planned way. Survey forecast is not what will actually happen, but what would happen in the existing trend of morbidity (chronic and acute infections) and environment deterioration through mortality may affect individuals, family and community at various stages of life be continued. The future development for health care must be planned on health survey basis on human health needs.

In this direction efforts must be concentrated on the prevention of waste. So long the treatment of sick was considered the primary purpose of medicine and henceforth medical care should be geared to for the promotion of health, prevention of illness, increased longivity, restoration of sick and rehabilitation. Health care cannot be taken for granted. It must be maintained and promoted through incessant activities—general education and health education represent the starting point of all health activities. Further, health is simply not the absence of disease. It is a positive, a joyful attitude towards life and cheerful acceptance of the responsibilities that life may put upon the individual.

The goal of family planning is to control the size of the family through conception control (by abortion, oral contraception, I.U.D. condoms, rhythm) and other chemical and biological methods and population control through abortion, other fertility control (social and biological control) and balancing fertility and mortality etc. A great number of health problems are associated with excess of fertility and increasing family size. Other problems are associated with increased fetal, neonatal and post-neonatal mortality rates, increased maternal mortality and incidence of infectious diseases among parents

*Biometry Research Unit, Indian Statistical Institute, Calcutta.

and children and poorer growth among pre-school and school children. Community medical care should include these in their planning of medical services and try to alleviate them in their stride.

However, many questions may not be answered adequately at the present time by conducting health surveys alone because we have not ascertained full facts yet nor have consequences been fully evaluated. The health of any population depends upon genetics, population composition, distribution and environmental factor and proper medical attention. The major implication of a large population on health is related to the impact of numbers on environment.

The demographic analysis community-wise would be of great help in planning medical services because costliest medical care is needed by the senior members of the community. Under this type of survey, it was possible to compute the total tax revenue production capacity of the population under different age structure conditions, so that data collection on each age basis is imperative and relevant no doubt.

As the fertility declines, the proportion of older people increases at the community level at the cost of younger group (moves towards to type 3), so that the community health needs and attention must be focused on senior members. By need based preventive medical care, it would be possible to postpone the onset of many diseases, then it would free resources in terms of medical care, skills, buildings, equipment at present tied down because of inefficient use of them in patching up ailing patients. Besides cost effectiveness through pension and retirement policies, productivity and leisure are considerable.

It frequently happens that many of the parameters that have relevance to a problem are not amenable to measurements or quantification. Although their relative values may be high but neglected in statistical analysis, interaction analysis (or morphological analysis), this problem can be taken care of.

Plan of Research

A cross-sectional analysis does not focus on life-cycle pattern but concentrates upon different cohorts of persons who are of different ages at given points of time and yields data which does not provide direct answers to questions about how the individual ages. Also it may lead to fallacious interpretation and erroneous inferring that differences among age categories in the society are due to the aging of the individuals. On the other hand, a longitudinal study involving the whole span of life of a cohort of persons is impracticable.

So as a compromise it is proposed for the present research that a linked cross-sectional statistical design (Rao and Rao, 1965) be adopted which involves studies of different cohorts of persons who are of different ages over a given period of time, say five years. This design would combine the advantages of both methods, cross-sectional and longitudinal. Interaction studies or morphological studies would be appreciated where qualitative and quantitative interaction is involved.

The following scheme would be adopted in collecting the required data:

(*a*) By means of an appropriate sampling design a random sample of households will be selected for a linked cross-sectional study. On every 'normal' (Das 1969) individual in the household will be observed various biochemical and physical variables and other indices that reflect growth survival and decay. Collection of data will be done by clinical methods in the laboratory attached to the Biometry Research Unit, Indian Statistical Institute, Calcutta.

(*b*) Periodic sample surveys will be carried out on the same community to investigate the prevalence and incidence rates of various diseases that affect the community. In addition climate as well as geographical condition, economic condition, social and status of health, distribution of population and variation of fundamental importance in Biochemical surveys. With a gap of one year and two years data will be collected and analysed in such a way (linked cross-sectional investigation) to economise on time, cost of efficiency. Data will be collected for 2nd year (first and 2nd year survey gap of one year), third survey data will be collected with a gap of two years and so on.

(*c*) Hospitalization rates of various diseases according to age and sex will be collected from records of hospital in the area of investigation noting the cases that come from outside the community under observation. Also will be observed the numbers of patients from the community under study that go to hospitals outside the area of investigation.

The data thus collected will be analysed by electronic computers using modern statistical techniques of multivariate analysis.

Level of Health

The measurement of the level of health of the community is the most fundamental problem that confronts the health administration. This is, in fact, what determines the medical care required by the community and nature and extent of the health facilities needed. The determination of the level of health is, therefore, the essential pre-requisite for all health planning. The concept of health cannot, in fact, be translated directly into objective measurements. It can be however negatively expressed through the measurements of diseases. Data collected on nature and extent of disease are nothing but data on morbidity—but these are of fundamental importance in health planning. The climate and geographical conditions also do affect this morbidity.

The structure of health services is largely determined by factors such as population density, the distribution of the population, conditions of health and transport facilities, and communications etc. Before any study of the morbidity of a community can be undertaken, data on the population of that community are clearly necessary. Significant changes in population distribution as between the various age groups may also occur.

Morbidity Data

The morbidity data used in determining health include data on total morbidity, data on acute communicable diseases and of certain non-communicable diseases, data on hospital patients, data on sickness with temporary loss of working capacity and data on morbidity and cause of death. Further morbidity data obtained by the mass screening of various groups of the population or representative sample of the population as a whole are of particular interest. Total morbidity is assessed on the basis of the number of first consultation. This index correctly reflects not only the nature and extent of disease, but also the day in which the disease pattern is tending to change. It is then possible to study the prevalence of disease among the population *i.e.*—the number of persons who seek medical care in any given year, both for disease as a whole and for specific disease.

Morbidity indices: First consultation for old illness, total number of recorded illness per 1000 population for which people have sought medical care.

First consultation for new illness (morbidity), the number of new illness per 1000 population with diagnosis established for the first time.

Exhaustive morbidity: number of illness for which a physician has been consulted plus the number detected during comprehensive medical examinations but for which the person concerned has not sought medical care during the course of the year.

Prevalence rate.

Infection rate (ratio of the number of detected cases to the number of persons examined).

Number of cases of illness involving temporary disability per 100 insured.

Number of days of illness with temporary disability per 100 insured.

Data on Morbidity with Temporary Loss of Work: These are very important in connection with industrial hygiene. The number of cases and number of days lost per hundred workers are an expression of the effect of the various diseases on working capacity, the economic loss resulting from disease etc.

Data on Morbidity and Cause of Death: Such data provide a measure of those diseases having total outcome. They are precise in character and are concerned with a previously measurable phenomenon. Morbidity data provide one of the most valuable means of assessing the level of health of the community.

Total morbidity: Total morbidity makes it possible to measure acute diseases as well as certain diseases following a prolonged course (choronic diseases). It is possible to obtain data on their development, the prevalence of disease among the population and the newly discharged cases of diseases in the year under consideration. Data regarding first consultation either in hospital or in outpatient clinics can be considered as incidence of diseases.

Reasons of Sample Screening

This helps to detect unrecognized diseases. Morbidity statistics provide information only on those patients who seek medical help. Those diseases which do not show symptoms such as anemia cannot be detected without screening. Some of the other diseases also come under this category. Information obtained by mass screening of supposedly healthy persons also serves health planning.

For the purpose of obtaining a complete picture of morbidity based on first consultations and the results of medical screening examinations of various age groups are of importance. The forecasting of progress of public health, a whole range of problems of which following are important:

Changes in the environment (housing, water supply, waste disposal sewerage, air and the soil and noise control).

For social well being of population (real incomes, work, leisure, diet and education etc).

Demographic shifts (birth rate, death rate, natural population increase and composition of the population by set, age, etc).

Forecasting the morbidity and its character, the eradication of communicable diseases or the reduction in their incidence, health status of population and of individual population groups, etc.

Characteristics of the Population's Health

1. Population at the end of each year (age, sex, social and occupational structure of the population.) 2. Birth rate. 3. General death rate. 4. Input morbidity (neonatal within four weeks of life, post-neonatal—2nd to 12 months). 5. Natural population growth.

Data from Hospital: It is possible to determine the diseases for which hospital treatment is required, the number of cases of such diseases, the characteristics of hospital patients (sex, age, etc.), morbidity, etc.

Occupancy of Hospital: Bridgman has shown mathematically on the basis of probability theory that optimum value of the average occupancy of hospital beds must be function of size of the hospital,

$$O_a = \frac{N}{N+3\sqrt{N}}$$

where O_a = average occupancy of hospital beds per year as a fraction of unity, N = average number of patients in a hospital,

$$D = \frac{365\,N}{N+3\sqrt{N}}$$

where D = average number of days on which a bed is occupied. The number of days spent by patient in hospital may be divided as follows—1st period, from admission to the begining of investigation by the intern, 2nd period, clinical and diagnostic investigation, 3rd period, treatment, and 4th period, discharge from the hospital.

Inter-relationship of Indices

The relation between the bed occupancy, average length of stay of patients in bed and the bed turnover, what is known as average turnover index, is very important both theoretically and practically. The average turnover interval is related to bed wastage or the time for which bed is empty.

Let X = bed occupancy (%), S = average length of stay of patient in bed (days), b = bed turnover (days), t = turnover interval (days), N = number of discharge and deaths.

Then NS = total number of occupied beds

$N(S+t)$ = total available number of bed days

Therefore,
$$X = \frac{100NS}{N(S+t)} = \frac{100\,S}{S+t} \qquad \ldots(1)$$

From this,
$$t = \frac{S(100-X)}{X}$$

In a similar way, the following equation for b can be obtained:
$$b = \frac{365}{S+t}$$

Substituting the value of t from equation (1), we get
$$b = \frac{3.65\,X}{S} \qquad \ldots(2)$$

Let D = average bed occupancy (days per year), P = average length of stay of patients in bed (days), F = turnover per bed, t = average length of time for which a bed stands empty (days), n = number of patients passing through hospital.

Then,
$$D = nP$$
$$365 = n(P+t) \qquad \ldots(3)$$
$$t = \frac{365-nP}{n} \qquad \ldots(4)$$
$$F = \frac{365}{P+t}$$
$$Ft = 365 - FP$$

Substituting for t from equation (4)
$$\frac{(365-nP)F}{n} = 365 - FP$$
$$365F - nPF = 365n - FPn$$
$$F = \frac{365n}{365} = n$$

Substituting in equation (3)
$$D = FP$$

Therefore $$F = \frac{D}{P} \qquad \ldots (5)$$

Substituting for n from (3) we get $$t = \frac{365 - D}{F} \qquad \ldots (6)$$

The above equation shows that the bed turnover and the average of time for which a bed stands empty be expressed in term of the average bed occupancy and average length of stay of patients in bed. The equation makes it possible to determine the turnover for any given value of the bed occupancy and the average length of time for which a bed stands empty.

Comparability of Indices

The availability of hospital cases and the efficiency of operation of hospital are compatible at both the national and international levels:

A = total number of hospitalized cases (per year), D = total demand = total number of hospitalized cases plus total number of unsatisfied applicants for admission to hospital, V = total number of bed-days provided, L = total number of bed average over the year, M = total number of deaths in hospital. Mh = total number of cases requiring hospitalization on medical indices, P = total size of population, average over the year, s = total number of patients discharged, K = average bed occupancy (days per year).

number of hospitalized cases per 1,000 population

$$F = \frac{A \times 1{,}000}{P}$$

demand for hospitalization

$$Fd = \frac{D \times 1{,}000}{P}$$

required for hospitalization

$$Fc = \frac{Mh \times 1{,}000}{P}$$

average length of stay of patient in hospital

$$Ls = \frac{V}{1/2(A + S + m)}$$

average % bed occupancy $$Om = \frac{j \times 100s}{365 \times L}$$

bed turnover $$T_o = \frac{1/2\ (A + S + M)}{L}$$

availability of hospital beds to the population

$$l=\frac{L\times 1{,}000}{P}$$

total number of bed days

$$j=j_1+j_2+j_3+\ldots\ldots$$

when j_1, j_2, j_3 ..... indicate bed-days in different hospital departments.

Calculation of Number of Hospital Beds Required

Such calculation is essential for health planning. Many formulae have been proposed by many investigators in different countries. These formulae are based on indices such as proportion of the population hospitalized, the average length of stay of patients in bed, the bed occupancy etc. In certain formulae account is taken of the variation in the daily number of patients seeking admission to hospital. Most of the formulae are suitable for short term planning:

$$Ka=\frac{N.R.P}{D.\ 100}$$

Where Ka = average annual number of beds required, N = size of the population, R = proportion of population K hospitalized, P = average length of stay of patients in bed (days), D = average bed occupancy (days per year).

The formulae considered here are suitable for use in short term planning, but do not take into consideration of variation in the daily number of patients seeking hospital treatment.

Formula Suitable for Long Time Planning

The first step is to determine the average daily number of patients expected to be admitted to hospital in the year for which the calculations are being made.

$$\text{Average daily number of patients expected to be hospitalized}=\frac{\text{Total number of bed days}}{365}=\frac{\text{Future population size}}{\text{Present population size}}$$

The number of bed required under the long term of plan is then,

$$Ka=\frac{\text{average daily number of patients expected to be hospitalized}}{\text{Bed occupancy (in \%)}}$$

The formula proposed, which takes the morbidity as expressed by the number of first consultation per year per 1,000 population its account is as follows:

$$K=\frac{A.R.P.}{D.\ 100}$$

Where K=average number of beds required per year per 1,000 population, A = number of first consultation per year per 1,000 population, R=proportion of patients selected for hospitalization (%), P=average length of stay of patients in bed (days), D=average bed occupancy (days per year).

In long term planning, of course, it is necessary to forecast the changes in morbidity that are likely to occur during the planning period.

This may be illustrated by the numerical example given below. If it is assumed that:

Number of patients admitted per day =5
Average length of stay of patients in bed =10
Bed turnover =10% *i.e.* 365 days
Then the number of patients admitted
during the year is =5×365=1,825.

The bed turnover is 365/10=36.5 *i.e.* one bed is used for the average by 36.5 patients each year. The number of beds required is given as follows:

$$\text{Number of beds}=\frac{\text{Number of patients}}{\text{Bed turnover}}$$

$$=1{,}825/36.5=50.$$

PART II

EDUCATION

A Brief Historical Survey of Educational Statistics in India

DURGAPRASAD BHATTACHARYA*
RAMA DEB ROY (MALAKAR)

Modern statistics, as Professor P.C. Mahalanobis has pointed out, is the result of the fusion of two originally distinct disciplines—"one primarily descriptive, concerned with collection of data; the other essentially analytic, associated with concepts of chance of probability."

Statistics originated as a technology of administration, and thus had an inherent social purpose.

The purpose of this paper is to make a very brief survey of the quantitative information on education in India since the early nineteenth century and to point out to some of the gaps.

Educational statistics is perhaps as old as education itself. At present, educational statistics of India cover, among other points, the following essential items:

(1) *Institutions*: number, type, location, name; (2) *students*: age-group, enrolment, wastage and stagnation, out-turn; (3) *finance*: budgetary allocation of the Union, States and Union Territories, sources of funds, heads of expenditure, pay-scales and emoluments of teachers, including fringe benefits; (4) *manpower*: number of job-seekers by education and skill on the live registers of employment exchanges, occupation of labour force by educational standards, technical hands; (5) *data on special category*: educational status of scheduled castes and tribes, and of persons with disabilities; (6) *special information*: reports of commission and surveys throw more information usually not available. Generally, the informations as outlined here are available in the publications of the union and local governments.

The status of education in the country as in 1974-75 is as follows:

*Indian Statistical Institute, Calcutta.

(1) *population* (in crores in 1974): total 58.2, 6-11 age group 7.7 or 13.2 per cent of the total, 11-14 group 4.2 or 7.2 per cent, 14-17 group 3.8 or 6.5 per cent, 6-17 group 15.7 or 27 per cent.

(2) *institutions* (1974-75): primary 4.3 lakhs, middle 1.02 lakhs, high and higher secondary 0.42 lakhs, colleges 3467, university 96.

(3) *enrolment* (1974-75): I-IV or 6-11 age group—82.7 per cent, VI-VIII or 11-14 group 36.0 per cent, IX-X-XI or 14-17 group 21.5 per cent, university education 3.7 per cent.

(4) *number of teachers* (1974-75 in thousands): pre-primary 19, primary 1230, middle 741, high/higher secondary 693, total 2683.

(5) *budget provision* (1974-75 in Rs. crores): 1570.56.

(6) *literacy as percentage to total population:* 1951-24.9 per cent, 1961—34.4 per cent, 1971—39.9 per cent.

Historical Survey: Upto 1830

Study was an essential component of occupation of three upper castes according to *Arthasastra* of Kautilya, but the *Sudras* or the overwhelming majority were totally deprived of this privilege. The application of the concept of probability in social phenomena is a relatively recent occurrence. The statistical system of India, so far as descriptive statistics is concerned, was perhaps considerably developed. In 1807, Francis Buchanan wrote, "A list called Khana Shumari, consisting a statement of number of the houses, families, tradesmen, castes, ploughs, looms, tanks and other public works, civil and religious, within the jurisdiction of the magistrate which is usually kept under all native governments and seems to be useful."

Buchanan himself conducted multi-purpose statistical investigation in seven districts of Bengal; one in UP now (during 1807-14). A micro-filmed copy of the full manuscripts was produced by P.C. Mahalanobis at the Indian Statistical Institute. For Purniya and Rangapur, he presented a number of males and females with different levels of education. In some other districts, he enumerated number of teachers according to the type of instruction. In some cases, he presented employment and unemployment statistics by levels of education. Colin Mackenzie, F.R.S., the first Surveyor General of India, following his Indian predecessors, compiled "Statistic tables or *Khana Shumaris,* Village Register or Dihizada . . ." in 1809-15 in ceded districts. The Survey of Travancore and Cochin States conducted by Lts. Ward and Conner from July 1816 to the end of 1820 contained in the *Dazajadda* Table number of public institutions in different districts to show a rate of one for every 3382 persons.

Walter Hamilton published the *East India Gazetteer* in 1815, a second edition of this gazetteer were published in two parts in 1828. The gazetteer is a mine of socio-economic data for the recent past including very rare and useful information on education. The two editions of the gazetteer were re-cast in a tabular form by Sm. Anima Bhattacharya of the Office of the Registrar General India around 1962-66. Enough glimpses into the pro-British era are there to have a preliminary idea of the status of education in India. Narendra Nath Law wrote on promotion of learning in India by early European settlers from 1600 to 1800 A.D.

An Appendix to the Report from the Select Committee of the House of Commons on Affairs of the East India Company (Vol. 1 Public) dated 16 August 1832 contains quite a good lot of relevant official data on education since 1781. The volume also contains a *Memoir* by Thomas Fisher (1772-1836) about the extent of Company's aid to establish native schools. The said *Memoir* dated 7 February 1827, "Compiled from the records of the *India* Governments at the *East-India* House, in pursuance of a Minute of the Committee of Correspondence, showing the extent to which Aid had been afforded by the local Governments in *India* towards the establishment of Native Schools in that country: *And*, a Supplement to the foregoing *Memoir*, dated 23 February 1832, containing a Narrative of the further proceedings of the local Governments in *India* relative to Native Schools in that country, to the date of latest records received from India" contains quantitative information on all the schools and societies having a link with the education in Bengal, Madras and Bombay. It starts with *The Calcutta Madrissa* giving the history, expenditure, subjects taught, pay scales of teachers, allowances per student etc., up to 1824. A similar account is also available for *The Benaras Hindu Sanscrit College* (founded in 1791), the old *Calcutta Charity School, the Calcutta Free School Society, Chinsurah Schools, the Calcutta School-Book Society* (founded in 1817). A General Committee of Public Instruction was formed at Calcutta in 1823 and a sum of one lakh rupees was placed at their disposal "with a view to better the instruction of the people. . . ."

The *Memoir* contains a vivid account of the educational status at Fort St. George and at Bombay. Thomas Munro is one of the early statistical investigators in India. Probably he was the first administrator to train field investigators every year with a view to obtain quantitative information on the condition of the land and people as early as 1807. Following this tradition, he issued a circular to several collectors accompanied by a blank form on the 25 June 1825. The form contained 27 columns calling for information on list of schools, number of scholars by sex and by type of instructions, by religion and caste, names of books generally read, monthly or yearly charge to the scholars and the sources of funds, etc.

Munro observed that reading and writing were almost entirely confined to the Brahmins and the Mercantile classes. Women of Brahmins and Hindus in general were, however, prohibited as learning was "regarded as unbecoming of the modesty of the sex. . . ." The answers to the circulars in original are available at the Tamil Nadu State Archives. In the then 20 collectorates of Madras having a population of 12.59 million (6.50 million males and 6.09 million females), there were 12,498 schools and colleges with 1,88,650 scholars, of which 1,75,089 were Hindus and only 13,561 were Muslims. It may be noted that 9,080 or about five per cent were females.

In the account for Bombay, a similar history with quantitative information is presented. A special committee of the Bombay Native School-Book and School Society was appointed in early 1824 to examine the system of education among the natives, and to suggest improvements necessary to be applied to it. In their report as recorded in the public proceedings of the 10 March 1824, a deficiency of text-book in local languages was enumerated as number one hindrance to education. In the proceedings it was also decided to call upon several collectors to report to the government about (*a*) number of village schools in their *zillas*, (*b*) proportion of school to villages, (*c*) allowances to school masters and sources of funds, (*d*) whether arrangements under, (*c*) could be extended to non-schooled villages, (*e*) if small salaries for teachers were deducted from revenues of villages, what allowances would be sufficient, (*f*) whether such charges might not be made from land granted from time to time, (*g*) whether any now-defunct religions allowances could be diverted to this purpose, (*h*) whether payment of money for this purpose might not be accepted in lieu of religions or other services for which land often held, and (*i*) finally, whether any inconvenience would arise from a rule that after a certain number of years no person should be entertained as a public servant, unless able to read and write.

"An abstract of the Returns from the Magistrate and Collectors of several districts subject to the Government of *Bombay*, of the State of Education of those Districts, recorded on the Public Proceedings of 26 January 1825, Nos. 21-24" containing nine heads and 12 columns was reproduced in the said *Memoir*. The table contains information for each collectorate on number of schools and scholars by caste, number of villages with schools and total villages, allowances of teachers and the present and future arrangements, possibility of making literacy a "must" for a public servant and likely reaction.

W.H. Sykes, the officiating statistical reporter to the government (later on a F.R.S. and President of the Royal Statistical Society), conducted a census in Candeish Collectorate in 1826 and collected data on number of schools under "stock" along with number of bullocks, ploughs and carts to show a district total of 85 schools in 66 *parganas* having one school for every 4,369 persons. In another return, he mentioned one school for every 3,357 persons in Poona and 2,452 in Darwar. In 1845, Sykes compiled a document entitled *Statistics of Education at Instructions of East India Company in India.*

The Memoir also contains a report on indigenous schools in the Delhi territory. Another report was on Calcutta School Book Society which published about 29,000 copies of books in 1828, of which 10,000 were in Bengali and 2,450 in Hindi. It also contained information on the state of education in some parts of the U.P. and Nagpur and further reports on Bengal districts.

Historical Survey: After 1830

Lord William Bentink appointed William Adam to enquire into the state of native education in Bengal and Bihar in 1835. In the first report, Adam covered 19 districts of Bengal and Orissa Proper or Cuttack. In the second report, Adam covered Rajshahye and in the third, he presented statistics of the city and District of Moorshedabad, of Beerbhoom, Burdwan, Midnapore, South Bihar and Tirhoot. He presented an "account of the plan of investigation adopted" as it might be useful for future statistical enquirers and also might render some explanation to sources of error in the results. His questionnaires were drawn in local languages and were changed on the basis of experiences. He himself intensively travelled in rural Bengal and also trained Pandits, Maulavis and Waquifkars who also canvassed schedules on his behalf. To ascertain the state of school instruction, he collected data on (*a*) the location of school; (*b*) name, religion, caste and age of teachers, sources and amount of his receipts, the extent of his instruction; (*c*) the number of his scholars—present or absent, their religion and caste, the present age and the probable age of his leaving the school, the progress made, books read and works if any written by the teacher.

On the state of domestic or adult instruction, he used another form: (*a*) number of families in a village or town with the name, religion, caste and principal occupation of the head of each family; (*b*) number of persons in each family by sex and by age group—below 5, between 5 and 14 and above 14; (*c*) number of families in each town or village giving domestic instruction to his children and number of children in each family (*d*) number of persons of adult age in each family (*i*) with learned education (*ii*) knows something more than mere reading and writing Bengali and Hindi accounts, Persian or the English language or any two or more of these (*iii*) who could merely read and write (*iv*) who could barely decipher or write their own name. He presented the summary of his enquiry in the first report which revealed a village school for every 400 persons and one school for every 63 children of school going age. There was a controversy over the figure and specially about the definition of schools. In Nattore, he found 65 schools in 485 villages for a population of about two lakhs giving one school for every 3,000 persons. This ratio approaches those given by W.H. Sykes.

The returns presented at the British Parliament from 1832 onward contain a massive volume of educational statistics giving schools and institutions with their location, number of scholars with their religion and caste, expenditure under various heads and sources. A full list of such papers is now readily available. The average annual expenditure on education by the Company was around Rs 2 lakhs during 1813-1830 and around Rs 7½ lakhs during 1834-35 to 1852-53. *Statistical Abstracts of India* began to appear from 1860 with data from 1840. These volumes also contained all types of important data on education. The Company was obliged to spend on education under the Charter of 1813 and of 1833. The Despatch of 1854 was the beginning of the second phase. The Hunter Commission was appointed in 1882 to enquire into the manner in which the effect had been given to the despatch of 1854. Centering the Commission, a volume of quantitative data came to the surface. A new serial under the title of *Progress of Education in India Quinquennial Review* made its appearance and continued for a long period. These volumes contain elaborate statistics on various aspects of education. The all-India census starting with

1881 began to throw a massive volume of data related to literacy and education. Regional census-type enumerations since the early nineteenth century also often contained useful information. Census data are still the largest single sources of information about the whole country.

Decentralization started after 1920's and continued. Data became gradually available with greater breakdown. Village level data are there in the district census handbooks with a limited purpose. Central, state and local governments maintain data relating to the activities in their own sphere. Educational commissions (the latest being the Kothari Commission of 1964-66) throw a volume of data in course of their deliberations to enable us to look into deficiency of both the system and of the available statistics.

Non-official writings on education with quantitative information were also flowing since the mid-nineteenth century, if not earlier, to form a series of illuminating treaties. Lal Behari Dey wrote his *Primary Education in Bengal* in 1869. *Tracts on Education* containing thoughtful pamphlets appeared in 1880's. Ata Husains' *Educational Statistics* appeared in 1928. He tried to explain the principles of statistics as applied to education and covered all aspects. *Swadeshi*, among other things, also produced educational treatise with statistical data.

Concluding Remarks

We have failed to abide by the Directive Principles of the Constitution regarding universal, free, compulsory primary education. Proportionately, more people are literates, but in absolute terms, illiterates are also on the increase. It is amusing to note that growth rates of literates came down from 78 per cent in 1951-61 to 52 per cent in 1961-1971; the growth rates of illiterates correspondingly rose from 10 per cent to 17 per cent. The latest all-India educational survey (1965-73) reveals a rise of 30 per cent in the enrolment of boys and girls over the numbers recorded in the previous survey, the rise is heartening because of the increasing share of girls on the one hand and the rural population on the other. The benefit of lasting literacy is still a difficult problem, as out of every 100 in class I, only 40 reach class V and 25 class VIII.

It is essential to find out the root cause of our failure to implement the Directive Principles even in three decades. Enrolment is now nearly 90 per cent at the primary level. Investigations should be conducted to find out the reasons of wastage and stagnation and the possible remedy with a better rational allocation of existing resources including idle man-power.

There is scarcely any data on living conditions of students and teachers. The conditions of the former group may indicate the root cause of wastage and stagnation while that of the latter will be helpful in many other respects. A survey on the standard of living of primary teachers was conducted by V.P. Pethe in the City of Sholapur in 1954-55 covering 76 per cent of teachers. In West Bengal, an enquiry into the general conditions of secondary teachers was conducted by one of the present authors in 1954. The survey covered 10 per cent of schools and 15 per cent of teachers in West Bengal. A preliminary enquiry into the conditions of college students was also conducted by us in 1951-53 on a small sample of 158 families. This survey was followed by another survey in late 1950's covering more than 1500 students of Calcutta at the instance of the University of Calcutta. All the four documents revealed a serious poverty casting its shadow on the academic life. In 1970's, conditions might have changed, but a broad-based enquiry at the national and regional level is urgently required.

A scientific spirit of enquiry was inserted in the newly amended constitution as a part of our way of life. It will be quite good to conduct investigations as to how our predecessors in the nineteenth century published volumes on science and technology in regional languages, often with a missionary zeal and visionary outlook, their quantity, quality and effect on public mind. This stream was not weak. Non-official efforts by scholars with the help of teachers' associations and literacy societies may be useful in this respect.

References

BHATTACHARYA, DURGAPRASAD. *ed.* Preliminary report on the enquiry into the general conditions of students in West Bengal, 1951-52. Calcutta, Pragati Prakasani, 1953. tables.

BHATTACHARYA, DURGAPRASAD. *Comp.* Provisional Report on the Enquiry into the General Conditions of the Secondary Teachers in West Bengal. Calcutta, ABTA, 1954. Tables.

BONTROS, An enquiry into the System of Education in British India. Serampore, 1842.

DAY, LAL BEHARI. Primary Education in Bengal. Calcutta, [—], 1869.

HUSAIN, ATA. Educational statistics. Lahore, Feroz Printing Works, 1928. Tables.

PETHE, V.P., A Survey of the Standard of Living of Primary Teachers of Sholapur City (1954-55). *In* Educational Studies and Investigation. New Delhi, NCERT, 1962.

SHAMASATRY, R., *ed.* Kautilya's *Arthashastra*. Bangalore, Govt. Press, 1915.

STARK, HERBERT ALIK. Vernacular Education in Bengal from 1813 to 1912. Calcutta, Calcutta General Publishing, 1916. Statistical Table on the Growth of Education in India 1855 and 1882. Calcutta, 1883.

SYKES, W.H. Statistics of Education at the Institutions of the East India Company. Calcutta, 1845.

Treatise on Popular Education in India, Calcutta, 1841, Parliamentary Papers HL 1845 Vol. 6; HC, 1845, Vol. 34; HC 1845 Vol. 60; HC 1846, Vol. 31; HC 1846-47 Vol. 48; HC 1852 Vol. 36; HL 1852 Vol. 11; HL 1852-53 Vol. 13; HC 1854 Vol, 47; HL 1854 Vol. 12; HC 1857, Vol. 29; HC 1857-58 Vol. 42; HL 1857-58 Vol. 11; HL 1859 Vol. 6; HC 1859 Vol. 24; HL 1859 Vol. 24; HC 1860 Vol. 52; HL 1861 Vol. 12; HC 1866 Vol. 52.

Statistics on Education in India

A.R. KAMAT*

In an earlier paper, we dealt with the sources of educational statistics in India, their limitations and comparability, and offered a few suggestions for their improvement.[1] Following that paper and its revised version, we shall, in the first instance, describe the data-collecting agencies and the state of the data, including its limitations. Later, we shall indicate the major gaps in our educational statistics and try to suggest ways and means of meeting them.

AGENCIES AND WHAT THEY COLLECT

There are three main sources of educational data:

1. Population census;
2. Annual reports of the Ministry of Education at the Centre, Departments of Education in the States, and the University Grants Commission; and
3. All-India educational surveys conducted periodically.

The census data gives the educational status of the entire population every ten years, the unit of study being an individual in a household or family. On the other hand the second and third sources are meant to reflect the operations of the (formal) educational system, the unit of information being an educational institution or an educational organization. The purpose of data collection under the second is to describe every year the current educational activity, in its different

*Gobble Institute of Politics & Economics, Poona.

[1]A.R. Kamat, "Indian educational statistics," *Data Base of Indian Economy*, Vol. II, Statistical Publishing Society, Calcutta, and The Indian Econometric Society, Hyderabad, 1975. A revised version "Educational statistics: sources, limitations and improvement," was presented to National Seminar on Social Statistics held at Delhi, March 17-22, 1975.

aspects. AIE surveys, conducted every few years, also have the same purpose (for the difference see below).

The 1961 Census of India was perhaps the most ambitious and imaginatively conceived effort of its kind and all its important reports are available. B-III A and B, B-VI and C-III are the main tables dealing with education. The first classifies population into workers and non-workers and by educational levels and industrial categories. The information is given for males and females, for rural and urban areas for all the states.

The educational classification used for rural areas has four levels: (*i*) illiterate, (*ii*) literate without educational standards, (*iii*) primary or junior basic, and (*iv*) matriculation and above. For urban population the classification is more elaborate where level (*iv*) is split into several sub-levels.

Table B-VI classifies persons at work other than cultivation by sex, four broad age-groups, occupation and by educational level as above for urban areas only. The third table (Table C-III) presents population figures by sex, age (ten age-groups) and educational levels as above for rural and urban areas.

The other important tables with education are Table B-VIII—A and B which classifies unemployed persons aged 15 and above by sex, age and educational level for urban areas, and by sex and educational level for rural areas; and Table D-IV which classifies migrants to cities and town—groups by sex, age, educational level and occupation (in the case of workers).

Another table, Table B-IX, which does not use educational level classification but classifies persons not at work by sex, age-groups and type of activity (one of which is the full time student) helps us estimate all full-time students in urban and rural areas in each of the above categories. Special tables (*e.g.* Table C-VIII) were taken out for the scheduled castes and tribes.

The 1961 Census also gives information on the distribution of scientific and technical personnel; this was collected by means of cards designed for this purpose and which the concerned persons were asked to fill and return by post. Some of the educational data is also available separately for districts.

The educational data for the 1971 census follows broadly the same lines of classification and tabulation as above. The educational levels are further split up in same tables. For instance, Tables B-III and C-III for urban areas have 14 educational level classes and for rural areas they have 8 such classes (instead of 4 in 1961), so far the following tables have become available: B-III, B-VIII, B-IX, C-III and C-VIII. All of them are based on one per cent sample. Tables of information about degree holders and scientific and technical persons have also become available. The data for this was collected by means of cards left with the eligible persons who were to mail them back. (The response rate is conjectured to be of the order of 50 to 60 per cent.)

The basic source of statistics about the educational system for India as a whole is the annual publication of the Ministry of Education, New Delhi: *Education in India*, Volumes I, II and II-A. Both the mode of collection of information and its statistical presentation have remained almost the same since they were first enunciated in 1949-50, with a few changes from time to time. Information is collected annually from every institution in the educational system through the agency of the state departments of education by means of forms A, B and B-1 designed for schools, universities and colleges respectively. Two more forms A-1, A-2 were introduced since 1964-65, collecting respectively information for the scheduled castes and tribes, and supplementary data required for educational planning. The data are compiled first at the State level and are then consolidated at the Centre for the whole country.

The Ministry's publication, *Education in India*, consisted, until recently, of Volumes I, II and II-A. The first (Vol. I) described the spread of education at different levels mainly in terms of number of institutions, enrolment and age-distribution of pupils, teachers, expenditure with broad sources, and examination results, supported with relevant tables giving figures for the states and for the whole country. At the end was a statistical survey giving all-India data on the main items for a few preceding years so that some idea of the trend could be obtained. Vol. II consisted of consolidated all-India tables (given in Vol. I separately for different levels of education and for different states). Finally, Vol. II-A gave scales of pay of teachers at different levels and under different managements.

The Ministry used to publish two more volumes: (*i*) *Education in States*, which was mostly a repetition of *Education in India*, Vol. I, and was therefore discontinued since 1963-64; (*ii*) *Education in Universities in India*, which was entrusted to the UGC which now publishes its annual volume of statistical data *University Development in India: Basic Facts and Figures*. (For the brief contents of these data see the Appendix on p. 232.)

The state governments publish annual volumes on the lines of *Education in India* with suitable modifications. Some States (*e.g.* Maharashtra) are also taking out annually, through their Directorates of Education, comprehensive *Statistical Abstract of Education*, and smaller volumes *Statistics at a Glance*.

For school education an important independent source of information is the series All-India Education (AIE) Surveys. The first survey was conducted in 1957, the second in 1965-66, and the third, which commenced in 1973, took out provisional figures on school data (reference date 31 December 1973) in small brochures since the middle of 1975. A comprehensive report has been outlined and is in the process of preparation.

The purpose of these surveys was (and is) to collect more systematically detailed information on school education and other data relevant for planning the spread and improvement of school education. The surveys have successively increased the items of information.

The Third Survey, for instance, which covers pre-primary, primary, middle, secondary and higher secondary (including P.U.C.) classes proposes to present data on: (*i*) schooling facilities, number of institutions, enrolment, teachers etc.; (*ii*) school buildings and hostel facilities; (*iii*) library and science facilities; (*iv*) ancillary services (*e.g.* mid-day meals, medical check-up etc.) and cocurricular activities (*e.g.* hobby clubs, cadets, etc.); (*v*) school finance; (*vi*) examination results; and (*vii*) facilities for scheduled castes and tribes.

The second and the third surveys were carried out by National Council of Educational Research and Training (NCERT) with the co-operation of state governments. The data were collected at the school level and consolidated at the block and district levels. The NCERT had earlier published *Educational Statistics—District-wise* giving data for 1960-61; later the Ministry of Education followed it up by publishing district-level educational data for 1965-66.

It is likely that a by-product of the Third Survey may be similar district-wise compilation of data for 1973-74. Finally it should be mentioned that the part of the Third Survey on higher education which was entrusted to the UGC has considerably lagged behind its intended schedule.

State of the Data: Lags, Limitations and Quality

Census Data. The importance of the census data is obvious: it is the only source from which one can get the educational status of the entire population, pursue the progress of literacy, and build up estimates of stocks of variously qualified manpower not only for India as a whole but also for smaller regions. Moreover, it can relate education to other important socio-economic variates— age, employment, occupation etc.

But its limitations are also obvious: apart from the fact that it cannot yield information on the working of the educational system, it is by its very nature too hurried an operation to ensure correctness of the response except on a few items.[2] Moreover, estimates of educationally qualified personnel built on sample basis may not be reliable for smaller regions because of sampling error. The census data on scientific and technical personnel, where the cards were left to the respondents for mailing back, would suffer from an unknown bias of non-response. Finally, as we have seen above, there is considerable time-lag in the publication of data, particularly in the case of 1971 Census.

Other Data. Before we take up the inordinate delay in its publication, let us consider other limiting features of the data collected by the Ministry of Education. There is the limitation arising inevitably because of the imposition of a common classification for all-India purposes on the different year-structures of school education in different States (*e.g.*, primary education may consist of class I to IV or class I to V, the total duration of the SSC course may be 10, 11 or 12 years etc.). Differences also existed, until recently, in the structure of higher education. With the acceptance of the 10+2+3 pattern in the next few years, and the possibility of education being considered a concurrent subject, a uniform structure may come into operation in the near future, after which this limitation will cease to exist. While the imposition of uniformity may be otherwise debatable it may bring happiness to those statisticians and others who like to think in terms of neat and tidy structures.

Then there are other limitations bordering on gross inaccuracies.

[2]See A.R. Kamat, *Progress of Education in Rural Maharashtra*, Gokhale Institute Studies No. 56, Asia, 1968; for our remarks on the correctness of village literacy figures given in the Census.

The figure for enrolment, which is taken from the school register as on the 31st March of the year, exaggerates the actual stabilized enrolment during the year. In addition to other factors which cause this inflation (often of an order of 20 per cent), one important reason is that the enrolment at the beginning of the year is mechanically carried over, month to month, to the end of the year; since elementary education is mostly free, there is no urge to strike off the names of habitually absent pupils from the register.

Another procedural limitation is that enrolments given under middle or secondary schools may not always correspond to middle and secondary stages of education because some of them also run lower classes; but the entire enrolment is shown under middle or secondary schools. While this limitation on the interpretation of enrolment data can be overcome by showing separately enrolments in primary, middle and secondary sections, it cannot be entirely got over for other purposes (e.g. relating institutional resources like buildings and expenditure to enrolment etc.).

A third difficulty arises while interpreting the figures given for the proportion of school-going children in a particular stage (e.g. enrolment in primary education, class I to V, as a proportion of age-group 6 to 10). This can be got over only by means of an improved classification using age-distribution.

But the most serious shortcoming of the Ministry's statistics is the long delay between the date of reference and the date when it makes a public appearance in print. (The procedural reasons are described in our earlier paper). At the time of the first meeting of the Advisory Committee on Educational and Cultural Statistics (April-May 1974), the published Ministry volume was that for 1965-66, those for 1966-67 and 1967-68 were in press and that for 1968-69 was being finalised. It was then decided to clear the backlog by (*i*) concentrating on the publication of 1973-74 on a priority basis and publishing it by June 1976, and (*ii*) creating special units to deal with the data for the four years 1969-70 to 1972-73. It was also decided to introduce a much simplified form, to be canvassed from 1975-76 (reference date 31 December 1975).

It has not been possible to check how much of this has been actually realized beyond noting that volumes for 1966-67 and 1967-68 are on the shelves of our library. An agreeable feature of the Ministry volumes for these two years is that they have combined old volumes I and II and have dispensed with much of the textual gloss of the earlier volumes.

It is clear that a time-lag of this order (six to eight years) makes this data lose its relevance except for archival or historical-research purposes. Realising this, the Ministry started issuing two short mimeographs on educational statistics: (*i*) *Selected Information on School Statistics*, and (*ii*) *Educational Statistics at a Glance,* which make available certain basic educational data within a much shorter interval, one to three years. This, however, does not solve the major problem of delay for which a three-pronged attack is necessary: (*i*) simplification of the schedules, and (*ii*) effective decentralisation of the collection of data by (*a*) activising the State Departments and creating a sense of urgency among them, and (*b*) strengthening the district level organisation.

Some States have also started publishing their educational data more expeditiously. For instance, Maharashtra has often published statistical abstracts on education within a period of two or three years, and publishes provisional summaries within a year. Besides, educational information is often compiled district-wise so as to be useful for district educational planning.

The AIE surveys, as mentioned above, provide much more information on (school) education, information which is also more relevant to educational planning. The quality of data is also better because of the difference in organization which can avoid (and also cut through) the usual administrative bottlenecks.[3] For the same reason the collected data can also become available more expeditiously.

The UGC volumes, *Basic Facts and Figures*, give data on enrolment and teachers as in August of the year of reference, but they sadly lack most other relevant information. For instance, they do not even provide data on expenditure or examination results. The UGC volumes have often appeared within two or three years of the reference year.

Gaps and How to Meet Them

Apart from the serious time-lag problem of our educational data, although much better than in many other developing countries, important gaps show up when examined from the point of view of plan-

[3]See e.g. discussion on comparability in our "Indian Educational Statistics." *op. cit.*

ning, both educational and socio-economic. To locate them it is best to approach the question from the other end. What should be our normal expectations in this respect—(*a*) about the functioning of the educational system, and (*b*) educational information about population? Taking into consideration the fact that educational planning is itself an important part of socio-economic planning, it may be useful for our purpose to think in terms of the following schema:

(*a*) General educational planning for (*i*) its (routine) expansion and (*ii*) improvement of functioning;

(*b*) Educational planning with general goals which are essentially socio-economico-political, such as (*i*) full (including adult) literacy, (*ii*) universal elementary education, and (*iii*) equality of opportunity at all levels of education;

(*c*) Educational planning with specific goals such as educational progress of (*i*) weaker sections—scheduled castes, scheduled tribes and other backward classes, (*ii*) women, (*iii*) religious minorities, mainly Muslims, and (*iv*) linguistic minorities; and

(*d*) Social and economic planning in which education plays an important role; in particular (*i*) economic growth with social justice, (*ii*) employment, (*iii*) occupational mobility, (*iv*) social change, and (*v*) cultural upliftment; all these to be sought for population in general as well as to its different sections, with special attention to those mentioned in *C* above.

When we think in some such a framework, or even otherwise, we can see that there are many gaps in our educational information (even if it were possible to collect and make it available much more expeditiously). For instance, we have no reliable figures on the expenditure and resource matrix which are necessary even for routine expansion mentioned in *A*; there is duplication in some times, like scholarships, and expenditure on non-teaching staff is not available separately. Moreover, the statistics fall far short when one comes to the question of *A* (*ii*), improvement, in the absence of information about attendance, physical resources (buildings, libraries and laboratory facilities, science teachers, etc.) which are available and their (even modest) normal requirements, and most of all about stock and flow of pupils for estimating drop-outs and repeaters.

These gaps in data, it is clear, will also affect *B* (*i*) and (*ii*). As regards *B* (*iii*), there is, no doubt, some information on scholarship programmes. But only some idea about the socio-economic profile of the student community at various levels, particularly at middle and higher levels, can assure us whether we are proceeding in that direction, and at what pace.

Considering *C*, while there is perhaps adequate data on (*i*) and some (less than adequate) on (*ii*), there is no data on *C* (*iii*) and *C* (*iv*) which, to my mind, are necessary for any effective planning for national integration. Clearly information relevant to *C* has to emanate both from the educational system (institutional data) as well as the data (census) about population. *D* obviously implies too tall an order for data; it was deliberately formulated in that manner to indicate the wide context in which education affects socio-economic development.

Shorn to its bare minimum, one still needs (*a*) the stock (and flow) position of qualified manpower at different levels, (*b*) the changing educational profile, (*c*) the changing requirements in the different sectors of the developing economy, (*d*) the employment-unemployment situation of the educated and its various sections, and (*e*) at least some broad educational indicators of social and cultural change. If the information from the census (and also other inquiries, like the NSS) is placed along side even these modest requirements, the large gaps between the available and desirable should become evident.

How are these gaps to be filled? Some within the framework of the present data-collecting agencies by means of changes and streamlining; for others, new investigations may be necessary, either on a continuing or ad-hoc basis, when they are not unfeasible. Still others, where desirable, may have to be written off because modest people cannot simply ask for the moon.

We start with the census. Considering the kind of operation the census is, it is hardly possible to prescribe additional items, except an occasional one, which they are already doing, anyway. But one can certainly ask for qualitative improvement in the collection, a more thorough coverage (about the incompleteness of which there were several complaints in 1971), and a quicker processing of data (on which no comments are necessary in view of the current position described well above).

The general scheme of the presentation of educational data (that is, its tabulation) appears to be adequate; but some marginal improvements are possible. For instance, tables for rural areas can do with a more detailed age and educational level classification; this has been done to a certain extent in the 1971 census, but it could be extended. Tables for different groups mentioned under *C* in our schema, where they are not already done today, should (and can easily) be taken out.

The coverage of degree-holders and scientific and technical personnel, which has improved in 1971 (almost 2.2 million out of the estimated 3.4 to 4 million), has much room for further improvement. The analysis can also be suggested in further depth for certain categories (e.g., among women), although the recent attempt at an inquiry of the Pune women graduates has not been a success. (Either graduate women of Pune are too tough for approach, or the investigators were unequal to their task, or both!).

The analysis of the existing material can be fruitfully extended in two other directions. First, analysis of bilingual or multilingual persons, classified by their knowledge of English and/or Hindi, can be further extended to classification by educational levels. Second, with the help of 1961 and 1971 data, changes in the educational profile in different sectors of economy, in different occupations, and different specific groups of population, should enhance our knowledge about the changes that are taking place around us.

The improvement of data on the working of the educational system (institutional data) is a more formidable task. Most attempts so far, in this direction, have proved ineffective, like the occasional stirring of a jar of jam which soon settles down to its old form. Even so, here is a fresh attempt, for what it is worth. The schema outlined in above suggest that, from educational institutions, information on the following broad items need to be collected:

(*1*) Level of institution (primary school etc.) with sections (and classes) taught, and type of management;

(*2*) Enrolment (by sex and age) in each class, attendance;

(*3*) Teaching staff: requirements, actual staff (sex, age, qualifications, emolument);

(*4*) Buildings: requirements, actual situation; hostel facilities, staff quarters;

(*5*) Library, science and other curricular facilities;

(*6*) Ancillary services (mid-day meals, free books, etc.) and cocurricular activities (scouting, cadets, etc.);

(*7*) Expenditure by main items; financial resources, scholarship programme;

(*8*) Output: examination results (by sex, levels, categories and specialization);

(*9*) Information on weaker sections (scheduled castes and tribes);

(*10*) Stock and flow statistics, drop-outs, repeaters;

(*11*) Information on other backward communities, Muslims and linguistic minorities; and

(*12*) Socio-economic background of (*a*) pupils, (*b*) teachers.

Out of these items, data on *1* to *9* may feature in the annual return which can be designed in a much more simplified form than the (45-page) one as at present. Even here information on items *4* to *6* may be collected every three years along with *10* and *11*; and that on *12* can be even less frequently canvassed, say every five or seven years.

It will be observed that the information mentioned above will be necessary to take stock of the status, to plan future expansion of education and to improve the working of the system; it also contains items which have socio-economic relevance. For making the information more useful for these purposes, in addition to simplification of the annual return, certain procedural changes may have to be introduced, as for instance, methods of maintaining stock and flow statistics, streamlining the procedure of maintaining accounts (so that double entries like scholarships and freeships are avoided, and items like salaries of non-teaching staff are clearly demarcated), etc. Moreover, with this data it may be possible to plan for progress, that is, improvement. For instance, reduction in the percentage of drop-outs and repeaters is obviously (along with examination results) an indicator of improvement.

With a little more effort—devising a literacy test and administering it periodically, every three or six months—it is possible to evaluate the achievement in primary schools in terms of the accepted goal of literacy. This will also help evaluate ameliorative programmes (like free mid-day meals). (I suppose it is not necessary to dwell on the importance of other items mentioned above for the planning and improvement of institutional functioning as well as for the realization of social objectives).

What is the agency for this data collection? The State education department is the only agency which can collect this information accurately and expeditiously if it can muster the will and organization to do so. With the possible concurrent control over education, it should be possible for the Centre to use its powers of persuasive coercion (aid and admonition) to activise lethargic state departments. The most effective unit of organization would be a district which usually has an education officer, strengthened by the addition of a statistical cell manned by a qualified statistician. (May this tribe multiply!). In fact, the district education office has to prepare a complete educational mapping of the district at all levels of education which not only indicates the present position, with its plus and minus points, but also, thereby, helps planning for the future expansion of education and improvement in its working.

The AIE surveys, however, should also continue. They will have a corrective, innovative and enlivening influence on the regular data collected by the state through its district units. In fact, in the concurrent set-up visualised for education, there is no reason why the AIE survey should not become a continuing organization with corresponding organizations at the state level. Besides conducting AIE surveys every few years, they can also undertake educational investigations, on sample or complete-census basis, on other important problems—functioning of single-teacher schools, functioning of public schools, working of rural colleges, evaluation of free-meal programmes, survey of educational facilities outside the formal education system, survey of coaching classes, etc.

Before concluding, let us have another look at the framework outlined above, particularly area D. That will convince us that there are many more gaps in our information of the impact of education on the socio-economic situation than one can reasonably hope to bridge either through extension or improvement of the census channel or the institutional channel. Moreover, as the saying goes, it is not possible to sew all the tears (or holes) in the sky. Even so, one may pick and choose a few of the most important gaps in our education data from the point of view of social and economic planning and suggest ways of meeting them.

I suggest that investigations be initiated on some of the following (and similar) questions: (*i*) an in-depth study of the educated unemployed, (*ii*) the changing educational profile in employment in (*a*) factories, (*b*) agriculture and (*c*) service sector, (*iii*) analysis of white-collar employment, with particular reference to weaker sections, (*iv*) a study of the relationship between income-levels and educational levels, (*v*) case studies of employment and educational level in certain public sector establishments (government service, LIC, banks, railways etc.), and similar studies in private sector concerns; and (*vi*) the changing educational profile of women in white-collar and other employment.

I am aware it is easier enumerating problems than solving them, suggesting investigations than carrying them out; even so, at least some of them should be immediately feasible from the point of view of money and personnel resources required to carry them out.

What are the appropriate agencies for such work? Tentatively one can think of the NSS and the State Bureaus of Statistics. But one need not rule out the possibility of a standing section in the census organization which can usefully undertake such investigations during the slack years between two successive censuses.

APPENDIX

The information available (*i*) In the Ministry volume (from 1966-67 onwards), (*ii*) In the UGC volume, and (*iii*) Information which is supposed to be collected by the Ministry from 1975-76 are given below for reference.

1. The Ministry volume (1966-67) gives information on the following:

(*i*) Number of educational institutions by management,

(*ii*) Enrolment by type of institution and management,

(*iii*) Enrolment in general education (collegiate) by courses, classes and stages; also for professional and other education; also by age-group for both these groups,

(*iv*) Enrolment in general school education by standards and age-groups,

(*v*) Age-distribution of pupils in classes I-V, VI-VIII and XI and above,

(*vi*) Enrolment in vocational/professional, special and other education, by type of education, by age-groups,

(*vii*) Statistics of compulsory primary education,

(*viii*) Number of teachers in institutions and pupil-teacher ratio,

(*ix*) Teachers by training and qualification in primary, middle and high schools; and in primary, middle and secondary stages,

(*x*) Direct expenditure on institutions by managements, sources, objects,

(*xi*) Indirect expenditure by sources; on buildings by type institutions and by sources; same on hostels,

(*xii*) Total expenditure on education by sources,

(*xiii*) Scholarships, stipends and other financial concessions,

(*xiv*) Education in rural areas,

(*xv*) Examination results,

(*xvi*) System of school classes and a few other minor items.

2. The UGC volume on university development in India (for 1969-70) gives information on the following:

(*i*) Universities,

(*ii*) Colleges and teaching departments,

(*iii*) University enrolment by faculties and stages,

(*iv*) Staff,

(*v*) Halls or residence and staff quarters,

(*vi*) Post-graduate enrolment.

Remark 1: The UGC statistics gives no information on the following important points: (1) Expenditure and resources; (2) types of management of educational institutions; (3) examination results; (4) non-teaching staff (administrative, library, laboratory etc.); (5) enrolment of scheduled castes and tribes; and (6) (some measure of) drop-outs.

Remark 2: The Ministry statistics (from 1966-67 onwards) also provides no information on (4), (5) and (6), although its previous volumes did so on (5).

3. The simplified form prepared by the Ministry for collecting institutional data (from 1975-76 onwards) would fetch information on the following:

(*i*) Educational institutions by type, management, stages, classes and courses offered.

(*ii*) Enrolment data,

(*iii*) Teachers by educational qualification and training,

(*iv*) Expenditure according to sources and objects,

(*v*) Fees, free studentships, scholarships etc.

Information on the scheduled caste and tribes enrolment was to be collected as a part of (*ii*), but only simple queries were to be asked on buildings, playgrounds, library, laboratory, hostels, mid-day meals, radio sets and mass media etc.

Statistics (so far collected) on (*i*) examination results and (*ii*) number of villages served by schools were to be dropped. On the following items information was to be collected on a sample basis: (*i*) more details on teachers e.g. age, emoluments, attrition rate etc., (*ii*) wastage and stagnation, (*iii*) class-wise examination results, (*iv*) average daily attendance, (*v*) age-distribution of students, (*vi*) distribution of classes/sections by number of pupils and teachers per section, (*vii*) multipurpose and various categories of professional and vocational schools.

Data Base for Elementary Education in Rural India

C. BAL KRISHNA*

It has been argued that in developing countries the problem of wastage at the elementary level of education continues to be serious and that it is due to implementation of educational policies which are of a "capitalist" variety.

Carnoy[1] holds the ruling bourgeois class responsible for its exploitative dominance on educational policies. Minhas[2] provides the empirical evidence that in India, during the third and fourth plan periods, there has been a neglect of the education sector--the per capita outlay (at 1960-61 prices) in the Fourth plan (of Rs 8.40) is less than the per capita outlay (of Rs 11.30) in the third plan. The distribution of outlays over all the plan periods have continuously and increasingly favoured the university education in the name of equality but often in fact as a bulwark of privilege, old and new.

Kamat[3], while describing the education situation in India, shows concern over the emergence of new type of elites different from the traditional ones as an outcome of the type of educational policies we have adopted especially after the political independence in 1947.

During the last decade there were a few (pilot) attempts to expand education facilities so as to improve in quantity rather than quality. Such programmes are covering the rural population of children as

*Indian Statistical Institute, New Delhi.

[1]Carnoy, M. *Education as Cultural Imperialism*, David Mckay and Co., New York, 1974.

[2]Minhas, B.S. "Objectives and Policy Frame of the Fourth Indian Plan," in Faber, M. and Seers, D. (ed.) *The Crisis in Planning*, Vol. II, Sussex University Press, England, 1972.

[3]Kamat, A.R. *Educational Situation in India; and Other Essays on Education*, P.P.H., New Delhi, 1973.

well as adults in an effort to achieve the goal of a literate society. Some of them are the following:

(*1*) The farmer's functional literacy programme, initiated in 1967 in 3 districts, was in action in 107 districts by the end of the fourth plan.

(*2*) Non-formal education programme for the children in the age group 6-15. Such children either did not go to formal school at all or dropped out due to economic and other reasons.

(*3*) Non-formal education programme for the adult in the age group 15-35. Both programmes 2 and 3 are quite new and their impact is yet to be felt.

(*4*) Satellite Instructional Television Experiments (SITE) was tried in 2400 villages in 6 different states for one year in 1975-76.

(*5*) The Scheme of development school under the Integrated Rural Development Programme in 20 districts.

All such programmes are supposed to be complementary to, rather than substitutes for, existing formal school education. Thus all such formal or non-formal programmes are aimed at the objective of achieving a literate society. This objective was laid down in the Constitution under the Directive Principles (Article 45), and it was to be achieved by 1960. But we are far from it. Though literacy has gone up in percentage terms, the absolute number of illiterates, both males and females, has gone up—at last up to the 1971 Census.

In this paper a data-base for providing indicators to tackle the perennial educational wastage problem has been suggested on the basis of a field survey view.

A Suitable Data-base

We could raise the question whether the above programmes along with the formal school system in rural India could provide us with data, (*a*) which help in measuring some performance-indicators, (*b*) which are useful to tackle the problem of heavy wastage due to stagnation and drop-out in elementary school, and (*c*) which could be collected with reasonable efforts in terms of monetary and time inputs so as to be useful for making worthwhile policy decisions.

Macro-negative vs. Micro-positive

So far efforts to collect data on education programmes, say, by NCERT, the Ministry of Education, NSS or the Census have been mostly for answering queries which help the administration make financial allocations to various states, districts within a state, tehsils within a district and, finally, schools within a tehsil. Usually it was the enrolement level in a school which was the indicator for granting inputs. There has been a consistent complaint that inflated figures of enrolements are provided so as to get as big a share of inputs as possible. There is some truth in it, but what is the solution when we have not developed any other bench-mark? In the words of Williams such macro-negative information rather than micro-positive information has been sought through data collection efforts; as quoted by McMeekin.[4]

The micro-positive indicates relationships e.g. between programmes and their effects, say, reduction in drop-outs resulting from a programme etc. The macro-negatives, on the other hand, merely include indicators of educated unemployment, differences in educational attainments, exessive drop-out etc. Nothing beyond that.

Outline of a Field Visit and some Observations

During 1975-76 a field survey was conducted to study education programmes at the elementary level through formal as well as non-formal methods in Udaipur district, Rajasthan. For this purpose about 40 villages in its 3 tehsils were visited over three months. Schools and a sample of households in these villages were contacted with the explicit purpose of studying the impact of, (*a*) school inputs (both hardware and software) on the efficiency of the school, (*b*) adult literacy (usually achieved through non-formal means of education) on the motivation to send the children to the formal school and retain them at least till they are literate by studying upto the lower primary level of elementary education, and (*c*) community efforts to improve the miserable condition of single-teacher schools (we have about one third of primary schools with a single teacher in the whole country).

It became quite clear after doing this survey that there is a lot of scope for improving on the existing data base by addition of new data, or even by altering it so as to get rid of some misleading data.

[4]McMeekin, Jr. R.W. *Education in Planning and Expenditure Decision in Developing Countries: With a Malaysian Case Study*, Praeger Publication, New York, 1975.

What we need could be put into following different heads:

(*i*) Single-teacher schools (whether full or part of primary).

(*ii*) School inputs and outputs.

(*iii*) Community involvement in the working of the village school to run it in a comparatively efficient way.

Single Teacher School

Quite a few such schools do have only a skeleton structure of just a room without any other hardware inputs. It seems as if the whole expenditure on such schools is on the salary of the single teacher as the other inputs are conspicuous by their absence (except, perhaps, rent). It will be worthwhile to collect at some time-interval data on: (*a*) hardware inputs like black-board and other teaching aids etc, (*b*) proportion of recurring expenditure and whether it is decreasing or increasing, and (*c*) the frequency with which such schools remain closed during the working session because of teacher's absence.

School Inputs and Outputs

Here it is of interest to know the level of hardware and software inputs. Since most of the lower-primary-level schools are managed by the panchayats, the supervision of such schools is extremely infrequent. The frequency of supervision depends upon such factors as the location of schools, especially its distance from highway—shorter the distance, the more frequent is supervision. Some schools have not been visited for supervision even once in five years because they are located in isolated places. On the other hand, other schools though few in number, are visited five times a year just because they are located near a highway.

The motivation not to retain the children as well as wastage due to drop-out and stagnation was observed to be less in the model schools with preferred inputs of both hardware and software, in quantity as well as quality. So here again it will be quite useful to know: (*a*) the level of expenditure on recurring items like teaching aids and other hardware inputs, (*b*) frequency of supervision, and (*c*) the software inputs (usually the teachers) (its quantity and quality).

At present, primary schools which are run by panchayat samitis in Rajasthan are allotted Rs 1.50 per 100 students per month for contigency expenses. This is a negligible amount by any standard of quality consideration.

Community Involvement

The community in villages contributes some amount through education cess per household. It is again about Rs 1.50 per year per household. But experience has been that due to some reason or the other it remains uncollected from quite a few houses. The teacher is usually from outside the village. This inhibits sufficient involvement of the teacher in the village community life as he has to shuttle to and from his place of residence a few villages away from the school, usually walking. The teacher, especially in the single-teacher school, practically remains out of touch with parents (and the community). He sometimes takes help from some educated youth of the village in running his school. This arrangement is voluntary and quite non-formal and usually not permanent. Elsewhere, I have explored the possibility of utilising this educated youth in the school of his village on formal basis.

CONCLUSIONS

In this short paper no rigorous and specific data base has been suggested. Rather, an effort has been made to point out the direction in which performance-oriented data, if properly collected, could provide us with indicators useful in arriving at policy decisions to tackle the problem of wastage due to stagnation and repetition. The importance of collecting the following data has been suggested: (*a*) software inputs (like pupilc-teacher ratio, frequency of supervision), (*b*) hardware inputs (teaching aids including black-board), and (*c*) single-teacher schools—their number in block or tehsil; other inputs from the community as well as the government.

Statistics on Vocational Education

S.N. GANDAM*

Expansion of vocational education is an accepted policy at national as well as other levels of educational planning. Vocational expansion has two aspects—to prepare trained personnel for various vocations in the economy and to improve the skills of existing vocational personnel by continued training.

Planning for vocational training is, no doubt, a difficult task. A planner has to match proposed training facilities with manpower requirements, and also face the task of achieving this with feasible finances. Thus, if detailed vocational education planning is to be done, it is essential to have information on (*i*) what are the existing facilities for vocational education and how they are utilized, and (*ii*) what are the manpower needs of the economy. With this information, and given the financial support, an educational planner would be able to chalk out vocational programmes.

Of the two items above, the latter is external to the system of educational statistics, and the data for studying it would visually be available in other sources. Indeed, it is the first one that forms the part of educational statistics. It is here that the paper suggests some modifications in the present data system.

Presently the major source of educational statistics at national level is *Education in India*, published yearly by the Ministry of Education. Few modifications are suggested in the data available therein.

In *Education in India*, we get enrolment and other statistics for vocational/professional education at three levels (*i*) school, (*ii*) undergraduate, and (*iii*) graduate and post-graduate. Presently data are available for the following categories at the three levels:

*Gokhale Institute of Politics and Economics, Poona.

School	*Undergraduate*	*Graduate and Postgraduate*
(*a*) Agriculture	(*a*) Agriculture	(*a*) Agriculture
(*b*) Commerce	(*b*) Commerce	(*b*) Commerce
(*c*) Fine Arts	(*c*) Fine Arts	(*c*) Fine Arts
(*d*) Medicine	(*d*) Medicine	(*d*) Medicine
(*e*) Physical Education	(*e*) Physical Education	(*e*) Physical Education
(*f*) Technical	(*f*) Technology, Engineering, and Architecture.	(*f*) Technology, Engineering and Architecture.
		(*g*) Law
		(*h*) Pharmacy
		(*i*) Veterinary
(*j*) Other Schools for Vocational/Professional Education.	(*j*) Other Colleges for Professional Education.	(*j*) Other Colleges for Professional Education.

The present format of *Education in India* has been made effective from 1966-67. Considering the period 1961-62 onwards, it is seen that the format has been changed twice, in 1964-65 and 1966-67. Till 1963-64, a break-up similar to present format was available; for two years, 1964-65 and 1965-66, a further break-up of some categories such as technical, medicine, and fine arts was available. But this was again given up when the format was revised in 1966-67. In addition to these categories, statistics for teacher training courses is available for (*i*) basic and (*ii*) non-basic.

Among the various vocational/professional courses, the technical category is most important on two counts—that it has a variety of courses, and that it has sizable enrolement. The following table gives enrolment for technical courses since 1961-1962 in terms of percentage to total enrolment for vocational/professional courses (including teachers' training).

(*i*) School and (*ii*) Graduate and post-graduate.

In the first three columns the figures are given with commerce included in professional courses whereas in the latter three columns are given the figures with commerce excluded. It may be recalled here that the Kothari Commission treated commerce as part of general education while computing their proportion in vocational courses.[1] It is seen from the table that the enrolment for technical courses is quite

[1]Education and National Development, Report of the Education Commission, 1964-66, Appendix I(vii), Reprint by NCERT.

TABLE 1 *Enrolment in technical courses as percentage to total enrolment in vocational and professional courses*

	Commerce included			*Commerce excluded*		
	School	*Under-graduate*	*Graduate & post-graduate*	*School*	*Under-graduate*	*Graduate & post-graduate*
1961-62*	43.24		18.35	51.71		26.14
1962-63*	40.20		18.49	50.51		26.12
1963-64*	43.90		19.36	53.50		27.52
1964-65	33.90	36.30	25.70	47.37	44.10	34.68
1965-66	42.20	37.40	24.60	51.10	44.62	34.09
1966-67	43.88	50.23	24.18	53.26	53.77	30.55
1967-68	42.43	51.07	32.87	52.59	55.24	29.99
1968-69	57.86	46.82	21.45	62.59	50.84	28.76
1969-70	58.25	46.10	19.59	62.30	51.03	27.22

*For these years enrolment is available only at two levels:
(*i*) School and (*ii*) Graduate and post-graduate.

high. If we consider the enrolment during 1969-70, it is seen that at school levels among the students offering vocational/professional course, 58.25 per cent students offered technical courses, the percentage at undergraduate and graduate levels being 46.10 and 19.59 per cent respectively. If commerce is excluded from vocational courses, the percentages are 62.30, 51.03 and 27.22 respectively.

The category of technical, with such a high enrolment, should be broken into sub-categories. It is proposed that for doing so the National Classification of Occupations may be used. This classification is available up to the three-digit level. The two-digit level would be helpful. The various courses available at industrial training institutes, polytechnics, industrial schools, technical schools, engineering colleges and other vocational institutions should be properly classified, using the National Classification of Occupations, and at least enrolment data be made available for these occupations separately. Our census data are available according to this National Classification of occupations and hence it is useful for manpower planning to have enrolment data classified similarly. A suitable scheme of classification should be formulated which may be used for all the levels.

Presently, area skill surveys are being done for number of areas. Analysis of the data by occupations has been found useful there. As a matter of fact, that becomes a must whenever manpower planning is to be done. Giving detail classified data would be a big task but it would be worth doing. At present we have very little statistics available on education compared to other fields; certainly we have a strong case to bring out more volumes than at present on educational statistics. In fact, a separate volumeon vocational/professional education may be planned.

The enrolment statistics given in *Education in India* relates to 31st March each year. This creates a difficulty for the vocational courses which are of less than one year's duration, say six months or three months, such as courses in catering and institutional management, practical weaving, etc. In these cases, only those students who are studying during March get counted. Others remain outside the statistics. Some modification to avoid this is necessary.

With 10+2+3 pattern being adopted by many states, the school statistics for higher secondary may be separated out. The students of 11th and 12th classes should be included in this category whether they are studying at school or college. At this stage also the data on vocational courses become crucial specially because of our target of diverting fifty per cent of the students after 10th class to vocational courses. To understand the proportions of students going in for various courses, it is necessary to have enrolment figures for the 11th class and also for the first year of various vocational courses where students are admitted after 10th class. Then only can we get a clear picture.

It is also necessary at all levels that we get an idea of the duration of courses. The investment for vocational courses is quite high, and the duration of course is an important factor influencing investmemt.

At present *Education in India* covers only recognized institutions. Data on non-recognized institutions are of equal importance. Quite often it is seen that non-recognized institutions take the lead in opening new courses which, later, recognized institutions follow. Computer programming, card-punching, television and refrigerator repairing, are merely few examples. In fact, these courses, started by non-recognized institutions, indicate the demand for trained personnel in the economy. Thus, it could be of vital importance to have statistics, at least of enrolment and duration, in respect of non-recognized institutions. The statistics may be collected periodically, if not every year.

For educational planning, it becomes necessary to conduct socio-economic survey, especially for vocational planning. The Education Commission did conduct such a survey in 1965. It is suggested that some important socio-economic information may be collected from each student after he takes admission for vocational courses. This information can be obtained and preserved by the concerned institutions. This would be of great use whenever the socio-economic surveys are conducted, may be locally, at national or state level. This stored information can be collected by the surveying agency on sampling basis or otherwise. The censal compilation of this information is not necessary.

An Appraisal of Educational Statistics in India

P.R. GOPINATHAN NAIR*

An appraisal of educational statistics can be attempted only in terms of the purposes for which they are collected. In present-day India, their purpose is mainly to serve as an aid to educational planning. Systematic educational planning does not seem, however, to have been attempted in this country, either at the national or state levels. The various five-year plan documents, prepared at the national level and in various states, do contain statements of educational objectives and targets as well as short-falls in performance, but they are too general to be termed planning in any meaningful sense of the term.

One of the reasons for the absence of systematic educational planning in this country is, perhaps, the non-existence of adequate techniques and tools for the purpose. Quantitative models of educational systems which could be used as bases of planning enrolment of pupils, employment of teachers, expenditure on education, etc. are of very recent origin. Even in advanced countries they are still in the early stages of development. In India, the process of constructing such models for educational planning for the country in general or for the different states has hardly begun. In such circumstances, an appraisal of the available statistics has to be attempted not in terms of the purposes for which they have been used in the past, but in terms of the data requirements for systematic educational planning.

NATURE OF EDUCATIONAL STATISTICS IN INDIA

Educational statistics available in India in recent years, in published form, fall into two broad categories: (*i*) statistics relating to the psychological aspects of learning, interaction of teachers and students, interactions among students, content of education, quality of teaching, media of instruction, policies of promotion, languages taught, the

*Centre for Development Studies, Trivandrum.

technology of education, etc., and (*ii*) statistics relating to the educational system. The latter category includes items like the number of students, teachers, institutions, expenditure and examination results. While the first category of information is obtained mainly through *ad hoc* studies at micro-levels, the latter is obtained from a regular system of data collection operated by the Union Ministry of Education. While the former type of data is relevant for planning the contents of education and the technology of teaching, the latter serves for planning the educational processes themselves.

Our discussion in this paper is limited to the latter category of statistics relevant for macro-planning of the educational systems and processes. This does not, however, imply that planning for the qualitative improvements of the educational processes is of any lesser importance. Further, we limit our discussion to the formal educational system comprising recognized institutions since data on informal education (such as adult education, educational services performed by voluntary agencies and unrecognized institutions, etc.) are not collected regularly in India.

The most important uses to which macro-level statistics could be applied include: (*i*) forecasting the future evolution of the educational system, (*ii*) estimating the consequences of current educational policies, and (*iii*) selecting optimal policies or paths of educational development. For these purposes information will be required mainly on; (*a*) student flows (within the various stages and branches of the system as well as between the system and the rest of the economy); (*b*) teachers, (*c*) class-rooms, and (*d*) costs.

The Present State of Educational Statistics in India

India has at present an elaborate system of collection, compilation and publication of educational data. Published statistics are available on various aspects of the educational system, mainly at three levels of aggregation: the district, the state and the nation. They include:

(*i*) enrolment of students (by stages and types of education and by sex);

(*ii*) number of institutions (by stages and classified into general special, professional, vocational etc.);

(*iii*) number of teachers, (by sex and classified according to qualifications, training, experience and emoluments);

(*iv*) expenditure (classified into direct and indirect, recurring and non-recurring, and by stages); and

(*v*) examination results.

Classification of institutions according to management (private, local bodies, government) is also available. Ratios like the pupil-teacher ratio, floor space per pupil, expenditure per pupil (and per capita) and student-population ratio are also available in published form. In some publications, information is supplied on drop-out rates for the country in general (based on calculations made from cross-section data or time-series data), by classes and sex, in school education.

Even though elaborate statistics are available, their present state is considered unsatisfactory both by official experts and private researchers. According to the *Expert Committee on Educational Statistics* the present situation is the following:

> "The existing arrangements for the collection, compilation and publication of educational statistics are unsatisfactory. The delays that occur render most statistics practically useless for planning purposes; the statistics that are collected do not provide sufficient information which can be used for formulating realistic educational programms for implementation; a meaningful analysis of even the information that is collected is seldom undertaken; and the way these are compiled leads to a large margin of error in educational statistics."[1]

It was further observed by the Expert Committee that the reason for the scant use made of much of the information being collected was, presumably, that they are not essential and relevant for policy and programme formulation.[2]

Similar views have been expressed in the *Fifth Five Year Plan Draft*. In discussing the problem of promoting education among the scheduled castes and the scheduled tribes, the following observation was made:

> "A major difficulty in assessing the progress of education among these sections of the population arises from the lack of firm data about their enrolment at the various stages of education beyond 1965-66 and the absence of sufficient number of in-depth studies about their educational status.[3]

Complaints about the defects of the educational statistics published in India have been raised by other agencies as well. For instance, in

[1]Government of India, *CABE Standing Committee Proceedings, June. 13, 1973*, Ministry of Education and Social Welfare, Delhi, 1973, p. 78.

[2]*Ibid*.

[3]Government of India, Planning Commission, *Fifth Five Year Plan Draft*, New Delhi, Part II, p. 205.

a recent study on *Educational Planning in India*, the following defects were pointed out:

> . . . the gaps in the educational statistics are serious; there are no serial data on enrolment by age and grade at the State level or on stagnation and wastages it is not known whether enrolment figures published relate to actuals on the date for which they are collected or to average attendance during the academic year; the relationship between parental occupation and pupil enrolment is practically non-existent.[4]

The Committee on Untouchability, Economic and Educational Development of the Scheduled Castes made the following statement in 1969:

> Much has been said about wastages involved in the education of the Scheduled Castes. However, the absence of detailed reliable data relating to the extent of stagnation and wastage at the various stages of education has limited the scope of making any thorough study of the problem. The Committee requested the Ministry of Education to collect data on the number of Scheduled Caste students enrolled in various categories of educational institutions. The Ministry was not in a position to furnish complete information state-wise as requested.[5]

The Committee which looked into the *Status of Women* in India has expressed their dissatisfaction with the educational statistics available in India in the following words:

> Since the quantum of grants for all educational institutions is linked to enrolment figures there is an inevitable tendency to attach undue importance to more enrolment. These statistics do not, however, indicate whether all children on a school register in fact attend school even for a short time.[6]

The reliability of the educational statistics in India has been called into question in other studies also.[7] We shall now turn to an examination of these aspects of the data—the process of collection, compilation and publication, the delays involved at each stage, the uses

[4]See M.K. Premi, *Educational Planning in India*, Sterling Publications (P) Limited, New Delhi, 1972, pp. 11-44.

[5]Government of India, *Report of the Committee on Untouchability, Economic and Educational Development of the Scheduled Castes*, New Delhi, 1969, p. 203.

[6]Government of India, *Towards Equality—Report of the Committee on the Status of Women in India*. Ministry of Education and Social Welfare, New Delhi, 1974, p. 225.

[7]See, (*a*) Amartya Sen, Agricultural Economic Research Centre, University of Delhi, New Delhi, *Primary Education in Rural India—Participation and Wastage* Tata-McGraw Hill Publishing Co. Ltd., New Delhi, 1971, p. 10.

(*b*) Amartya Sen, *The Crisis of Indian Education*, Lal Bahadur Shastri Memorial Lectures, 1970, (mimeo.) pp. 12-13.

(*c*) A.R. Kamat, *The Educational Situation*, People's Publishing House, New Delhi, 1973, p. 312.

made of the available data, and their adequacy and limitations – in some detail.

PROCESS OF COLLECTION AND PUBLICATION OF DATA

The main agency responsible for the collection of educational statistics in the country is the Ministry of Education, Government of India. Statistics are collected through state governments and the universities. Besides the Ministry, the Planning Commission, the National Council of Educational Research and Training (NCERT), and the Commissioner for Scheduled Castes and Scheduled Tribes are also engaged to a lesser extent than the Ministry in their collection and publication.

The Ministry of Education collects information as on March 31 every year. Till the end of 1975, the practice by Ministry was the following: At the state level data are collected by the Department of Education and the universities. Data on elementary school education (classes I to VII/VIII) collected by the respective schools are sent by the heads of institutions to the educational officer at the sub-district (taluk/tehsil) level who, in turn, pass them on, after scrutiny, to district educational officers. The heads of secondary schools and of the teacher training schools send the data relating to their respective institutions directly to the district officers. The district officers compile the data at the district level and send the consolidated returns to the state directorate. The directorate collects data directly from colleges and other departments under the state government. After scrutiny, the data received from the different sources are sent in consolidated form to the Ministry of Education. The universities collect data from their own departments and from the affiliated institutions, and send them in consolidated form directly to the Ministry of Education, with copies to the University Grants Commission.

From 1964-65 to 1974-75 the practice has been to compile the data in forms A, A1 and A2.

Form A is the main set of the data compiled at the state level and sent to the Ministry. The major items contained in this form were:

(*i*) institutions (for boys and for girls separately);
(*ii*) enrolment (age-wise, sex-wise and class-wise);
(*iii*) teacher (sex-wise and according to general qualification);
(*iv*) expenditure;
(*v*) education in rural areas; and
(*vi*) examination results.

Form A-1 contains data relating to scheduled castes and scheduled tribes. Information in the following items are included in this form:

(*i*) Number of students in attached hostels and residents in attached hostels:

(*ii*) Number of students receiving general education (collegiate) by courses, stages, and classes;

(*iii*) Number of students receiving professional and other education (collegiate) by courses and stages;

(*iv*) Number of students receiving general (school) education by classes;

(*v*) Number of students receiving professional, vocational, special or other education (school) by type of education; and

(*vi*) Scholarships, stipends, other financial concessions and freeships to students.

Form A-2 is designed to furnish information particularly relevant for planning purposes. The main items of information contained in this form are:

(*i*) pupil-teacher ratios, separately for primary, middle and high schools/sections,

(*ii*) number of teachers according to training, emoluments, age and sex in primary, middle and high schools/sections; and

(*iii*) progress of compulsory education;

(*iv*) number of Repeaters at the Elementary stage (Classes I to VII/VIII);

(*v*) number of villages with and without schools according to population.

From the above list of items it is clear that they together covered, on a census basis, a large number of important aspects of the formal education system in every state. This method of data collection has, however, been suspended recently in the light of the discussions made by the Central Advisory Board of Education.

The Committee of Experts on Educational Statistics, referred to earlier, which met in 1973, came to the conclusions that data collection in future should be of three types:

(*i*) data to be collected annually on census basis from institutions, which will include class-wise and sex-wise (but not age-wise) distribution of enrolment, and number of teachers (trained and untrained separately);

(*ii*) data to be collected annually on the basis of sample surveys; and (*iii*) data to be collected periodically (say, once in five years or so) comprising information on problems which have implications for the formulation of educational plans.

Subsequently, in February 1976, an all-India conference of state educational officers was held in New Delhi which gave approval to the conclusions drawn by the expert committee. In that conference, a decision was taken to vest the entire responsibility for compilation of data collected from the various institutions (including universities) with the state education departments. This decision was taken in the light of the fact that the existing system of collection and compilation of educational data was unsatisfactory.

The number of items on which information is collected has been, therefore, considerably reduced; the emphasis since February 1976 has been on the clearance of the backlog of educational statistics on a priority basis. Teams of officers from the Ministry of Education have been visiting the states for on-the-sport finalisation of the data in collaboration with state officials. Proformas for the regular collection of data are still being simplified and revised even though the earlier decision was to collect information, on the basis of revised forms from the first year of the fifth five-year plan. A decision has since been taken to start collection of data in revised forms only for the year 1976-77 onwards. The progress of the efforts to clear the backlog of statistics (that is, statistics upto the end of 1975-76) through collection of data in what are known among the officials of the statistics wings of the education departments as "arrear forms," is still in its early stages. It is understood that in most states in India, the last year for which data have been collected and submitted in "arrear forms" is 1972-73.

The Ministry of Education used to publish educational statistics mainly in two volumes: *Education India* Vol. I and *Education in India* Vol. II. Statewise data were published in Vol. I and national data in Vol. II. The last year for which these volumes have been published is 1965-66. In view of the long delay involved in their publication, periodical publication of provisional educational statistics (in mimeograph) on different aspects of the educational system was in practice during the last few years. Some such publications are listed below:

Provisional Educational Statistics in the States (1966-67); *Selected Educational Statistics* (1969-70 to 1970-71); *Educational Statistics at a Glance* (1970); *Expenditure Shown in the Annual Budgets of State Governments* (1970-71 to 1972-73).

The annual publication entitled *Education in the Universities in India* (containing information on the number of universities and their teaching departments, the number of colleges by type of education, enrolment, number of teachers; examination results; income and expenditure; etc.) was also being published by the Ministry of Education till 1968-69. From 1969-70 onwards its publication has been the responsibility of the University Grants Commission. The last year for which this publication was made is 1965-66.

The Ministry of Education has also published district-wise educational statistics for all states for 1965-66. Earlier, district-wise statistics for 1961 had been published by the National Council for Educational Research and Training (NCERT). In addtion to the data on enrolment, teachers and institutions, the district-wise data contain information on ratio of enrolment to population; proportion of trained teachers to the total number of teachers, and per capita expenditure on education.

Data collected by the NCERT

In 1957 the Ministry of Education conducted an all-India survey to identify "habitations" with and without schools with a view to planning the location of new schools, particularly in the rural areas. The report of the survey was published by the Ministry in 1960; separate reports were published also by different states.

The NCERT, which came into existence in 1961-62, has also been engaged in the collection and publication of educational data. Its main focus has, however, been the qualitative aspects of education. Among the publications by the NCERT relating to the quantitative aspects of educational system, the following are the most important: *The Indian Education Year Books,* and the *Report of the Second All-India Educational Survey* (1965).

The first year book published in 1961 is a review of the development of the educational systems in the various states from 1947 to 1961; the second year book (1964) dealt with both the quantitative and qualitative aspects of elementary (classes I to VII/VIII) education; the third year book (1967) was on problems of educational research, and does not contain much quantitative information.

The Second All-India Educational Survey conducted by the NCERT in December 1965 updated the results of the first survey, conducted in 1957, and collected some additional information as well. The enquiry was confined to school education. Information on school facilities, enrolment, number of teachers, etc., was collected and published in this survey.

We noticed earlier that the Central Advisory Board of Education and the Planning Commission felt that the available educational statistics were inadequate, for a variety of reasons, for purposes of educational planning. It was, therefore, decided that the NCERT should conduct a quick all-India educational survey with the following main objectives: (*i*) to make up-to-date the data collected in the first and the second educational Surveys, and (*ii*) to obtain data for educational planning in the fifth five year Plan and for taking decisions on educational policies.

The survey was intended to cover the entire field of education, both school and collegiate, in the country. The data to be collected were on enrolment by sex and age, number of teachers by qualification and experience, and subjects taught, number of educational institutions, physical facilities and expenditure by type and state of education, as on 31 December, 1973.

It is understood that this survey (The third All-India Educational[1] Survey) has been completed only in respect of school education, and that the survey of higher education is still in its early stages. On scrutiny of the final tables designed (53 categories of tables are designed) for presenting the data collected at the school education stage, it is seen that they include the following categories:

(*i*) Habitations according to the availability of schools within them;

(*ii*) Villages according to the scheduled caste and scheduled tribe population and educational facilities;

(*iii*) Habitations, villages and schools according to languages spoken, media of instruction, first language, second language and third language taught;

(*iv*) Schools according to introduction of work experience programme;

(*v*) Schools running on the shift system, having parent-teacher organisations;

(*vi*) Age-wise distribution of students in schools;

(*vii*) Distribution of pupils according to distance walked to attend school;

(*viii*) Distribution of schools having clubs and societies and according to activities of outsiders;

(*ix*) Number of pupils having text books;

(*x*) 'Other' schools;

(*xi*) Schools for the handicapped; and

(*xii*) Sources of income and pattern of expenditure of school.

From the above it is obvious that most of the information collected through this third survey would have been available had the annual returns in Forms A, A-1 and A-2 been collected regularly. It is also obvious that the data obtained from this survey (which, it is learnt, has been completed only for the school education stage), will not be of much service for educational planning during the fifth Plan of which more than half the period is already over by now.

The NCERT has also made several *ad hoc* studies on sample survey basis mainly on problems of wastage and stagnation in elementary education.[8]

Data Collected by the Planning Commission

Another agency which collects educational statistics on an *ad hoc* basis is the Planning Commission. For instance, in 1967 the Programme Evaluation Organisation of the Planning Commission conducted an all-India study on sample survey basis on the problems of "Extension of Primary Education in Rural Areas."[9] Occasionally it has also compiled and published them, for instance it published in 1969, *Selected Educational Statistics at a Glance*, which contained data upto 1967-68.[10]

Before passing on to a detailed examination of the coverage, uses and limitations of the available data, we may briefly refer to their reliability, particularly the reliability of data relating to primary school education.

The Reliability of Educational Statistics in India

In recent years doubts have been expressed by researchers on the reliability of the educational data, particularly those relating to primary education, published by the Ministry of Education. For instance, in a

[8]See, for instance, S N. Mukerjee, *Wastage and Stagnation in the Primary and Middle Schools in India*, NCERT, New Delhi, 1969.

[9]Planning Commission, Government of India, *Problem of Extension of Primary Education in Rural Areas*, Programme Evaluation, New Delhi, 1967.

[10]Government of India, Planning Commission, *Selected Educational Statistics at a Glance*, (Plan and Non-Plan). Education Division, Planning Commission, New Delhi, 1969.

study of *Primary Education in Rural India* conducted in 1967-68, the following observation is made: "much trust cannot be put on the Ministry's enrolment figures as representing the actual number of school students."[11] The observation was repeated in 1970[12] and in 1973.[13] The main weaknesses in the Ministry figures are reported to be the following:

(*a*) they contain an element of over-reporting, of more than 20 per cent;

(*b*) the degree of over-reporting varies from state to state;

(*c*) the highest degree of over-reporting is in the states which are educationally more backward; and

(*d*) over-reporting is larger in the case of girls than in the case of boys.

The criticism was based on a comparison of the enrolment figures for 1961 and the data on full time students in the age group 0-14 in the 1961 census. A careful examination of these two sets of data shows that discrepancy between them hardly works out to even 2.5 per cent (see Appendix 1).

There are, however, reasons to suspect that the enrolment data for primary classes are inflated to some extent, particularly in a few states. For example, the enrolment of boys, belonging to the age-groups 6-7 and 7-8 in Jammu and Kashmir, Tamil Nadu and Uttar Pradesh, and that in the age group 6-7 and 8-9 in Karnataka, seem to have been more than 100 per cent in 1968-69. This discrepancy could have been due, on the one hand, either to false reporting of age by pupils, or to errors in the estimation of the population in single age-groups or both. On the other hand, it could have arisen from an over-reporting of enrolment. In the absence of conclusive evidence, we are not however, in a position to draw any inference.

Delay in Publication

We have already noticed that the two publications of the Ministry of Education, (*Education in India,* Vols. I and II, *District-wise Educa-*

[11]Amartya Sen, Agricultural Economic Research Centre, University of Delhi, *Primary Education in Rural India—Participation and Wastage*, Tata-McGraw Hill Publishing Co. Ltd., New Delhi, 1971, p. 10.

[12]Amartya Sen, *The Crisis of Indian Education*, Lal Bahadur Sastri Memorial Lectures, 1970 (mimeo) pp. 12-13.

[13]A.R. Kamat, *The Educational Situation*, People's Publishing House, New Delhi, 1973, p. 312.

tional Statistics, and *Education in the Universities in India*) have not been published for any year since 1965-66. For later years, only provisional statistics are available. Educational data in summary form are available for the period till 1972-73 in the *Statistical Abstract of India* 1974 published by the Central Statistical Organisation. Thus, it is clear that long delays are involved at each stage—collection, compilation and publication.

Data Collected, but not Published

A significant shortcoming with the system of publication of statistics is that many items of information collected are never published. It is understood that data have been collected from the various states in Forms A, A-1 and A-2 for 1964-65 to 1970-71. In the publications by the Ministry of Education, many of the items of information contained in these forms are omitted. For instance, the age-wise, class-wise and sex-wise enrolment of students at all levels of education are collected from each State; the age-wise details are furnished, however, only in *Education in India*, Vol. II, which furnishes information for the country as a whole. Education—particularly school education—being a state subject, the educational policies for this stage are framed at the state level—policies for reducing the age heterogeniety of students enrolled in class I, reducing drop-out and stagnation rates, etc. For the formulation of policies for reducing the age heterogeniety of the class I cohort the crucial information required will be the current state of affairs in each state with regard to the age composition of the class I cohort.

Another information which is of great usefulness for planning is that on repeaters in each class. This information (which was collected for the years upto and including 1970-71) for the elementary stage (classes I to VII/VIII) is contained in Form A-2 (Table 4). Distribution of pupils in each of these classes is furnished according to the number of years spent. This item of information for any year which, if combined with the data on class-wise enrolment in that year and in the previous year could be used to calculate the transition ratios of pupils from class to class and to the rest of the economy. By such an exercise, it will also be possible to calculate the average drop-out and stagnation rates in each class at the elementary stage.

A very serious shortcoming of the data published for the states is that it gives enrolment figures only for each stage of education (like pupils in classes I to V, pupils in classes VI to VIII, and so on); publication of the class-wise (and age-wise) statistics of enrolment would have been much more useful for understanding the proportion of pupils entering the education system belonging to each age-groups in each class and the proportion attaining functional literacy etc. The lumping of enrolment figures for entire stages has led to serious misconceptions about the proportions of population in each age group enrolled in schools and about the educational progress that the different States have been making over the years.

USES AND LIMITATIONS OF THE PRESENT EDUCATIONAL STATISTICS

Educational statistics published in India are made use of mostly by the planning bodies both at the Centre and in the states. They are used to forecast future enrolment and expenditure as well as output of the educational system. Enrolment projections in the fifth Plan draft of the Planning Commission has given estimates for 1973-74 and targets for 1978-79 of the proportion of population in the age groups 6-11, 11-14, 14-17 and 17-23 who will be enrolled in primary, middle and secondary schools and in colleges respectively. One of the shortcomings of expressing enrolment in a stage of education as the proportion of the population in the relevant age groups (for example, enrolment in classes I to V are shown as enrolment of pupils in the age groups 6-11) is that the public, including researchers and sometimes planners too, lose sight of the fact that these two are entirely different propositions.

As an example, we wish to point out the analysis made on the basis of such mistaken notions, the recent study on *Primary Education in Rural India* in which enrolment in classes I to VIII is taken to be identical with enrolment of children in the age group 6-14.[14]

By lumping together enrolment at a stage of education, the planners also delude themselves into distorted notions of educational growth. For example, the increase in the proportion of enrolment in classes I to V to the population in the age group 6-11 is taken to be an index of the country's progress towards the realisation of the objective of universal enrolment at the primary stage. The Planning Commission has made the following statement in the fifth Plan draft: ". . . full time facilities will be provided for 97 per cent of the children in the age group 6-11 and 47 per cent in the age group 11-14 by the end of the

[14] *Primary Education in Rural India, op. cit.*

fifth Plan. . . . if these targets are realised in full, it should be possible to fulfil the constitutional obligation largely by the end of the Sixth Five-Year Plan."[15] Needless to point out, this is a misleading statement because, even if the total number of persons enrolled in classes I to V forms 100 per cent of the population in the age group 6-11, the number of pupils actually belonging to this particular age group attending primary school will be much less than and the bulk of the enrolment at the primary stage will be in the earlier classes, namely classes I and II, so that the proportion of those initially entering the system in class I who complete the minimum number of years of schooling required for gaining functional literacy will be much smaller still.

The constitutional obligation is clearly not to make the total enrolment in classes I to V (irrespective of the age composition of those enrolled) equal to the total population in the age group 6-11, but to ensure functional literacy to all children, which means that all the children belonging to each age group should complete at least four years of schooling. In fact, the constitutional obligation goes beyond this and stipulates seven to eight years of schooling to children belonging to each single age group.[16]

[15]*Fifth Five-Year Plan Draft*, *op. cit*, Part II, p. 194.

[16]The total enrolment in class IV and the enrolment of children belonging to the age group 10-11 in schools as percentage of population in the age group 10-11, and the enrolment of children belonging to the age group 6-11, as percentage of the population in the same age group, in 1968-69 are furnished below (all figures in percentage):

	Enrolment in class IV as proportion of population in the age group 10-11, 1968-69		*Enrolment in schools of children belonging to the age group 10-11, as proportion of population in the age group 10-11, 1968-69*		*Enrolment of children belonging to the age group 6-11 as percentage of population in the age group 6-11, 1968-69*	
	Boys	*Girls*	*Boys*	*Girls*	*Boys*	*Girls*
Andhra Pradesh	58	37	60	32	74	49
Assam	59	36	50	29	70	44
Bihar	44	13	51	13	69	23
Gujarat	72	42	77	45	75	46
Jammu & Kashmir	63	27	69	29	94	38
Karnataka	70	46	57	32	85	62
Kerala	113	107	88	74	95	86

The Planning Commission has calculated the dropout rates for the country as a whole, in the various classes at the school stages. Such calculations are made, however, by comparing the enrolment in the higher classes in the subsequent years with the enrolment in Class I in a given year.[17] This method of calculation is, obviously, defective for a variety of reasons: (*i*) the enrolment in class II and above in a year is determined by the size of enrolment in class I and the dropout and stagnation rates in the various classes during a period extending to a number of years immediately preceding the year of study; it will represent the actual extent of dropout only if enrolment in Class I over the years and the dropout and stagnation rates in the different classes were constant, and (*ii*) this method does not serve to estimate the rate of stagnation.

One of the consequences of the practice of making enrolment projections on the basis of inadequate and defective information is that in India the divergence between projections and performance has been widening over the years. For instance, the Census data placed in juxtaposition with the educational data for the period 1951-1971 show the following paradoxical results:

(*1*) the growth rate of literacy has been declining in India in recent years, though the growth rate of enrolment at the primary stage has been rising;

(*2*) the percentage of illiteracy among the lower age groups of the population has been showing tendencies of stabilising at a level of around 50 (40 among boys and 60 among girls);

(*3*) the rural-urban difference in literacy rates has been widening although the rate of enrolment at the beginning of the primary school in the rural areas has been as high as in the urban areas;

(*4*) the male-female differences in literacy rates have not been decreasing in the rural areas in spite of the fact that in rural areas

Madhya Pradesh	55	20	63	24	60	25
Maharashtra	86	49	87	58	72	50
Orissa	58	25	42	15	63	32
Punjab & Haryana	64	39	66	36	66	37
Rajasthan	53	17	65	17	65	21
Tamil Nadu	94	65	80	50	98	72
Uttar Pradesh	69	36	72	30	95	53
West Bengal	61	35	71	39	90	54

[17]See, *Selected Educational Statistics at a Glance* (Plan and Non-Plan) op. cit.

enrolment of girls in class I has been increasing at a faster rate than that of boys;

(*5*) the degree of inter-State variation in the level of literacy has not been narrowing down despite the fact that there have been special enrolment drives and large increase in expenditure on primary education in the educationally backward areas;

(*6*) the rates of dropout and stagnation have not fallen from their previous high levels;

(*7*) the enrolment of girls at the first year of the primary school is only about 40 of the total enrolment in that class; and

(*8*) the higher levels of education—particularly the tertiary level—are comparatively better developed in many States in which the base of the educational pyramid is narrow and the dropout rates are high;

We may note that none of the above paradoxes can be convincingly explained by looking at the type of enrolment projections contained in the several plan documents and the results of the many private researches made into this problem.

The poor state of information on the extent of dropout in the educational system of India and the wild guesses rendered possible as a result of such a state of affairs is reflected in statements like the following: "But in our system, the wastage averages around 60 per cent at all levels from the first standard to the post graduate. . . . This 60 per cent educational wasters are coterminus with the 60 per cent of our people living at or below the poverty line and 80 per cent of our school and college survivors come from the top 20 per cent of our middle and upper classes."

Such statements do not seem to be based on any careful analysis of data. The available evidence indicates, on the other hand, that even in states in which dropout rates are the highest in the early classes of school education they are much less in the higher classes. Further, there do exist wide differences among states, which are placed on comparable levels of per capita income and comparable degree of skewness in income distribution, with regard to dropout and stagnation rates at the various stages of education. Even granting that 80 per cent of the school and college survivors belong to the middle and upper income classes, the conclusion does not follow that, therefore the dropouts belong entirely to the lower income classes at the higher stages of school education and at the college education stage.

Another misconception, arising again from the paucity of relevant and adequate data seems to be that the state of illiteracy in the different states more or less corresponds with the rate of enrolment in primary schools. This statement is only partly true; it is seen that in some of the States which are the most illiterate, like Uttar Pradesh and Jammu and Kashmir, enrolment in class I is among the highest in India.[18]

Owing to the non-existence of reliable estimates on the rates of dropout and stagnation in the different classes at the stage of school education, it has not been possible for the planners to work out operationally meaningful estimates of the expenditure required for achieving the defined targets of educational development. In fact, the allocations of educational expenditure have been made by the rule of thumb both in the states and at the Centre. Occasionally, however, one comes across cost estimates of education worked out by multiplying the additional number of pupils proposed to be enrolled by the per pupil expenditure incurred due to dropout and stagnation, and expenditure incurred by private agencies.

[18]Enrolment in class I as percentage of population in the age group 6-7 and the percentage of literacy in the various States in India are shown below (all figures in percentage).

	Enrolment (of first year students) in class I as percentage population in the age group 6-7 (1968-69)			*Literacy rate (1971)*	
	Boys	*Girls*	*Men*	*Women*	*Persons*
Uttar Pradesh	106	112	31.8	10.2	21.6
Tamil Nadu	126	106	51.7	26.8	39.4
Jammu & Kashmir	153	70	26.4	9.1	18.3
Kerala	111	101	66.5	53.9	60.2
Maharashtra	118	89	51.3	26.0	39.1
Karnataka	103	89	41.9	20.8	31.5
Assam	113	77	37.7	18.9	28.8
Gujarat	113	71	46.12	24.6	35.7
Andhra Pradesh	113	73	33.3	15.7	24.6
West Bengal	103	69	42.8	22.1	33.1
Bihar	115	44	30.6	8.5	19.8
Rajasthan	121	37	23.7	5.8	18.8
Punjab & Haryana	96	54	Punjab 40.0	25.8	33.4
			Haryana 37.2	14.7	26.7
Orissa	87	54	38.4	13.8	26.1
Madhya Pradesh	92	39	32.8	10.8	22.1
INDIA	119	75	39.5	18.4	29.3

The present educational statistics do not provide information on the value of the physical capital already in existence in the educational system—in terms of land and buildings equipment and furniture, etc. This also constitutes an item of information essential for calculating per pupil costs at the different stages of education.

Shortcomings are also met within the several forecasts made by different agencies—both official and non-official—of the outturn of the educational system from its different stages in the different states. It should be obvious that estimates based on inadequate and defective understanding of the system in existence are not likely to yield realistic results in this direction either.

SUGGESTIONS

To simplify the process of data collection, it is desirable to divide the process into (*a*) annual collection and (*b*) periodical collection.

In the category (*a*) the following items may be included: (*i*) class-wise and sex-wise enrolment of students separately for all levels and types of education; (*ii*) the number of institutions (recognised and unrecognised separately) by level and type of education, with the number of classes, teachers (sex-wise) and pupils (sex-wise) in each; (*iii*) examination results separately for each examination and for boys and girls; and (*iv*) educational expenditure, item-wise and according to sources of funds.

The second category of statistics may be collected in more minute detail at longer intervals than a year. The purpose of this set of data should be the formulation of educational plans. For this purpose, it is necessary to obtain information on the pattern of flows—of students, teachers and finance—within the system and between the system and the rest of the economy. The statistics now being collected relate to a particular date of the year, March 31.

As we have shown in the exercise given in Appendix A, it is possible, by combining data on age-wise, class-wise and sex-wise, composition of students, to convert the stocks and into flows, if information is available on grade repetition, mortality, transfers, and readmission of pupils during the period between March 31 in a year and March 31 in the next year.

The practice which was in existence till recently was to collect age-wise, class-wise and sex-wise statistics on enrolment at all levels and types of education (in Form A); and to furnish the details of grade repeaters according to the number of years spent in each class and according to sex for the elementary school (classes I to VII/VIII, in Table 4, form A2). It is necessary to include in this Table information on the age of pupils as well. Further, instead of limiting this information to the elementary level, data may be collected for all levels and types of education. Examination, results may also be furnished by the year and month of the examination the class in which the examination is held, the age of students who pass, and their sex-wise distribution.

In India, no attempt has been made till now to collect information on mortality transfers and readmission of students. These items of information also may be collected according to class, age and sex for all levels and types of education. The two consecutive years for which such data are collected may be conveniently fixed as the first and second years of a five year Plan so that the calculations made on their basis could be made available by the end of the third year of that plan period when the process of preparing the plan for the next five year period will be underway. Information on the entry and exit of teachers at the various levels and in the different types of education, say, due to first appointment, promotions, retirement, and death, may also be collected so that flows of teachers could also be calculated. It should be possible on the basis of these two flows and of the flow of finance to prepare much more realistic plans than are prepared at present for educational development.

The responsibility for the collection, compilation and publication of these two sets of statistics may be vested primarily with the Ministry of Education. It is to be pointed out, however, that there should be a much higher degree of promptness in these aspects than has been evinced so far.

One of the frequent complaints of the officials of the state education departments has been that the state governments do not give funds even for typing or stencilling the educational data they process and the studies on educational planning they undertake. Since it is now the accepted national policy that the basic unit of planning should be the district, the state departments of education should be instructed to compile the data at the district level and publish them promptly for use by educational planners, both official and private. At the same time, it should be the responsibility of the Ministry of Education to publish all the information mentioned under categories (*a*) and (*b*) for each State. Educational statistics, however elaborate, aggregated at the national level for a country of India's dimensions will be, to say the least, totally unserviceable for the formulation of any realistic and operationally meaningful educational plans.

In addition to the above items of information—the responsibility for the collection of which may be assigned to the Ministry of Education—a lot more of information on the educational system will have to be collected—preferably through sample surveys—on a continuous basis. They will include items like the physical plant in education, the qualification, experience, training and emoluments of teachers, the parental background (occupational, educational, income, caste, etc.) of pupils, the structure of the educational system, the timing of schooling and the content of education. Ideally, the responsibility for the conduct of such surveys and the publication of their results should be vested with an institute like the NCERT. It is desirable to have a continuous programme of such surveys (on the lines of the surveys conducted by the NSS) each surveys concentrating on the specific topic of enquiry.

In the foregoing discussion we have not discussed the type of statistics other than the planning. It is obvious that without them—for example, the need (or demand) for personnel with levels and types of education and the availability of funds—educational planning cannot be attempted. A discussion of these and related questions will, however, take us beyond the scope of the present exercise.

Appendix I

Reliability of the Educational Statistics in India

In recent years certain doubts have been expressed by researchers on the Economics of Education about the reliability of the Ministry figures. For instance, in a study on Primary Education in Rural India conducted by the Delhi School of Economics during 1967-68, we come across the following statement: "trust cannot be put on the Ministry's enrolment figures as representating the actual number of school students.[19] Amartya Sen repeated the same assertion in 1970.[20]

[19]Agricultural Economic Research Centre, University of Delhi, (Amartya Sen, Honorary Director), *Primary Education in Rural India, Participation and Wastage*

The main weaknesses in the Ministry figures are reported to be the following:

(*a*) they contain an element of over-reporting, of more than 20 per cent;

(*b*) the degree of over-reporting varies from State to State;

(*c*) the highest degree of over-reporting is in the States which are educationally more backward; and

(*d*) Over-reporting is larger in the case of girls than in the case of boys.

These are indeed serious objections destroying much of the validity of exercises done on the basis of data supplied by the Ministry of Education. It is, therefore, necessary to examine whether the objections raised are in fact valid.

(1) *Disparity between the Ministry figures and the Census figures*

In the two studies cited, it is held that difference of 7.1 million pupils is observed for 1961 between the 1961 Census figures of fulltime students in the age group 0-14 and the Ministry of Education figures relating to pupils studying at the primary and middle school stages during 1960-61. The conclusion drawn after scrutiny of the two sets of data, is that the Ministry figures contain over-reporting to the tune of 20 per cent or more.

The above conclusion is arrived at on the implicit assumption that the 1961 Census figures relating to the number of students are more reliable than the Ministry figures. The validity of such an assumption is not, however, beyond doubt. When data are collected about age and occupational status in a vast country like India with its high degree of illiteracy and numerous diversities in social and economic characteristics and that too within a short period of a fortnight through the agency of untrained investigators as a small part of a much larger scheme of enquiry, errors of a not too insignificant magnitude are likely to creep in.[21] The age reporting is likely to be

(The McGraw-Hill Publishing Co. Ltd., New Delhi, 1971, p. 10.)

[20]Amartya Sen; *The Crisis in Indian Education*, Lal Bahadur Shastri Memorial Lectures, 1970 (Mimeo) pp. 12-13.

[21]Pravin Visaria, Employment and Unemployment in India : A review of selected Statistics in the *Report of the Committee of Experts on Unemployment Estimates* (Planning Commission, Government of India, 1970) p. 44.83.

particularly unreliable. The Census authorities have recognised the fact that an overwhelming majority of the informations on behalf of the households are illiterate. These individuals are said to have a tendency to report the age in some round number like 5, 10, 15.[22] Taking this possibility into account, the Census authorities smooth the figures using approved statistical techniques and publish the 'adjusted figures' along with the actual census count. In these circumstances, it is unreasonable to place too much faith on the accuracy of the estimate relating to the number of students belonging to the age group 0-14 furnished by the Census. In fact there is a good reason to doubt even the estimate of the total number of fulltime students as reported by the 1961 Census. It is well-known that the 1961 census definition of workers resulted in an upward bias in the number of persons reported as workers. Any person engaged in a seasonal activity such as agriculture, animal husbandry and household industries, who had worked for at least one hour a day throughout the greater part of the working season, was considered a worker. In the case of "regular employment in any trade, profession, service, business or commerce," any quantum of gainful work performed on any of the fifteen days preceding the data of enumeration would entitle him to be classified as worker. As a result of the adoption of such definition, the magnitude of non-worker population according to the 1961 Census was smaller than that obtained from alternative estimates. It is therefore also likely that many children in the age group 0-14, who might have been involved along with other members of the family in the dominant activity of agriculture in rural areas were classified by the Census as workers. The number of fulltime workers in the age group 0-14, as reported by the Census was 14.5 million. The Census category of 'fulltime students' who, it may be noted, are one of a large number of divisions among non-workers. Since the over-reporting of 'workers' implies, *ipso facto*, as under reporting of 'non-workers' the division 'fulltime students' would also be, in all probability, an underestimate.

The foregoing discussion is not intended, however, to advance the point of view that the figures supplied by the Ministry of Education are not over-estimates. It is possible that they are. Some of the reasons have been mentioned in the Delhi University study referred to earlier: In many States, there are compulsory education laws and sometimes

[22] *Primary Education in Rural India*, op. cit. p.6.

the Government's assistance and subsidy for expansion of lower elementary education is linked with the growth of enrolment at the lower elementary stage.[23]

Fortunately we do not have to argue about the cooperative reliability of these two sources of information on a *priori* grounds. A careful examination of the two sets of data would show that discrepancies of the magnitude indicated in the two studies referred to earlier (that is around 20 per cent) do not in fact exist between them.

(*a*) *The Ministry figures*

The total enrolment at the elementary stage in India, in 1961, according to the Education Ministry, was 41.7 millions. This figure constitutes the total number of children in the lower primary and upper primary (or higher primary or the middle school) stages of education; it does not constitute the number of children in the age group 6-14 since large number of children below the age of six and above the age of fourteen are also found at the elementary (i.e. lower primary plus upper primary) stage of education in India. This is a fact which has been repeatedly pointed out in a number of studies. For instance, the report of the Second All India Education Survey says: "The enrolment in Classes I to V constitute 74.36 per cent of the estimated population in the age group 6 to 10. It is necessary to clarify this statement.*As is generally misunderstood this does not imply that 74.35 per cent of the children of the age group 6⁺ to 10⁺ are attending school.* What this statement implies is that the enrolment in classes I to V is 74.36 per cent of the estimated population in the age group 6⁺ to 10⁺. The enrolment also includes children from age group below and above this range." Further, the enrolment in classes VI to VIII is equal to 30.15 per cent of the estimated population in the age group 11⁺ to 13⁺ . . . . . *This should not be interpreted to mean that 30.15 per cent of the population in the age group 11⁺ 13⁺ are enrolled in classes VI to VIII.* What it implies is that the total enrolment in classes VI to VIII irrespective of the age of every child, is equal to 30.15 per cent of the estimated population in the age group 11⁺ to 13. Table 1. reproduced from "*Education in India, 1963-64*" published by the Ministry of Education gives the order of magnitude of the children in the appropriate age group and those below and above

[23]*Primary Education in India, op. cit.* p. 11.

TABLE 1—*Pupils belonging to the age groups below 6, 6 to 11 and 11 to 14 in India in Classes I to V, 1957-58 to 1962-63*

Year	*Enrolment in Classes I to V (in lakhs)*			*Pupils below 6 and above 11 in classes I to V (in lakhs)*			*Percentage of pupils below 6 and above 11 in classes I to V (in lakhs)*		
	Boys	*Girls*	*Total*	*Boys*	*Girls*	*Total*	*Boys*	*Girls*	*Total*
1957-58	194.04	87.66	281.70	46.14	18.20	64.34	23.8	20.8	22.8
1958-59	210.15	97.42	307.57	48.68	19.46	68.14	23.2	20.0	22.2
1959-60	222.96	105.24	328.19	51.66	21.41	73.07	23.2	20.2	22.3
1960-61	234.68	113.47	348.15	54.00	23.05	77.05	23.1	20.3	22.1
1961-62	259.84	131.18	391.62	60.45	27.14	87.69	23.3	20.8	22.4
1962-63	276.37	142.35	418.72	63.73	29.58	93.31	23.1	20.8	22.3

Source: Government of India, Ministry of Education, *Education in India 1962-63*, (Publication No. 706, Delhi 6. 1968, Vol. I., Table CL) p. 239.

this group in classes I to V during the six years from 1957-58 to 1962-63.

The total enrolment of children, in classes I to VIII and belonging to the age group 6-14 in the different States in 1961 is furnished in Table 12 (pages 673 and 674) of the *Second Indian Year Book of Education, 1964*. Out of the total enrolment of 41.7 millions in classes I to VIII only 36.3 belonged to this age group, 3.0 million being below 6 years and 2.4 million above 14 years of age. However, if we want to find out the total number of pupils in this age group attending classes I to VIII, the total enrolment in pre-primary schools and the number of pupils in secondary schools who are less than 14 years of age. These two items are furnished in the supplementary Volume II of the Report of the Education Commission. According to this document, there were 178,642 pupils in the pre-primary Stage (see page 11) and 496, 635 pupils in secondary schools (see page 26) who were below 14 years of age in 1961. Thus we get the total number of pupils below 14 years of age in 1961 attending various stages of education according to the Ministry of Education.

Children in the age group 6-14 attending classes I to VIII	:	36.3 million
Children below the age 14 attending secondary schools	:	0.5 million
Children below 6 years of age attending primary schools	:	3.0 million
Children attending pre-primary schools	:	0.2 million
Total	:	40.0 million

These discrepancies may be due either to under-reporting of the number of students in the 1961 Census (for reasons explained earlier) or to over-reporting in the Ministry figures (for reason attributed in the Delhi University study on Primary Education in Rural India). In the absence of more accurate information it is not right to trace errors in estimation wholly to one or the other to place the source of the discrepancy of these two sources of data.

(*b*) *Discrepancy between the estimates of the Ministry of Education and of the Planning Commission.*

Amartya Sen has mentioned that discrepancies are also found between the estimates of the Ministry of Education and of the Planning Commission regarding the percentage of enrolment in the lower primary stage of education to the population in the relevant age group. He points out that, according to the Draft Fourth Five-Year Plan, the percentage of enrolment in 1960-61 was 62, while it was only 55 according to the Report of the Education Commission. One obvious reason for differences, it is noted, is that the Planning Commission gives the enrolment ratio for classes I to V, whereas the Education Commission figures refer to classes I to IV. Since this should have made the Planning Commission ratio lower rather than higher. Sen seeks the explanation elsewhere and finds it in the definition of "what is called pre-primary class," and "what is called Class I in primary education." According to him, "the Education Commission classified the earliest year or two as pre-primary in the States with 11 year or 12 year schooling, while the Planning Commission does not drew any firm conclusion from this line of thought since he concludes that the matter can be settled only after checking the exact content of education in the early school years in the long schooling States about which no definite study exists.

(c) *Census figures*

According to the 1961 Census, the total number of fulltime students among non-workers in the age group 0-14 is 34.6 million. Workers reported in this age group numbered 14.5 million: it is possible that a sizeable proportion of this group were also attending school. If we accept the estimate of 4.4 millions for the latter (this is upper limit suggested in the Delhi University study on Primary Education in Rural India) the number of students in the age group of 0.14 comes to 39.0 millions.

(d) *Discrepancy*

The discrepancy between the two sets of data is thus reduced to 1.0 million. If we compare the number of fulltime students among non-workers as reported by the 1961 Census, and the number of students in the age group 6-14 attending the elementary stage of education as reported by the Ministry of Education (36.3 millions) the discrepancy is 1.7 million; it will also seen from Table 2 that the Union Ministry figures are lower than the Census figures for a few States like Assam, Kerala, Orissa and the Punjab.

TABLE 2—*Estimated Number of Students under 14 years of age, 1961*

States	*Ministry of Education figures of students in the age group 6-14 attending the elementary stage of education in 1961*	*1961 Census figures fulltime students among non-workers in the age 0-14*	*Differences*
1	*2*	*3*	*4*
Andhra Pradesh	2,979.5	2,549.4	+430.1
Assam	1,039.3	1,101.0	− 61.7
Bihar	3,224.2	2,780.9	+243.3
Gujarat	2,098.1	2,060.6	+ 37.5
Jammu & Kashmir	245.3	184.6	+ 60.7
Kerala	2,854.8	2,901.8	− 47.0
Madhya Pradesh	2,003.2	1,804.7	+198.5
Madras	3,551.2	3,552.6	+198.5
Mysore	2,216.9	2,175.9	+ 41.0
Maharashtra	4,107.5	3,933.6	+173.9
Orissa	1,193.4	1,381.1	+187.7
Punjab	1,638.2	1,840.3	−202.1
Rajasthan	1,130.8	1,072.1	+ 58.7
Uttar Pradesh	4,401.8	3,609.4	+792.4
West Bengal	3,148.7	3,023.3	+125.4
INDIA	36,342.2	34,595.8	+ 1746.4

On a close examination of the percentage figures supplied by the Education Commission and by the Planning Commission, one does not find the discrepancies pointed out by Sen. In the supplementary Vol. II of the Report of the Education Commission, enrolment in Classes I to IV in 1960-61 is given as 68.9 per cent of the population in the age group 6-9 and in class I to V as 62.4 per cent of the population in the age group 6-10 (p.16). In the *Draft Fourth Five-Year Plan,* enrolment in classes I to V in 1960-61 is given as 62.2 per cent of the population in the relevant age group (pp. 329-330). This clearly shows that the educational data published by the different official sources in India fairly tally with one another.

Gaps in Educational Statistics

R. K. BHANDARI*

The importance of statistics for efficient administration, policy decisions and successful planning can hardly be over-emphasized; but the need of accurate and timely collection of educational statistics is still greater because it involves an element of human resources vital for national development. In education we do not need only current data on any reference data, but also projected data for perspective planning, because planning of human resources is long-term. What we need is not only stock educational statistics but also flow statistics, demographic projections, manpower requirements and other related economic and social indicators with a view to linking educational development with the economic and social development of the country.

The explosion of population coupled with explosion of knowledge on one hand and the democratic aspirations of the people on the other has put the present educational system under a great strain; and the task of eduactional administrators and educational planners has become more difficult, particularly in the present difficult position of financial resources in the country. Our country cannot afford to prepare plans with unrealistic targets, or plans which do not utilize the resources optimally.

For this, the first requirement is availability of adequate basic statistics which, then, must be analyzed and used most effectively for formulating educational plans. In every aspect of planning, which is indeed a powerful instrument of development, you need statistics. There are statistics needed to determine the goals which can be realistically aimed; statistics of different types are required for formulating the plans. When it comes to implementation of plans, again a great deal of information and data of proper realiability and speed

*Statistics Unit, Ministry of Education and Social Welfare, New Delhi.

are necessary. Implementation has to be monitored and project execution made more efficient by a feedback process which has its own requirement of data, having the characteristics of speed, accuracy and comprehensiveness. It is seen that planning in its comprehensive sense is a complex interconnected process in which statistics play a major role, although they never appear to be too conspicuous.

Apart from the importance and need of statistics for the purpose of planning, educational statistics are needed even for running efficiently the day-to-day administration of the educational system in the country. The statistics required for administration are broadly grouped under: (*a*) institutions, (*b*) enrolment, (*c*) teachers and other personnel, (*d*) equipment and buildings, and (*e*) finances.

The collection of up-to-date data even on these few items is quite a heavy and complicated task in our country, which has a large student population and decentralized democratic system of education involving multiple bodies and agencies managing educational institutions. But all the same, it is necessary to collect educational data for running the educational system efficiently.

Historical Reviews

The systematic collection of educational statistics began with the report of the Indian Education Commission (1882). This document, with its appendices, contains very valuable statistical data on the growth of education in India after the middle of the 19th century. In subsequent years, reports on educational statistics were collected and published in the quinquennial reviews of the 'Progress of Education in India' for 1886, 1892-97 to 1932-37 and the decennial review 1937-47. Since 1913-14, annual statistics also began to be collected and published.

The main difficulty with the statistics of the pre-independence period is that the area covered by them varies from time to time—up to 1937 the statistics of India included British-Burma. Educational statistics of some erstwhile princely states were included till 1911-12, and were totally discontinued with effect from 1916-17. Owing to these changes in the area covered, the statistics of this period are not strictly comparable. Nor do they cover the entire country at any time.

In the post-independence period, Form 'A', which was introduced in 1949-50, is the most significant landmark and contained the most comprehensive and complete set of statistics ever collected in India.

Educational statistics in this form began to be collected annually and published with appropriate analysis in *Education in India*, Vol. I & II, which is the most important publication of the Ministry of Education and Social Welfare. With the adoption of this form, the distinction between annual and quinquennial educational statistics disappeared. But the annual data collected in Form 'A' was more comprehensive than that collected quinquennially before independence.

The statistics of the British period as well as the Form 'A' of 1949-50 were designed essentially to assess the progress of education in India. With the adoption of planning in 1951, the situation changed completely, and the system of educational statistics evolved in the past appeared to suffer from two main defects: (*i*) the data collected were rather too inadequate and lacking in a good deal of significant information, and (*ii*) there was generally a very long time-lag, about three to four years, between the date to which the statistics related and their publication. These deficiencies seriously reduced the utility of these statistics for purposes of educational planning and day-to-day administration.

The Ministry of Education, therefore, made the first exercise in revising Form 'A' in 1957-58, and a new form was designed which covered much larger ground. The new form was discussed with the state governments, but it could not be adopted for two main reasons—first, fearing that the adoption of the new form would further increase the time-lag in the publication of educational statistics, and second, state governments felt that they would not be able to collect the data in the new form unless the staff of their statistical units was substantially increased. The matter was, therefore, shelved.

Towards the end of the Second Plan, however, the subject was taken up again in the first national seminar on educational statistics, held in September 1962. The seminar examined the whole problem in detail and on the basis of these discussions the following principles were adopted for the revision of Form 'A'.

(*a*) The total volume of educational data required should be divided into Form 'A', Form 'A-1', Form 'A-2' and periodical studies and the compilation of the data should be staggered over the whole year.

(*b*) The new Form 'A' should contain the minimum essential data which would be broadly comparable with that now collected in the existing Form 'A'.

(*c*) Form 'A-1' should contain the essential educational data in respect of children of scheduled castes and scheduled tribes, as those are badly needed for planning the educational development of the weaker sections of the country.

(*d*) Form 'A-2' should contain the supplementary data which is needed for purposes of planning and studies.

These new forms were accepted by the states and were introduced from the collection year 1964-65. The scope and coverage of collection of data in education was much enlarged and included, *inter alia*, all the details of educational institutions by managements; the number and enrolment of attached classes and departments; enrolment by type of institutions and level of instruction with break up of courses at different levels and ages, etc.; expenditure both by sources of income and by objects or details of items on which it was spent, teachers both by type of institutions in which they were employed and the level at which they were teaching; the output by courses of examinations at various levels; institutions located in rural areas and details of scholarships; stipends, etc.

Besides these essential items on which data was collected in Form 'A' and 'A-1,' relevant data began to be collected in Form 'A-2' relating to some of problems of qualitative improvements in education—wastage and stagnation. Teachers by qualifications and age-groups, attached classes and departments to various institutions, single-teacher schools, age group composition of school classes etc.

These revised forms remained in force from 1964-65 till 1975-76. Of course, some modifications were introducted from time to time as recommended by the national seminars or conferences of educational statistics held periodically to review the position.

Present Position

While the idea of collecting information in these comprehensive forms was a laudable one, the present administrative set-up and machinery for collection of educational statistics in the states could not cope with the heavy task involved in the collection of educational statistics in these forms. The collection of statistics in these forms fell into arrears, and the time-lag in the collection of educational statistics increased tremendously. It was seriously felt that in the day-to-day administration of the educational system as well as for formulating annual plans, some vital statistics should be made available with a minimum time-lag so that they may serve the purpose for which they are collected. It is because of this situation that the sixth national conference on educational statistics was convened in September 1975 to consider, *inter alia,* the revision of these forms with a view to designing some simple forms containing a minimum number of items for collecting data on census basis.

As per recommendation of this conference, the forms were totally revised and introduced from 1976-77. The data proposed to be collected in the revised forms include the number of educational institutions, enrolment therein by type of institutions as well as by levels of education, the number of teachers by qualifications and type of institutions, and the income and expenditure data. To reduce the time-lag, the revised schedules have been bifurcated into three parts—(*i*) to collect data on institutions, enrolment and teachers, (*ii*) to collect financial data, and (*iii*) to collect examination results. A time-schedule has been prepared to collect these data according to the convenience of the source from which it is collected, and according to the time by which these data can be made available by the primary sources. It is hoped that with the introduction of these simplified forms, some current data will be available for the use of educational administrators and planners.

With the decision to collect some minimum data in the revised schedules, the centre has not forsaken the idea of collecting mass data required for micro-planning, perspective planning and research studies. These data will, however, be collected with a periodicity of 3 to 5 years, according to needs, and also on a sample basis. A standing committee on educational statistics at the national level has been set up to advise the Ministry of Education and Social Welfare on collection of educational statistics as well as in deciding the items on which the data is to be collected.

Machinery for the Collection of Educational Statistics

Education is a state subject, but the Central government is responsible for planning, coordinating and guiding educational activities in the country. To discharge this responsibility, the Centre has to collect the necessary data in respect of educational institutions spread all over the country.

Now, in a country like India (with a large area and population, with nearly seven lakhs recognised educational institutions of different types, and under different management and control), it becomes difficult to centralise the collection of these data.

Further, the state governments, who have to administer their educational institutions, also need more or less similar data. So, in consultation with state governments, the Centre has designed comprehensive schedules for the collection of the data. The main sources of supply is, therefore, the states and Union Territories. Besides, data are also collected from universities and colleges relating to higher education.

For collection of the educational data from the primary source—the educational institutions—state governments have established statistical units in the offices of the directorates of public instruction/education. The Centre has liaison with these units. These units are normally headed by a statistical officer or an assistant director of education, and have a small contingent of investigators/statistical and other ministerial staff, according to the requirements. Complementary staff is supposed to exist at the district level in the offices of the district education officers of various states. This staff is supposed to collect and consolidate statistics in respect of their districts for onward transmission to the state statistical units. In some states some staff is working at the block/taluk level for the collection and consolidation of the educational data in respect of primary and middle schools.

Starting from the educational institutions and before reaching the national level, educational data have to pass through a long channel. The different authorities in between have to handle them in varying degrees, according to their responsibilities. A part of the data is collected by statistical units at the state level, while the rest are collected at the district or taluk level. In a few states, there is an additional office between the district office and the state headquarters, called the regional or the divisional office. This office shares responsibilities with either the district office or the head office or both.

Although the procedure of collection of educational data in states differs, generally the following is adopted at different stages of collection:

A set of basic proformae for the collection of information from various categories of educational institutions, is designed by the Centre on the basis of the main forms of collection—so far known as Forms 'A', 'A-1' and 'A-2' and now ES I, ES II, ES III, ES IV. The institutional proformae are printed by the state Governments (in local languages in case of primary schools) and supplied to the institutions.*

To the universities and colleges, and institutions under the control of other Departments such as Health, the proformae are supplied by the state headquarters (previously it was supplied by the Centre), to high/higher secondary schools by district offices and to elementary schools (primary and middle) by block/taluk offices. Generally the authorities responsible for the supply of blank proformae are responsible for the collection and compilation of information. An up-to-date list of institutions is maintained by the respective agencies every year for the supply of blank proformae to ensure cent-percent coverage. While the block/taluk authorities send the consolidated information to the district authorities, the district authorities in turn add the information collected by them and send the consolidated information to the state headquarters who, in turn, consolidate the information for the state as a whole, fill them into national forms, and supply them to the Centre (Ministry of Education).

A full-fledged division of statistics and planning exists at the Centre, which is responsible mainly for the collection, consolidation and publication of educational statistics at the national level on the one hand and the formulation of the five-year and annual plans of the Centre and the states, and their analysis, etc., on the other. Two deputy directors, five research officers/assistant education officers and about 25 investigators/statistical assistants, besides the ministerial staff, are manning the division.

*FORM E.S. I relates to selected basic information about all types of educational institutions, enrolment by type of institutions and by level/stages of education, teachers by type of institutions and institutions in rural areas etc.

(*Ref. date is 30th Sept.*)

FORM E.S. II relates to similar information in brief about studies belonging to scheduled castes and scheduled tribes.

(*Ref. date is 30th Sept.*)

In FORM E.S. III information about Income by sources and expenditure on various items incurred by various educational institutions is collected.

(*Ref. date is 31st March*)

In FORM E.S. IV information about selected important Final Examination conducted by Universities and Boards of Examinations is collected.

(*Ref. date is all examination conducted during the year under report*)

SCOPE AND COVERAGE OF EDUCATIONAL STATISTICS

The growing needs of our educational administrators and planners have created a great problem for the decision with regard to the coverage and scope of collection of statistics. On the one hand the need is growing for more and more statistics, on the other the time involved in the collection of data becomes more and more with the increase in the number of items on which the data are to be collected. The answer again revolves around the provision of a complementary machinery required for collection. Considering the constraint resources of the country, it may perhaps be difficult to build such a large-scale machinery. The task of the educational statistician in deciding the scope of cellection of statistics within the limited means thus becomes difficult. He is to decide whether he is to collect the details of all types of institutions existing in the country, or on a selected few, according to minimum needs. Again, he is to decide whether the information required by the administrator will be forthcoming within the time-schedule. He will then have to report to the administrator the type of information that he could collect within the present infrastructure and within the time-limit and it is on the basis of the decision of the administrator that he will decide the scope and coverage of his collection.

Educational statistics are needed for (*a*) educational administration (*b*) educational planning, and (*c*) educational research. The requirements of all these using agencies are important, pressing and voluminous. Considering the practical situation of limited financial resources and infrastructure, the educational statistician is to draw priorities of items on which the data are to be collected. Even in the limited scope of the collection of educational statistics required for day-to-day administration, detailed data is to be collected in respect of (*a*) educational institutions, (*b*) enrolment, (*c*) teachers and other personnel, (*d*) equipment and building, and (*e*) finances. The collection of the data on these items is vital.

Apart from annual data collection programmes of the Ministry of Education, the all-India educational surveys carried out by the NCERT are another source of educational data. The first and the second surveys were carried out in 1956-57 and 1965-66, and the third survey is in progress (at time of writing). In this survey, detailed data on institutions, teachers and students, etc., are collected on complete enumeration basis. In the third survey, some 24 schedules have been canvassed by the NCERT, and data on practically all aspect of education have been collected. Even pre-primary schools, coaching institutions, schools for physically handicapped, schooling facilities for tribal areas, non-formal education programmes, educational finances, technical education and higher education have been covered.

Gaps in the Collection of Educational Statistics

Although a good deal of data are being collected annually, there are several important items which are not covered in the regular data collection programme. Some of the items on which statistics should be collected but are not collected are as follows:

(*a*) *Data on non-formal education.* These days, when there is a considerable emphasis on out-of-schools education, partly because of the limited capacity of schools to accommodate the increasing number of students and partly because of the suitability of this type of education for working classes, many programmes of non-formal education are being offered in various states. These include, *inter alia*, correspondence courses and evening courses. It is important to collect adequate data for all courses and programmes of non-formal education.

(*b*) *Data on flow students in the school system.* At present data collected on students and teachers give us stock statistics only. The flow statistics, which help in finding out what percentage of students repeat grades or drop out from the school, or go to different streams each year, are not available. Such flow statistics are required to be collected for educational planning and evaluation studies.

(*c*) *Data on average daily attendance.* A few ad-hoc studies suggest a big gap between enrolment and the average daily attendance for which the data is not collected regularly. Collection of this data is extremely important for planning and diagnosis of the faults of the educational system.

(*d*) *Data on unrecognised institutions.* Large number of standard, unrecognised institutions provide educational facilities in big cities and towns, but no account of them is taken while assessing the extent of educational facilities in the country and expansion of education. The collection of data about these institutions is, therefore, important.

(*e*) *Data on private expenditure on education.* At present no data are collected about the expenditure incurred by students or parents on education. This information is vital to work out the actual cost of education.

(*f*) *Data on health and home back-ground of children.* No data on this subject are available. It is important to study why some children show poor performances in schools in spite of having normal intelligence, and highlighting other needs of the children which possibly require greater attention than their education.

(*g*) *Data on utilisation of existing facilities.* These data, essential for planning, are not collected. These data will be helpful in nationalisation of the existing facilities and optimum utilisation of the scarce resources.

(*h*) *Data on attrition rate of teachers.* From the data at present collected about teachers, it is not possible to know how many teachers leave their jobs each year for various reasons; this is required for balancing the demand and supply of teachers.

(*i*) *Administrative and non-teaching staff.* These data, though easy to collect, are not at present included in the annual schedules. The collection of the data on this item, with all details of salaries, qualification, etc., is necessary for manpower planning.

(*j*) *Data on ancillary services.* Data on extra-curricular activities, midday meals, transportation of students, health-care centres, sports and other youth welfare activities, which are vital for planning and administrative purposes, are not at present collected. It is necessary to collect these data once in 2 or 3 years, if not annually.

Besides the above gaps, some details of the data so far collected have been dropped from the new forms introduced from 1976-77 with a view to reducing the time-lag in collection. These will, however, be taken care of when the Ministry of Education decides to collect comprehensive data on different aspects of education either once in 3 or 5 years or on sampling basis.

DEFICIENCIES AND PROBLEMS OF COLLECTION OF EDUCATIONAL STATITICS

Apart from the gaps in the data collection stated above, the deficiencies which have been pointed out time and again by various people, and which happen to be a major handicap in the utilisation of statistics for planning, administration and research purposes, can be briefly listed as follows:

(*i*) *Time-lag.* There is a considerable time-lag in the collection and publication of educational statistics, which is mainly due to the existence of inadequate machinery in states for the collection and compilation of educational statistics. The institutional, proformae are not printed and supplied in time to institutions, nor are these collected according to time-schedule at the block/taluk and District, levels. Either the exclusive staff for this work does not exist at these levels, or they are not trained. All these factors result in the present time-lag.

(*ii*) *Unreliability of data.* The reliability of data on some items is questionable. Age-wise data are not accurately compiled, nor is a proper record maintained. Enrolment figures of primary schools particularly in rural areas are inflated. Income and expenditure data from private institutions are generally not very reliable. Adequate arrangements do not exist for scrutiny and reconciliation of the data at almost all levels of the collecting agencies.

(*iii*) *Lack of data for micro-planning.* Data on strategic plan programmes are not adequately collected to help monitoring and evaluation of plan programmes and for perspective planning.

(*iv*) *Inconsistencies in data from different sources.* Data on more or less similar items are at present collected by the Ministry of Education, the UGC and the NCERT (educational surveys). The data produced by these three agencies do not tally—serious inconsistencies are found which make it difficult for users; planners particularly find it difficult to formulate enrolment targets based on the variety of figures produced by these different agencies.

Suggestions for Improvement

Following are some suggestions for improvement in the collection of statistics:

(*i*) *Reduction of time-lag.* The time-lag in the collection and consolidation of statistics upto district level, which is the main problem, can be reduced by according due priority to this work and provision of necessary staff at the block and district levels. Further, the channel through which data at present travel from institutions up to the state headquarters should be reduced. With the creation of different directorate of various types of education in the states, agencies collecting data at the state headquarters are also being multiplied. This is a retrograde step and is against the recommendation of the seminars and conferences on educational statistics. Inadequacy of staff is the main reason of the time-lag and should therefore be removed.

(*ii*) *Reliability of data.* Data can become reliable if coverage is complete and inconsistencies and comparability are thoroughly checked at all levels of collection and consolidation. To ensure this, adequate and trained staff is required. Data should be scrutinised according to instructions given in the 'Manual of Educational Statistics', and discrepancies removed before consolidation. The staff appointed for this work has to be trained periodically to ensure reliability of data.

(*iii*) *Better coordination.* Collecting agencies should establish coordination in the collection work. The differences in the reference data and the concepts and definitions of the terminologies used in forms should be removed. As far as possible, responsibility of collection work should be demarcated.

(*iv*) *Periodical collection and Sample Survey.* A programme should be drawn up to collect information on items not at present attended to, either periodically, with a gap of 3 to 5 years, or on sampling basis, to remove the gaps in the collection of educational statistics.

Improving Educational Statistics

TRILOK N. DHAR*

Information—statistical and other—is essential for making well-informed decision. Intuitive judgements of significant individuals, based on personal experiences, may have some significance in situations where the variables involved are limited, time horizon not too distant, and the scale of operations somewhat narrow. The alternative use of resources, determination of priorities, formulation of projects to fulfil the designated goals and evaluation of performances are all complicated processes and require considerable inputs of information. Educational planning requires information which is both qualitative as well as quantitative. The planners and the administrators need information to determine the extent to which educational benefits are reaching the designated groups and fulfilling the specified objectives. Information also allows a timely correction of the distortions that occur in the implementation of projects.

Agencies for Collection of Educational Statistics

A number of organizations collect and publish educational and other statistics which are used, in one form or the other, in educational planning. These organizations or agencies can broadly by categorized into (*a*) those which are directly involved in educational decision-making, and collect facts and figures about the educational system as part of their regular function; and (*b*) those which are not involved in any educational function but collect information which is utilised in educational planning.

Some of the agencies falling in the first category include the Ministry of Educatian and Social Welfare, the University Grants

*Joint Director (Education), Planning Commission, New Delhi.

Commission, the Education Division of the Planning Commission, National Council for Educational Research and Training, and the State Education Departments; those which fall into the second category include the Registrar-General's Office, the Directorate General of Employment and Training, and National Sample Survey.

A brief description of the type of educational statistics, that the organizations of the first category collect and report, follows:

(*i*) *The Ministry of Education and Social Welfare*. This is the main agency which collects, compiles and publishes educational statistics in India. The statistics reported are varied and voluminous. Apart from the data on institutions, enrolments, teaching personnel and expenditures, the Ministry's publications provide information on the changes that have taken place over the years and also on qualitative indices like the proportion of children attending schools, percentage of trained teachers, pupil-teacher ratios etc. Most of the information is collected on its behalf by the state governments on a census basis, from educational and training institutions, which numbered over 700,000 in 1974-75. Although firm statistical data become available after a considerable lapse of time, the Ministry of Education brings out "provisional" statistics which are generally up-to-date although confined to selected items. The delay in the availability of firm statistics reduces their utility considerably. The Ministry of Education also brings out analysis of State and Central budgets, a directory of institutions of higher education, prevalent salary scales, fees charged in various types of institutions, educational structure and so on.

(*ii*) *Planning Commission*. Educational statistics in the Planning Commission are the responsibility of the education division. Apart from five-year plan projections, information is obtained from the states annually on selected items like enrolments at various stages of education, institutions of various types, teaching personnel and so on. The states are also required to indicate the expenditnre incurred or likely to be incurred on specific educational programmes. The statistical information asked from the states is generally future-oriented in the sense that the emphasis is on finding out what the State propose to do although statistics indicating the base-year position is also obtained.

(*iii*) *University Grants Commission*. This organisation collects information from universities and colleges. The main statistical publication of the Commission is *University Development in India*—Basic Facts and Figures. Its annual reports to Parliament also contain statistical information about various developments in the field of university education. The reports of its visiting committees, which assess the financial and other needs of the universities and findings of the expert groups which it sets up to consider specific issues relating to higher education, contain considerable statistical information which is valuable for the planning of higher education.

(*iv*) *National Council of Educational Research and Training*. The Council has a full-fledged unit for surveys and data processing. The unit has recently completed the third all-India education survey. The various departments of the Council also engage in surveys of the facilities available in educational institutions. Instances of this type are surveys of teacher training institutions and of the state institutes of education undertaken by the Council's department of teacher education. These surveys indicate the deficiencies in the facilities available in these institutions and help planners to include specific programmes to remove them.

(*v*) *The National Staff College for Educational Planners and Administrators*. This has, as part of the third education survey, conducted a survey of educational administration in various states. The memoranda that the college prepares for its training courses/seminars also contain statistical information although much of it is taken from documents brought out by other organizations.

(*vi*) *The State Education Departments*. These remain the main suppliers of statistical data for the Ministry of Education, the Planning Commission and other central agencies. It is through the states departmental machinery that education statistics are collected from institutions. The statistical wings of these departments check the accuracy of information supplied by institutions and consolidate it before passing it on to the Ministry of Education and Social Welfare. While the state departments also provide the personnel and machinery for special surveys, like the third education survey, the expenditure on these may be borne by the Central Government. The state education departments bring out statistical publications indicating the state of education in their respective jurisdictions; many of them containing information which is not published in the Education Ministry's documents. By providing time series data at one place these publications turn out to be quite useful for preparing state profiles and examining the projects that the state governments propose for inclusion in their plans. To the extent these publications provide district-wise, data, they indicate the disparities that exists within the states.

(*vii*) *Educational institutions*. These remain the primary suppliers of information. They also provide personnel for special surveys. For instance, in a number of states primary school teachers have been deployed for the enumeration of non-attending children. As the basic unit, from which information is and can be gathered, educational institutions are also subjected to a large number of questionnaires and survey schedules; their contribution to educational research, however, remains unrecognised.

Agencies other than those directly involved in the educational process which nevertheless collect, compile and report statistics useful for educational planning are indicated briefly along with the type of information that they report:

(*a*) *Census Reports of the Registrar General's Office* provide vital data on a number of items useful for planning, such as the total population, its breakdown into sexes, specific age groups and rural-urban component, educational and literacy status of the people, occupational structure, distribution of villages/towns by different population slabs and so on. The special studies, such as that of scientific, technical and professional personnel carried out as part of the 1971 census, also provide valuable information for planning of facilities for education in professional areas.

(*b*) *The Directorate General of Employment and Training* collects information from employment exchange about educated personnel registered with employment exchanges and also of teachers seeking placement assistance. Although the data have serious limitations, they are nevertheless indicative of the trend in the employment of educated personnel. Special studies conducted by the organization, like those on the pattern of graduated employment, the employment status of persons belonging to scheduled tribes and the area skill surveys, have provided useful information to educational planners.

(*c*) In addition to the education division, other divisions/sections of the Planning Commission generate and/or compile important statistical data. The programme administration division compiles information about plan outlays and expenditure and the quantum of Central assistance given to the states. These data provide indication of the relation of education to the total economy as well as the likelihood of resources becoming available for educational development in the States. The manpower division carries out studies of the requirements and utilisation of manpower in different sectors; the perspective planning and the economic, finance and resources divisions compile data which are useful for educational planners. Only part of the data generated, compiled and utilised in the Planning Commission is published.

(*d*) *The Institute of Applied Manpower Research* has carried out a number of specific studies on the requirement and utilisation of manpower of specific categories. These have enabled the Planning Commission to identify surpluses and shortages of critical manpower and make necessary adjustments in the intake of and out-turn from training institutions. The Institute's analysis of expenditures on engineering institutions has provided useful data on unit costing. It has, as part of the third education survey, made a survey of technical institutions.

(*e*) *Although the National Sample Survey* data on education are very limited, some of the information collected—employment status of the population by educational levels is a case in point—are helpful to educational planners. The data on households, although they have not been utilized to the desired extent, can help to relate educational development to the socio-economic conditions.

(*f*) The statistical data published by the Ministry of Finance—development and non-development expenditure, revenue and capital budget for instance—provide useful information on educational expenditures.

(*g*) The data on State's and national income published by the Central Statistical Organisation are used to determine the relative emphasis that education is receiving in the country as a whole and in various States. The Central Statistical Organization also brings out statistical abstracts which present in one place informatlon on various aspects of national life.

The above analysis indicates that a number of agencies collect, compile and publish statistical data which is either educational in character or has a bearing on educational decision-making. The data collected are voluminous; a substantial part of them may not be used because it is outdated, not very reliable or because the purpose for which they have been collected are not the purposes for which data are needed. Little coordination exists between various agencies that compile educational statistics. Consequently, there is considerable duplication of effort. The multiplicity of agencies has led to a dispersal of qualified staff, each agency having less than the required number of people to look after educational statistics. Fewer agencies with, delimited responsibilities, would allow concentrated input of staff, both in terms of number and in expertise, and of equipment.

GAPS AND DEFICIENCIES

The inadequacy of the educational data for planning purpose and the deficiencies of the system for collecting educational statistics have often been commented upon. For instance, the expert committee on educational statistics, which the Planning Commission constituted when the draft fifth five-year Plan was being formulated, observed:

The existing arrangements for the collection, compilation and publication of educational statistics are unsatisfactory. The delays that occur render most of the statistics practically useless for planning purposes; the statistics that are collected do not provide sufficient information which can be used for formulating realistic educational programmes for implementation; a meaningful analysis of even the information that is collected is seldom undertaken; and the way these are compiled leads to a large margin of error in educational statistics.

Among the more important reasons for this state of affairs appear to be the large number of items on which information is collected each year many of them not of any direct use for planning; the large number of institutions and organizations from which information is obtained, many of them not possessing the requisite resources in staff or competence; the number of levels from which data are obtained; and the general non-recognition of the importance that accurate and reliable statistics have for any worthwhile and realistic planning.

The evaluation of the adequacy of statistics for planning purposes must be on the basis of well-defined criteria. These criteria, in their turn, should be derived from a study of the objectives and processes of planning. Planning means the direction of effort to reach predetermined goals. An educational plan must include both a statement of the objectives and an indication of the means that will be adopted to reach these objectives. If a larger number of institutions than intended have come to be established and many more students than visualized enrolled in these institutions, one would be justified in saying that the directional effort in educational development is lacking.

That educational planners and administrators have not been able to promote the growth of education in desirable directions and/or prevent its growth in unwanted areas is known, although the reasons for it may not be quite explicitly stated. The gaps in educational statistics and lack of educational information necessary for planning can partly be explained by the lack of planners control over events and partly by the inordinate emphasis that is placed on the intuitive judgement of the decision-makers. However, without digressing on the process of educational planning as it has emerged in India, one can identify some of the important gaps in statistical information. These are briefly discussed in the paragraphs that follow:

(*i*) *Lack of flow statistics*. The data that are collected on students and teachers represent their availability in the system at a particular point of time. How many students from one grade to the other or from one stream to the other flow is not known. This information is required by planners to determine the transition proportions on the basis of which additional places have to be created in the next higher grade/stage to accommodate students flowing to it from the lower grade/stage. The flow data also help to determine the internal efficiency of the educational process itself. A large proportion of students repeating a grade or dropping out of the system altogether points to the inefficient manner in which educational enterprise is being run. Although under the present system, which is largely aggregative, it would be difficult to collect flow statistics easily, it should be possible to do so by collecting data on repeaters and on the activity status of each student for the previous year. This could be done if for each student a data card providing information on some significant points, like socio-economic status of the family, date of birth, promotion through grades etc. is evolved and maintained.

(*ii*) *Who benefits?* If equality of educational opportunity is a major objective of educational planning, information about who benefits from education is essential for developing programmes which will ensure a more equitable distribution. The statistics on education do not provide any information about the socio-economic composition of the student body or of those who receive state subsidy in the form of scholarships, free studentship and other fee concessions. Information is also required to indicate social, economic and other handicaps which prevent certain sections from sending children to schools or their performing well in the school system although in their innate ability they compare favourably with other students in the group.

(*iii*) *Utilization of facilities*. Planning requires the creation of additional facilities only after the existing facilities are optimally utilized. Data are not collected as part of the regular statistics on the extent to which the existing facilities, in the form of teaching personnel, building space and equipment, are adequately utilized. Even the data collected through surveys—such as by the education survey in respect of schools with particular student-teacher ratios—do not provide information which helps in projecting the requirement of new places; for, pupil-teacher ratios do not indicate the availability of space and equipment which in fact will determine how many more students an institution can accommodate. The need is to collect data on the distribution of institutions by capacity and size and of classes by size and space. Related to this are the data on average daily attendance. That there is considerable gap between enrolment and attendance is well-known. Attendance statistics are important for indicating the extent of actual utilization of facilities and the extent to which new enrolments can be provided for with appointment of more teachers or construction of additional classrooms.

(*iv*) *Unrecognized institutions*. A large number of instructions, which do not fulfil the criteria for recognition and grant-in-aid, have come into existence in metropolitan and other urban areas. Although not recognised, they cater to the educational needs of certain sections of the population. In many of these institutions, the standard of facilities and instruction provided may be substantially higher than available in institutions maintained with public funds. In Delhi, for instance, a large number of pre-primary and primary schools have been established under private enterprises; these are being maintained primarily from fees charged from parents. Similarly, a large number of coaching institutions, which help people to pass various examinations privately, have also come into existence. Although they do not figure in the official educational statistics, these institutions nevertheless fulfil the felt needs of the community. To the extent that they ignore these institutions, the official statistics do not indicate the total educational effort of the community. The disregard of the enrolment in privately maintained primary schools, for instance, has tended to give a false idea of the burden that the State has to bear in universalizing primary education. The third Education Survey has attempted to collect data on and from unrecognized institutions; the coverage is, however, not complete.

(*v*) *Expenditure data and its linkage*. The Ministry of Education publications report expenditure from various sources—government fees, endowments, municipal and district board and others. They also break down expenditure into direct (constituting primarily the salaries of staff) and indirect which has both recurrent and non-recurrent components. These expenditures are reported by types of institutions. A number of limitations of these data prevent their meaningful use. Except for fees, which constitute part of the private expenditure on education, no information is available as to what it costs parents and students to obtain education of a particular type and level. A very significant omission is the contribution that communities make to education—for instance, in the form of land, labour and materials for the construction of classrooms. With an idea of private and community expenditure on education, the total effort of the country in supporting education cannot be determined. The absence of this information tends to underplay the role of private investments in education when plans are formulated; more often than not the plans tend to provide for the entire cost of education, with marginal adjustments being built in by taking into consideration the contribution from fees. It is also difficult to relate expenditures to enrolments. While enrolments are given by stages and schools, expenditure is reported by institutions. Since an institution is designated by the highest class it teaches many institutions have more than one stage; for instance a high school may have primary, middle and high school classes. The expenditure incurred on this school, therefore, is for all the three stages. It is difficult to determine precisely the per student cost of education at various levels of education. The Ministry's publications also report expenditure incurred by institutions by sources. One fails to understand how institutions are able to make a distinction between sources while spending money that they receive from various sources. After all, while meeting contingent expenditure for instance, an institution does not predetermine which rupee to spend from government grants and which from District Board grants. In some cases the reported educational expenditure may lead to double counting. Take for instance scholarships part of which a student uses for paying institutional fees. Thus, part of the expenditure enters government account twice, first as disbursements and later as "expenditure met from fees."

(*vi*) *Attrition rates of teachers*. While information on sex and educational and training qualifications are collected annually for teachers, no data are available to indicate how many teachers are replaced annually. Data on desertion, death and retirement are very important to determine the net annual replacement of teaching personnel. These help in determining the additional training facilities that will need to be created during a plan period. That this data may not be collected on an annual basis nor from all institutions is recognized. Carefully designed surveys can indicate the attribution rates in the teaching profession and any variations in these rates among various localities.

(*vii*) *Ancillary facilities.* In addition to providing instruction, educational institutions cater to many other needs of the children. They make arrangements for co-curricular activities, provide mid-day meals and free books and stationery, arrange for transportation of students, arrange for their health inspection etc. With greater emphasis on the promotion of education among the weaker sections, some of these, like mid-day meals, free books and uniforms, have assumed significance. Apart from the time of the teaching and other personnel, provision/organization of these activities costs money. Except for expenditure on hostel facilities, the Ministry of Education publications do not report any detailed data on these either in terms of the expenditure incurred or numbers benefited. Many of these items are, however, being covered in the third education survey. A definite programme of data collection on these and related items is called for.

(*viii*) *Administrative and non-teaching staff.* Although not very difficult to collect, details on the administrative and non-teaching staff are not collected annually. The non-availability of information on clerical and supporting staff provided in educational institutions, particularly secondary schools and colleges, makes it difficult to determine the total personnel requirements—and, consequently of financial requirements—of educational institutions.

(*ix*) *Measures of output.* The only measures available to determine the output of the educational system are the examination results which indicate the total number of students successfully passing the various final examinations and their proportion to the students appearing in these examinations. Considering the substantial element of subjectivity involved and the various means adopted by students to pass examinations—many of them neither fair nor educationally desirable—the examination results do not indicate the true output of the educational institutions. No information is also available as to the relationships between the various inputs and outputs of the education system. This lack of any simple measure of determining the success of a school or a college makes it difficult for the planners to decide where the scarce resources should be invested to maximize returns from the system. Among other things, it should be possible, as a first step, to design and administer standardized achievement tests in various subjects which can help in rating the relative effectiveness of institutions in developing some cognitive abilities among the students. Research undertaken for the purpose of determining the relationship between inputs and outputs should also be sponsored.

(*x*) *Educational disparities.* Equitable distribution of educational provisions is an important objective of educational planning. The extent to which educational disparities have been reduced as a result of planned effort is difficult to determine in the absence of precise and detailed data. The Ministry of Education publications provide statistics on the porportion of children of various age groups enrolled in different levels of education by States. These, along with the data on institutions and expenditures, which can provide some information about statewise disparities in respect of institutions available per 10,000 of the population, per capita expenditure incurred on education and so on. Educational disparities are, however, larger within the States than among the states. In addition to spatial disparities there are disparities between groups such as the scheduled castes and scheduled tribes. District-wise data on the availability of institutions, of facilities for education at various stages, of teachers, the expenditures incurred per capita and per student, etc., can provide information on disparities within the states. The ministry had at one stage initiated the compilation of district-wise data. The third all-India education survery is likely to provide some information on district-wise disparities as well as on the extent of the benefit that weaker sections are taking of educational provisions. District data have become particularly significant for educational planning at the regional and sub-regional levels.

A brief reference may, in passing, be made to other problems of educational statistics in India. Firstly, as was indicated earlier, there is considerable time-lag in the availability of firm and detailed educational statistics. Although provisional statistics on selected items are available for 1975-76, published statistics from the Education Ministry have become available recently for the year 1969-70.

Secondly, statistics collected by various agencies show considerable variation. A case in point are the variations in the enrolment in classes I-V and VI-VIII reported by the state governments to the Planning Commissiom for 1973-74, indicated for the same year in the provisional statistics brought out by the Education Ministry and revealed by the third education survey. The extent of variation is large as is indicated below:

Enrolment in 1973-74 (in lakhs)

	Classes I-V	*Classes VI-VIII*
Reported in the draft fifth Plan	638	150
Reported in the provisional statistics of the Education Ministry	632	147
Revealed by the third education survey	611	141

The all-India statistics tend to hide some glaring variations in the State figures. For instance, in respect of Uttar Pradesh, the third education survey has revealed the enrolment in classes I-V to be 95 lakh in 1973-74 which is 24 lakh less then 119 lakh indicated in the draft Fifth Plan and 21 lakh less than reported in Education Ministry's provisional statistics; incidentally the enrolment of 95 lakh in 1973-74 in Uttar Pradesh is even less than the enrolment of 104 lakhs reported in the Ministry of Education publication, *Education in India* for 1969-70 for this state. Although not as large, variations in enrolment exist in the case of other states also. Such large variations cannot be explained merely on the basis of the reference dates being different viz., in the case of the survey December 31, 1973, and March 31, 1974, for the statistics supplied to the Planning Commission. Such large variations even in respect of 1973-74 figures make the reliability of educational statistics suspect.

SUGGESTIONS FOR IMPROVEMENT

The analysis of the major gaps and deficiencies indicates broadly the items/areas on which statistics need to be collected for any meaningful planning of educational development. Information on many of these items cannot be collected through channels traditionally required to collect educational statistics; nor would it be feasible and worthwhile to gather information on all the items annually and from each and every institution. The expert committee on educational statistics of the Planning Commission gave considerable thought to the problem. Considering the difficulty as well as the undesirability of collecting them on all items annually, the Committee recommended that the educational statistics collected should be of the following three types:

(*a*) *Minimum data to be collected on census basis.* The information will be collected annually from each institution; among others, these data will include classwise and sexwise distribution of enrolment, trained and untrained teachers, educational expenditure on specific items and from various sources, etc.

(*b*) *Selected statistics.* Information on selected items to be collected annually through surveys.

(*c*) *Periodical theme oriented.* These will attempt to collect information on specific problems, particularly these which have implications for the formulation of the plans for educational development.

The National Advisory Committee on Educational and Cultural Statistics, which the Ministry of Education has constituted for advising it, endorsed the recommendations of the expert committee. The forms under which statistical information in collected were revised in the sixth all-India conference on educational statistics, held in New Delhi from August 21 to 23, 1975. The Ministry of Education is going ahead with the collection of statistics under the revised scheme.

While the revision of the forms may speed up the compilation and reporting of essential educational statistics—because of the lesser number of items and entries involved—the danger that information on the items deleted, on the assumption that they will be covered by "theme oriented studies" and "special surveys", may never get to be collected. The statistical machinery available, either with the Ministry of Education or in the State Education Departments, is too deficient in strength and technical competence to be able to undertake studies and surveys. Annexure to this paper indicates the extent of deficiency in personnel at the State and district levels. Unless, therefore urgent step are taken to develop suitable mechanisms, the volume of educational statistics will be reduced without any corresponding gains.

A few suggestions are for consideration:

(*i*) The most important step that needs to be taken is the strengthening of the statistical machinery all along the line, more particularly at the district and the state headquarters. Apart from recruitment of competent staff in adequate numbers, this strengthening should include computerization at the Central level and mechanisation at the state and district levels. The strengthening of the statistical machinery was an essential component of the package of reforms suggested by the Planning Commission's expert committee. In order to make them useful for educational planning the committee had visualized the arrangements for collection and compilation of educational statistics to be a part of the overall machinery for educational planning at the State and district levels.

(*ii*) There is need for coordination in the collection and compilation of educational and related statistics. Suitable administrative arrangements may be evolved at district and state levels for pooling the resources of personnel trained in statistical methods. That the Bureaus of Economics and Statistics should also take over educational statistics is a suggestion that has been advocated with the purpose of providing the necessary technical inputs.

(*iii*) Suitable programmes for financing educational research and surveys by competent individuals and organisations should be provided for. Such research will help to generate information which can generally not become available through the convassing of regular forms from educational institutions.

(*iv*) The financial and other resources of various organisations—the Indian Council of Social Science Research, the Zakir Hussain Centre for Educational Studies, the National Council for Educational Research and Training, the National Staff College for Educational Planners and Administrators, the various university Departments of Education, the training colleges, State Institutes of Education etc—shoud be utilized to generate information useful for educational planning. It may be worthwhile to identify significant areas of educational research and finance them on a more coordinated basis than is done today.

(*v*) Since the services of the existing personnel cannot be dispensed with, it is necessary to develop suitable programmes for upgrading their competence in analysing educational statistics. The Central Statistical Organization, the Indian Statistical Institute, the National Sample Survery and other competent organizations should be assisted to undertake education-cum-training courses for existing personnel.

As stated earlier, the analysis of gaps indicates the items on which information is not available and needs to be collected. It also indicates the use of this information for planning purposes. In summary, some of the important areas are highlighted again.

Educational Statistics in the Census and the National Sample Survey

MAHENDRA K. PREMI*

Although collection of statistics on education—educational institutions, enrolments, teaching personnel, expenditure and type of management, which are required for administration, policy planning and decision making—by the Ministry of Education was initiated in 1947, the Indian census has been collecting and publishing educational data from the census of 1872, when information was collected through two questions—(*i*) ability to read and write, and (*ii*) youths up to age 20 attending school, college or under private tuition.

Depending upon the requirements of the economy, the questions relating to literacy and educational attainment in the various censuses have undergone changes from time to time as is revealed by Appendix which provides information on the census questions on literacy and education, concepts and definitions used, and the tabulations generated from them.

From the Appendix, it is noticed that prior to 1941 the census collected information on the level of literacy only, and the same was cross-tabulated by sex and age, and occasionally by religion/caste/tribe/race. Information on the number of persons able to read and write in English was also collected in the censuses from 1901 to 1941. Although information on actual examination passed was collected in the 1941 census, the same was not tabulated due to severely curtailed tabulations of that census.

The three censuses of indepeudent India have provided useful information relating to the stock of literate and educated persons by their levels of educational attainment. With the launching of the five-

*Centre for the Study of Regional Development, School of Social Sciences, Jawaharlal Nehru University, New Delhi.

year plans, the need for data on educational attainment of the working population and on educated unemployment was recognized in the census, and therefore these tables were generated in the 1961 and the 1971 censuses besides tables on educational attainment of the population by sex and age in rural and urban areas. Special tables were generated in the 1961 census to provide information on level of educational attainment of each scheduled caste and tribe at the state level.

The Census Commissioner for the 1961 census introduced a special card in that census to collect information on the exact degree obtained, pattern of employment and unemployment and earnings of "scientific and technical personnel" and covered all those persons who had a degree in physical sciences, or in engineering, technology, medicine, etc. The scope of this inquiry was enlarged in the 1971 census by including all persons who had completed their graduation or possessed a degree or diploma in a technical field. The tables on degree holders and technical personnel providing information on level of education by subject field and type of employment and, in case of unemployed persons, by duration, have proved very useful for manpower planning at higher levels.

Beginning with the 1951 census, certain basic data at village urban-block level giving area, number of households, size of population by sex, literate and educated persons, scheduled castes and scheduled tribes population and workers classified in broad industrial categories have been published for each decade by the census organisation in the District Census Handbooks of each state/union territory. Data have also been published in the 1961 and 1971 District Census Handbooks on the amenities available in each village which include educational institutions by level. These data have been found very useful for micro-level analysis although they suffer in terms of their accuracy.

The National Sample Survey (NSS) was launched by the Government of India in 1950 as a multipurpose inquiry at the instance of the then Prime Minister the late, Jawaharlal Nehru, to collect independent data on various socio-economic aspects of the Indian economy. Since then, this survey has been conducted in the form of rounds. Data on literacy and educational attainment of the population have been collected in a majority of rounds, either in the schedule on "population, births and deaths," or on "employment and unemployment." In collecting this information, record has been made of the highest level attained in terms of set cutting points—primary, middle, matriculation/higher secondary, degree, etc., and in the case of students, the class in which studying has been recorded. It may, however, be noted that in the NSS, priority is given to an individual's status as "worker" over all other statuses as was done in the 1961 census; by this process we always get an under-estimate of school going children from this source.

Data on household expenditure on fees, books, etc. have been collected in the "consumer expenditure" schedule but this expenditure has usually formed part of the miscellaneous group. However, in the 17th round, data on household expenditure on education have been separately published.

It is important to note that the NSS is canvassing, for the first time, a separate schedule on "education" in its 31st round covering such items as current enrolment by grade, problems of school attendance against the socio-economic background of children, problem of children not at school, household expenditure on education, and activity pattern of children and youth. These data are being collected for the four eastern states of Arunachal Pradesh, Manipur, Tripura and Nagaland, covering both rural and urban areas in the first three states and the urban areas alone of the last state. The information collected in this schedule will help in analysing school enrolment by socio-economic categories, stagnation and dropouts, number of "students workers," etc.

Tabulation of Data in the Census and the NSS (and the Purpose They Serve)

The last column of Appendix I provides information on the tables that have been generated in each census by using "literacy and educational attainment" as one of the variables. In the censuses upto 1931, literates were classified by sex, age, religion. Tables were also given separately cross-classifying literates by caste/tribe/race, etc. Tables on persons attending school or under private tuition were generated in the censuses of 1872 to 1891.

One of the basic tables of the Indian censuses from the very beginning relates to distribution of population by sex, age and literacy and educational attainment. The educational classification used for rural areas in the 1961 census has four levels: (*i*) illiterate, (*ii*) literate without educational standards, (*iii*) primary or junior basic, and (*iv*) matriculation and above. Age was classified into ten intervals, these being quinquennial upto 30-34, followed by 35-44, 45-59 and 60-plus In the 1971 census the educational categories were increased to eight, but the age categories were reduced to seven only, the last one being "35 and above."

In the urban areas, also educational categories in 1971 became different from those of 1961. This created a number of other problems, besides those of comparability. For example, in the 1961 census it was possible to analyse and associate the educational attainment of women in child-bearing ages or of workers in the age group 15-59 with many other variables. Such analysis is not possible utilizing the data of the 1971 census. However, since these tables are available at the district and, sometimes, at the tehsil/taluk level, they have proved useful for economic planning.

Considering the requirement of economic planning the Commissioner for the 1961 census generated a number of tables providing information on industrial and occupational classification of workers by their educational attainment (Tables B-III A and B and B-VI: see Appendix). Special tables have been generated for the scheduled castes and the scheduled tribes giving industrial classification of workers by their literacy and educational attainment. In the 1971 census tabulations of workers cross-classified by literacy and educational attainment and broad industrial categories (Tables B-III A and B), and occupational categories (Tables B-VI Parts A (ii) and B (ii)) have been made. However, because of changes in the educational categories and in the concept of worker between the 1961 and 1971 censuses, a good deal of comparison is lost.

The classification of "unemployed" 15 years and over by sex, age-groups and educational levels in urban areas (B-VIII Part A of 1961) and by sex and educational levels in rural areas (B-VIII Part B), and a similar classification of "others" among non-workers in the 1971 census provide the stock of unemployed by the level of education they have already secured.

While classifying the population according to its economic activity in the 1961 census, status of a person as "worker" was given preference over all other statuses. This led to an under-estimate of the school-going population in that census. However, a comparison of these figures for the age group 5-14 with the enrolment data for the same age group for that year provided an estimate of "student workers" in that year. In the 1971 census, since the population was classified on the basis of "main activity," we believe that the census will provide a reasonable check in respect of school enrolment in different age groups. It was expected that the information on "secondary work" of persons whose main activity was different from "worker" will help in estimating more accurately the population of student-workers but, because of slackness of the census enumerations in collecting information on secondary work, the above estimation has been ruled out.

As indicated earlier, the Census Commissioner for the 1961 census introduced a special card on "scientific and technical personnel." The response rate in the case of medicine (degree or above—modern and other indigenous systems) and engineering and technology (degree or diploma equal to degree or post-graduate degree) turned to be 61.14 and 65.33 per cent respectively. Data collected through this card were used to provide information on the strength of scientific and technical personnel by each branch, marital status, activity, nature and sector of employment, income, and age and period of unemployment, of these highly qualified persons. In the 1971 census the scope of this inquiry was enlarged by covering all degree holders and technical personnel even with diploma level qualifications. The tabulated data of this census (Tables G-I to G-XII) again provide valuable information in respect of highly qualified manpower of the country.

Migrants to cities with population 1,00,000 and over have been classified for the first time in the 1971 census by sex, age, educational level and occupation of the workers. These data provide the present educational levels of the migrants to the cities which though useful in themselves do not indicate whether the particular educational level was attained by the migrant before or after migration.

In the NSS, information on literacy and educational level has either been classified to analyse the fertility/mortality/migration differentials or the differentials in educational attainment of the workers by various industrial/occupational categories. The educational levels generally used for such cross-classifications are: (*i*) illiterate, (*ii*) literate but below primary, (*iii*) primary, (*iv*) middle, (*v*) metric, and (*vi*) graduate and above. The information has been specially used in analysing impact of education of wife/husband on the size of the family. In the field of employment and unemployment, this classification has helped in understanding the current situation in the country. It may be noted here that although the NSS has so far brought out more than 270 reports in published and draft form, but none of them have been devoted specifically to "education."

REQUIREMENT OF DATA FOR ECONOMIC AND SOCIAL PLANNING

The requirement of educational data in the context of social and economic planning can be looked from three major viewpoints—(*i*) future educational projections to analyse the supply of skilled man-power, (*ii*) analysis of educational data to understand the extent of regional disparities, and (*iii*) analysis of educational data to discern the differential attainments of different social groups, e.g., scheduled castes and scheduled tribes, various religious and minority groups, women and other deprived sections of the population. In this section we look at the specific requirements for each of the above view points.

No strategy of future educational planning can be worked out without projections of school enrolment for which at least four general types of basic information is needed; the first relates to population of school age, the second to pupil enrolment, the third to various rates and ratios derived from the first two types of data, and the fourth to questions of administrative policy affecting education in general and school enrolment in particular. Since the last type of requirement is purely dependent on administrative policies and decisions, this hardly has any direct relationship with educational statistics. The third type of data requirement is derived from the first two and hence it does not require any special treatment. In what follows we have, therefore, discussed the first two types of data requirement for educational projections.

Under the first category we need size of population by sex and single year age separately for rural and urban areas at the district level. These data become available from a population census and population projections for future dates. Under the second type of requirement we should ideally have serial statistics on number of pupils enrolled in schools by sex, age and grade according to those who are new entrants, who have been promoted from the previous grade and those who have stagnated in the same grade, and number of pupil who drop out of the school system each year. These data are required for rural and urban areas at least at the state level if the considerations of costs preclude such tabulations at the district level.

In view of the presence of a large number of unrecognised institutions and to account for their role in imparting formal educa-tion, we also need regular data on number of unrecognised institu-tions, their enrolment by sex, age and grade. These data are not brought out in any publication of the Ministry of Education or in the reports of the Directors of Public Instructions in the States since they cover only the recognised institutions.

The unit of area in terms of which data are available is of crucial significance in regional analysis. National and state aggregations are obviously inadequate and do not permit any meaningful spatial analysis. This is particularly so in the light of the fact that the district is being increasingly adopted as a unit for area planning, and developmental activities are increasingly operationalized at the level of the block/tehsil. Keeping this in view, Moonis Raza and Premi, in their paper presented at the third data base seminar of the Indian economy held at New Delhi, 1974, indicated the geographical units at which the tabulations of educational statistics are required. At the national seminar on social statistics, New Delhi, 1975, Naqvi drew attention to certain important dimensions with regard to education in our villages, and adult literacy which have been entirely missing from our educational statistics and which are necessary for social and economic planning.

One of the major objectives of social and economic planning is to provide equality of opportunity, particularly in obtaining formal education, for various groups of people, viz., scheduled castes and scheduled tribes, other minority groups and economically deprived sections of the population, and women. To evaluate the progress of school enrolment and educational attainment of these categories of people, we need these data in a serial form year after year. We also need informations on occupation and income of parents of pupils studying in different levels of education so as to understand the differentials in educational attainment of pupils coming from different backgrounds.

In India, we have generally looked at educational data from an individual's point of view. However, it has been increasingly felt that tabulation of educational data on school enrolment, type of school in which studying, and educational level attained by treating household as a unit of analysis and cross-classifying the same by size and type of family, and by other characteristics of the households will provide very useful information for social planning. Since it is believed that there are important differentials in the educational attainment of the children belonging to land-owning households, agricultural labour households, households of traditional craftsmen and factory workers, and urban households it is necessary to have relevant tabulation in this respect. Analysis of educational performance of the younger children in relation to the educational attainment of their father/brothers and mother etc. is also important.

Data used by additional tabulations (extent)

Besides the time-lag in the publication of educational data by the Ministry of Education, their reliability has been questioned by researchers on several scores. There is no agency in India which has till now made any attempt to check the reliability of the educational data. The third educational survey which has endeavoured to provide independent information is being examined critically in the ministry.

Although the census data also suffer from various types of inaccuracies and deficiencies which more glaring at the micro-level, still they constitute an independent source of information. In the 1971 census economic activity of every individual was determined on the basis of his "main activity." We therefore expect that the 1971 census provides reasonably good statistics of student population by sex and age right upto the district level by rural/urban residence. The data on students from the census can be cross-classified by marital status, religion or any other significant variable.

Further, since the census is the only source, besides sample surveys, of information on the migration status of every individual and his present activity, it should be possible to obtain information on "migrant-students" by place of origin and place of destination. All this requires generation of special tables from the 1971 census data which are now available on tapes for 20 per cent urban sample and 5 per cent rural sample. As a minimum, census data can be utilized to generate the following tables at the state level separately for rural and urban areas as they are considered important for social and economic planning:

(1) Population 5-24 years of age by sex, single year age, and school attendance.

(2) Population aged 5-24 by sex, quinquennial age groups, marital status and school attendance.

(3) Population aged 5-24 by sex, school attendance and place of last residence.

(4) Educational attainment of the total population by sex, broad age groups and religion.

Obtaining other data through the Census and NSS

Here we recognise that census operations are huge, and it is not possible to collect detailed data on different aspects. Secondly, whenever efforts have been made in a population census to collect complex data, the results have not been encouraging because of the indifferent quality of such data. However, as indicated above, census data on school attendance are important from many considerations and we recommend this question for inclusion in the 1981 cenus.

It may be mentioned here that the United Nations, in their *Principles and Recommendations for the 1970 Population Censuses*, made "school attendance" as one of the important items for data collection. Further, in the 1969 pretest of the 1971 census individual slip a question "if studying in any institution now" was tried out. Here, the term "institution" left a certain degree of vagueness. The enumerators were not clear as to what to include and what not to include. If we decide to introduce a question on "school attendance" in the 1981 census, it would be useful to make the difinition of school/institution very specific. It would be helpful to record the exact grade in which the particular person is studying while collecting data on school attendance.

From the viewpoint of educational strategy for social and economic planning we need household data providing information on problems of education against the socio-economic background of the parents, problems of children not at school, reasons for dropout household expenditure on education, and activity pattern of children and youth, etc. Such data can be collected only through household survey. In the third all-India educational survery, "institution" was regarded as the basic unit for data collection and all the 26 schedules were devoted to one aspect or the other of different types of institutions. Thus, it is either the NSS alone or some other similar agency which, by conducting household survey on education, can provide relevant data on above aspects.

We wish that the schedule on education introduced in the 31st round of the NSS for the four states of eastern zone only, will be modified suitably on the basis of this pilot study and canvassed at the national level in the next round.

REFERENCES

Up to the thirteenth, the National Sample Survey rounds were of three to six months duration. From the 14th round which started in July 1958, the duration of each round was made one year which coincides with agricultural year, i.e. from July to June. The 31st round started in July 1976.

M.K. PREMI, "Student Workers in the Age Group 5-14: A Socio-Demographic Analysis," *the Manpower Journal*, VIII (4), January-March 1973, pp. 68-84.

CENSUS OF INDIA, 1961 Volume I, *India*, Part II-C (i)—*Social and Cultural Tables*, Delhi, Manager of Publications, 1965.

M.K. PREMI, *Educational Planning in India*, New Delhi, Sterling Publishers (P) Ltd., 1972, p. 81.

MOONIS RAZA AND M.K. PREMI, "Scale of Data for Studies in Regional Development—A Few Observations," Paper presented at the Third Data Base Seminar of the Indian Economy, New Delhi, December 1974.

S. NAQVI, "Some Areas of Darkness in India's Social Statistics," Paper presented at the National Seminar on Social Statistics, New Delhi, 17-22 March, 1975.

A.B.L. SRIVASTAVA AND K.N. HIRIYANNIAH, "Educational Statistics in India —Deficiencies and Suggestions for Improvement," paper presented at the National Seminar on Social Statistics, New Delhi, 17-22 March, 1975, pp. 1-23. For example, they write:

"... the reported enrolment figures in primary schools of rural areas are often inflated. The age data of students are notoriously inaccurate. Income and expenditure data from private institutions are generally not very reliable. There are many other items on which correct data are not supplied either due to non-availability of accurate information, carelessness or deliberate attempt to distort the figures" (p. 7)

UNITED NATIONS, *Principles and Recommendations for the 1970 Population Censuses*, Statistical Papers, Series M, No. 44; New York: United Nations, 1967, pp. 40, 58.

Appendix

Census Questions on Literacy and Education, Concepts and Definitions used, and the Tabulations Generated from them by taking Literacy/Education as one of the variables, 1872-1971

Census Year and Forms of Questions	*Concepts and Definitions*	*Tabulation*
1	*2*	*3*
1971 (*i*) Literacy (Loro) (*ii*) Educational level (*iii*) Graduate Card	*Definition of Literate*: "A person who can both read and write with understanding in any language is taken as 'literate'. A person who can merely read but cannot write is not a literate. It is not necessary that a person who is literate should have received any formal education or should have passed any minimum educational standard". If a person claimed to be literate in some other language, the respondent's word was taken as correct. "An Illiterate" is a person who can	(1) C-I Part A Age, Sex and education in all areas. (2) C-I Part B Age, Sex and education in urban areas only. (3) C-VIII classification by literacy and industrial category of workers and non-workers according to main activity among (*i*) scheduled castes, (*ii*) scheduled tribes. (4) B-III Part A—Classification of workers and non-workers according to main activity by educational levels

1	2	3
	neither read nor write or can merely read but cannot write in any language". All children up to 4 years of age were treated as illiterate even if the child was going to school and had picked up reading and writing a few off words. Ability merely to sign ones name was not adequate to qualify a person as being able to write with understanding.	in urban areas only. (5) B-III Part B—Classification of workers and non-workers according to main activity by educational levels in rural areas only. (6) B-VI Part A (*ii*)—Occupational classification of persons at work according to main activity other than cultivation classified by sex and educational levels in urban areas only.
	(*ii*) *Educational level*: The highest educational level attained by a person was ascertained and recorded against this item. For a person who was still studying in a particular class, the highest educational level attained by him/her was the one that he had actually passed not the one in which he/she was studying. In doubtful cases such as whether a person has passed primary, middle, higher secondary or other definite levels, the actual standard passed such as, say, IIIrd standard, VIIIth standard, 1st Year,	B-VI—Part B (*ii*): (7) Occupational classification of persons at work according to main activity other than cultivation classified by sex and educational level in rural areas only. (8) B-VIII persons classified non-workers according to main activity cross-classified by sex, age—groups and type of activity. (9) B-IX Part A: Non-workers categorised as others aged 15 and above

1	2	3
	B. Com., etc. was recorded. When a person had both general and technical qualifications, the technical education level was given perference. Whether the general educational level was higher than the technical educational level or where it was not possible to decide which of the two levels was relatively higher, the highest level of education as returned by the person concerned was recorded. In recording the highest educational level of a graduate or a post-graduate subject of specialisation was also recorded. . . . Like previous census detailed information in respect of Graduates or Post-Graduates or those with a technical Diploma or Degree was collected. For this purpose especially designed card known as "Degree-holder and Technical Personnel Card" was given to each graduate and others at the time of enumeration. The persons concerned were requested to fill the details and hand it over to the enumerator.	classified by sex, age groups and educational levels in urban areas only. (10) B-IX Part B: Non-workers categorised as others aged 15 and above classified by sex, age groups and educational levels in rural areas only. (11) D-III: Migrants to cities classified by sex, broad age groups, educational levels and, in case of workers, by occupational divisions. *Special Tables for Degree Holders and Technical Personnel* G-I Distribution of degree holders and technical personnel in each subject filed by level of education. G-II Distribution of degree holders and technical personnel in each subject field by status and level of education. G-III Distribution of degree holders and technical personnel by level of education and emoluments classified by sector of

1	2	3
		employment.
		G-IV Distribution of degree holders and technical personnel by subject fields, age-groups, sector of employment further classified by emoluments.
		G-V Distribution of employed (other than self-employed) degree holders and technical personnel by type of organisation of present employment classified by levels of education and subject fields.
		G-VI Distribution of unemployed technical personnel with engineering and technology qualifications classified by degree and diploma levels and by subject of such degree and diploma.
		G-VII Distribution of degree holders and technical personnel who are unemployed and seeking employment in each subject field by duration of unemployment level of education and sex.
		G-VIII Distribution of unemployed degree holders and above in Arts, Humanities and Commerce classified by degrees

1	2	3
		and their subjects.
		G-IX Distribution of unemployed degree holders and above in Sciences and other selected subjects classified by degrees and their subjects.
		G-X Distribution of unemployed persons having qualifications in Technical/vocational trades by subjects.
		G-XI Degree holders and technical personnel engaged in research by subject field and levels of education.
		G-XII Distribution of degree holders and technical personnel by country of education, subject field, levels of education and sex.
1961 (*i*) Literacy and education (*ii*) Card for scientific and technical personnel.	(*i*) *Literacy and Education*: It was recorded whether a person was literate or illiterate. The test for reading was ability to read any simple letter either in print, or in manuscript. If the person could read one of the examples in the Enumerator's Hand-	C-III Part A. Age, Sex and Education in all areas. C-III Part B. Age, Sex and Education in Urban areas only. C-III Part C. Age, Sex and Education in

1	2	3
	book with facility he was taken to have passed the test for reading.	Rural areas only. Appendix to Table C-III.
	The test for writing was ability to write a simple letter. The test for literacy was satisfied if a person could with understanding both read and write.	Union Table I—Distribution of Scientific and Technical Personnel by each Branch and sub-branch of Science or Technology.
	An illiterate person was defined as one who could neither read nor write or could merely read but could not write in any language.	Union Table II—Age composition of persons in each branch of Science or Technology. Union Table III—Permanent addresses by branch of education.
	(*ii*) *Standard of Education*: If the person could both read and write and also had passed a written examination(s) as proof of an educational standard attained the highest examination passed was also recorded.	State Table I—Distribution of Scientific and Technical Personnel by each branch and sub-branch of science or technology.
	In addition to the data relating to the Scientific and Technical Degrees and Diplomas collected through the individual slips, it was found desirable to undertake a more detailed investigation not only into the full spectrum of scientific and	State Table II—Type of Activity and Marital status of Persons in each Branch of science or technology. State Table III—Year of obtaining Post-graduate degrees in Physical Sciences and Graduates and Doctorates in Engineering, Technology, and Doctorates

1	2	3
	technical disciplines but also into certain conditions of work and service obtaining among scientific and technically trained personnel. This was accomplished through a specially designed Business Reply Post Card called as the "B and T". During his visit to each household between 10 and 28 February, 1961, a census enumerator was required to leave these special cards, one for each of the members of such household which contained person or persons trained in Science or Technology with a request that the card should be completed by the person himself and kept ready for collection by him when he visited the household again during the revisional round on 1-5 March, 1961. Cards which have been filled in the meantime were collected by the enumerator during the revisional round for onward transmission to the Registrar General. In case of those which have not been filled in, the person was requested to fill it carefully and post the card in the post office as early as practicable.	in Engineering, Technology and selected Branches of Medicine. State Table IV—Persons holding Degrees in Engineering, Technology and selected Branches of Medicine and also Degrees in selected Branches of Physical Sciences. State Table V—Nature and Sector of employment of persons in each Branch of Science or Technology. State Table VI—Total monthly by income of persons employed in each Branch of Science or Technology classified by sector of employment. State Table VII—Tenure and sector of Employment of persons in each Branch of Science or Technology. State Table VIII—Age and period of unemployment of unemployed persons qualified in any Branch of Science or Technology. C-VIII Part A—Classification by literacy and Industrial category of workers and

1	2	3
		non-workers among Scheduled Castes.
		C-VII Part B—Classification by Literacy and Industrial category of workers and non-workers among Scheduled Tribes.
		B-III Part A—Industrial classification of workers and non-workers by educational levels in *Urban areas* only.
		B-III Part B—Industrial classification of workers and non-workers by educational levels in *Rural areas* only.
		B-VI—Occupational Division of persons at work other than cultivation classified by sex, broad age-groups and educational levels in *Urban areas* only.
		B-VIII Part A—Persons unemployed aged 15 and above by sex, age-groups and educational levels in *Urban areas* only.
		B-VIII Part B—Persons unemployed aged 15 and above by sex and educational levels in *Rural areas* only.
		D-IV—Migrants to cities classified by sex, broad age groups, educational

1	2	3
		levels and in case of Workers also by Occupational Divisions and Groups.
		STC-III Part A(*i*)—Education in Urban Areas only for Scheduled Castes.
		STC-III Part A(*ii*)—Education in Urban Areas only for Scheduled Tribes.
		SCT-III Part B (*i*)—Education in Rural Areas only for Scheduled Castes.
		SCT-III Part B (*ii*)—Education in Rural Areas only for Scheduled Tribes.
		SC-I—Persons nor at work classified by sex, type of activity and educational levels for Scheduled Castes.
1951 Literacy and Education	(1) *Literacy and Education* The literacy of a person was recorded under the following categories:	C-IV—Age and Literacy.
		D-VII—Livelihood classes by Educational standards.
	(*i*) A person who could neither read nor write; or a person who could read but could not write was regarded as 'illiterate'.	D-V (*vi*)—Special tabulation for displaced persons. Distribution by age and literacy.

1	*2*	*3*
	(*ii*) A person who could both read and write was regarded as 'literate'. The test for reading was ability to read any simple letter either in print or in manuscript. The test for writing was ability to write a simple letter. Children bellow the age of 4 years were regarded as illiterate. (2) *Educational level* If a person who could read and write and had also passed any examination(s) the 'highest examination passed' was recorded.	
1941 (1) Can you both read and write? If so, what script do you write? Can you read?	Literacy was defined as the ability to write a letter to a friend and read the answer to it but not otherwise. In the case of persons who were able to read and write, the name of the script was also noted. The information was also collected separately for those persons who were only able to read or were unable to read.	Age and Literacy

1	2	3
(2) How far have you read? Give any examination passed	If a person could both read and write, the highest examination that he had passed was recorded against this item. When the person had not attended any school or college, the class or standard of education attained was indicated.	
(3) Are you literate in English?	Information was also collected for those persons who could both read and write English.	
1931		
(1) Whether literate (i.e., able to write and read a letter)	Information relating to literate and illiterate was recorded. Literacy was defined as the ability to write a letter and to read the answer of it. It excluded those who could read but could not write. All the children below the age of 5 years were treated as "illiterate".	
(2) Whether able to read and write English?	Information in respect of those persons who could both read and write English was collected.	(1) Literacy by Religion and Age, Summary figures of literacy. Part I—General Table. Part II—Distribution by provinces

1	2	3
		and states. Part III—Cities. (2) Literacy by selected castes. (3) Unemployment of Educated Persons.
1921 (1) Literate or Illiterate	Information was collected for literate and illiterate in respect of each person. Literate was defined as one who could write a letter to a friend and read the answer to it. Information in respect of those persons who could read but could not write was also collected separately. All those persons who could neither read nor write and children below 5 years of age were treated as "Illiterate".	(1) Literacy by Religion and age: Part I—General Table for India. Part II—Details by Provinces and states. (2) Literacy by Selected Castes, Tribes or Races.
(2) Whether literate in English?	Information was also collected for those persons who could both read and write a letter to or from a friend in English.	

1	*2*	*3*
1911		
(1) Literate or Illiterate	Information in respect of 'literate and Illiterate' was collected under the following categories: (*i*) All persons who could write a simple letter and read the answer to it in any language were treated as 'Literate'. (*ii*) Those who could not read and write any language were treated as 'Illiterate'.	(4) Education: Part I—General Table for India. Part II—Details of provinces and states. (5) Education of Selected castes, tribes or races.
1901		
(1) Literate or Illiterate	The information was collected into the following two broad categories: (*i*) All persons who had the ability to read and write merely their own name were treated as 'Literates'. (*ii*) All persons who could not both read and write were recorded as 'Illiterates'.	(3) Education: Part I—General Table. Part II—By provinces, states and by main religions. (4) Education by selected castes, tribes or races.
(2) Know or does not know English	Information was collected for literates in English which included all persons who could both read and write English whether they were still learning or had left.	

1	2	3
1891		
(1) Learning, Knowing or Illiterate	The information in respect of each person whether grown-up child or infant was recorded under the following categories: (*i*) Persons under instructions either at school, house or college, were recorded as 'Learning'. (*ii*) Persons who could both read and write some language but were not at the movement under instructions were treated as 'Knowing'. (*iii*) 'Illiterate' was recorded for those persons who were not under instructions and were not able to read and write any language. It included also those who could read but could not write or could sign their own name but not read.	(1) Education, by Religion and Age. (2) Castes, Tribes and Races Education.
(2) Foreign languages known, if any	Information was collected of foreign languages of those persons who could both read and write any foreign language. English was also recorded	

1	2	3
	for a person who could read and write English.	
1881 Education (1) Under instruction (2) Not under instruction but able to read and write	The information was collected on "Education" as follows: (*i*) *Under instruction*: All those persons who were under instruction either at home, school or college were recorded as 'Under Instruction' (*Sikhte*). (*ii*) *Not under instruction but able to read and write*: Those persons who were not under instruction but were able both to read and write were treated as 'Known' and recorded under the head 'Not under instruction but able to read and write'. (*iii*) *Not under instruction and not able to read and write*: Those persons who were neither under instructions nor able to read and write any language, or who were able to read but could not write or could sign their own names only but could not read were recorded under the item 'Not	Distribution of Population according to Education.

1	2	3
	under instruction and not able to read and write'.	
1871 Education (1) Able to read and write	The information on education was collected under the following categories: (*i*) Those who could both read and write. (*ii*) Those who could not read and write or those who could only sign their names.	(1) Number of persons who were able to read and write or under instructions by three specified periods (12 years of age, 13 to 20 years, and 21 years and above) by sex and their percentages.
(2) Youth upto age 20 attending school, college, or under private tuition	Information was also collected for youths upto age 20 attending school, college or under private tuition.	(2) Exactly similar Tables were generated by religion, namely, Hindus, Muslims, Buddhists and others'.

Manpower Statistics in India

Q.U. KHAN*

Manpower planning can be defined as determining goals for the development and utilization of human resources as part of policies for general economic and social development, and specifying measures for achieving these goals. It involves optimizing investment decisions in terms of employment and the calculated adjustment of the existing supply of and demand for manpower at different levels of education, training and skills with a view to ensuring the highest level of productive employment consistent with long-term goals of economic development. Manpower situation for any given area or country at any stage of socio-economic development can, therefore, be seen as an outcome of the demographic, educational (including all types and forms of training) and employment market conditions.

The aim of this paper is to make a survey of the state of manpower data at present along with agencies collecting them. The paper will also highlight the major gaps in data from the point of view of social and economic planning, and list the new items of data that could be profitably collected in the near future to facilitate effective manpower planning. This paper, however, does not analyse these data. It merely presents an inventory of what is available and in what shape and form.

An Inventory of Manpower Data

An inventory of manpower data required for planning purposes can be considered under four broad heads as follows: (*i*) Economic indicators, (*ii*) demographic statistics, (*iii*) educational and training statistics, and (*iv*) employment market data.

*Head of Research Division, Institute of Applied Manpower Research, New Delhi.

(*i*) *Economic indicators*. As manpower planning is derived from and determined by the national economic perspective, certain minimum data on the economic situation of the country are essential for effective manpower planning. A few economic indicators on which manpower planning is generally based relate to: (*a*) Gross value added, (*b*) investment targets, and (*c*) processes of production, levels of technology and rate of tranfer of technology.

Information on these items should be available for the recent past by industry and area (such as rural-urban, provinces, regions, etc). There should also be sufficient clear indications as to how these indicators will move during the next ten to fifteen years.

(*ii*) *Demographic statistics*. Demographic statistics relevant for manpower planning relate to labour force and its various characteristics. As the size and composition of labour force is dependent on the size of base population and the vital rates, manpower planners require the data on these aspects also to have an idea of the future labour force. In brief the information on labour force should be available in terms: (*a*) age specific activity rates by sex (for females additional information by their marital status, motherhood and economic activity) for different areas; (*b*) economic structure of the labour force in terms of occupations, industrial sectors, educational levels, experience and productivity rates; (*c*) length of expected working life at birth and at age 15 (the information may be separated into net years of active life and net years of inactive life); (*d*) replacement rates i.e. new entrants, retirements and deaths by sex, industry, occupation and education; (*e*) size and structure of families and households; and (*f*) projections of labour force for the next 20 years by age, sex and rural-urban or provincial areas (highlighting the trends in migration).

(*iii*) *Educational and training statistics*. Educational and training statistics are required to facilitate the assessment of the supply of educated and trained manpower. A detailed information about the stock of educated and trained personnel by age, sex, levels of education and its distribution in different regions and industries is, therefore, basic for any manpower planning exercise. Similarly, a continuous flow of data on intake, enrolment and out turn from the educational and training institutions by sex, level of education, field of specialisation and rural-urban or provincial location is equally important in any manpower exercise.

(*iv*) *Employment market information*. The employment market information acts as a barometer of the demand for manpower. Under this category surpluses and shortages of manpower, rates of unemployment and under-employment, waiting period and internal migration and brain drain are some of the crucial items of information required for efficient and effective manpower planning.

SOURCES OF MANPOWER DATA IN INDIA

The number of agencies involved in the collection, tabulation and dissemination of manpower data is quite large and it is neither feasible nor very relevant to list them all individually. It is thuoght sufficient to mention the important ones. Most of these organziations are, however, not primarily charged with the collection of manpower statistics and many a time the data collected and tabulated in specific forms by an organization are to serve certain other specific purposes as identified by the organization. Some of the important organizations and the data collected by them useful in manpower planning are briefly discussed below:

(*i*) *Central Statistical Organization.* Under the Department of Statistics of the Ministry of Planning the Central Statistical Organization (CSO) is charged with compiling and publishing national income accounts and other statistics, such as industrial statistics, price statistics, etc. From manpower data point of view, the data generated through the Annual Survey of Industries are of great importance. The Annual Survey of Industries (ASI) covers the entire factory sector except to defence installations and oil distribution and storage units.

The CSO publishes the following: (*a*) Statistical Abstract of India —annual and monthly, (*b*) Statistical Pocket Book of the Indian Union—annual, (*c*) Estimates of National Product*—annual, (*d*) Sample Survey of Current Interest in India—annual, (*e*) Basic Statistics Relating to the Indian Economy—annual, (*f*) Annual Survey of Industries—annual, (*g*) Monthly Statistics of the Production of Selected Industries of India—monthly, (*h*) Bulletin on Index of Industrial Production—monthly, and (*i*) Retail Price Bulletin, Consumer Price Index Number for Urban Non-manual Employees—monthly.

(*ii*) *Directorate General of Technical Development* (*DGTD*). Since 1951, the development wing, which was redesignated the DGTD in 1962, supplies data on installed capacity, production ex-factory value,

*Since 1973 this is brought out as "Estimates of national product saving and capital formation."

stocks, employment and number of shifts worked about organizations mainly in the private sector. The CSO publishes its bulletin "Monthly statistics of the production of selected industries of India" on the basis of these data collected by the DGTD.

(*iii*) *National Sample Survey Organization* (*NSS*). The NSS has been conducting sample surveys on a nation-wide basis regarding production, labour and other aspects of economic life. These multi-subject surveys are conducted in the form of successive rounds. The following subjects have been covered regularly in the various rounds: (*a*) Household income and consumer expenditure; (*b*) Rural retail prices of selected commodities; (*c*) Employment and unemployment particulars; (*d*) Labour force statistics; (*e*) Demographic statistics; and (*f*) Crop surveys.

(*iv*) *The Office of the Registrar General of India* (*Census Office*). The population census is a statistical operation of great value for economic and social planning. It provides detailed data on labour force and its characteristics over a long period of time. It also provides information on literacy and the educational standard of the population. In India, the first census was conducted in 1872, but systematic work started only in 1881 since when it has been repeated once in every ten years.

Apart from being a decadal enquiry, the census has not adhered to uniform definitions and concepts, thereby making the task of preparing comparable time series too difficult. Even the data of the latest two censuses (1961 and 1971 Censuses) are not comparable for a number of items.* The scheme of classification of data has similarly not been uniform throughout.

(*v*) *Council of Scientific and Industrial Research* (*CSIR*). The Division of Scientific and Technical Personnel of the CSIR maintains the following three registers for scientific and technical manpower: (*a*) the general register; (*b*) the Indians abroad register; and (*c*) the specialists register.

(*a*) *The General Register*. Persons with a minimum qualification of post-graduate degree in science, degree in engineering and technology and degree in allopathic medicine are enrolled in this register.

(*b*) *The Indian Abroad Register*. This register was started in 1957, and persons with foreign qualifications or work experience in science,

*For example the number of workers counted in 1971 Census fell short by eight million to that counted in 1961 although there was an increase of four points between 1951 and 1961.

engineering, technology, medicine, management or social sciences are enrolled in this register. The enrolment can be made when a person is abroad or immediately after his return to India.

(*c*) *The Specialists Register*. This is a relatively new register and enrols persons with specialists knowledge or experience, and is more or less the same as those contained in the general register. Registration in all these registers is voluntary. It is, therefore, very difficult to give a precise estimate of the extent of coverage. Only a rough idea of the relative distribution of persons with various subjects/specialisations over time can be made.

(*vi*) *Ministry of Education and Social Welfare*. The Ministry of Education is the oldest, most comprehensive and important source of information on a variety of educational items. The systematic collection of statistics by the Ministry dates back to 1882 when the Report of the Indian Education Commission was released. Since then educational statistics for all levels and types of education have been published in the Quinquennial Reviews of the Progress of Education in India from 1892-97 to 1932-37 and the Decennial Review 1937-47. Since 1913-14, annual statistics also began to be collected and published but they were not so detailed as the quinquennial statistics. Since 1949-50 the Ministry has been collecting statistics in 'Form A' which is very comprehensive and detailed. These statistics have been published in the annual publications "Education in India" and "Education in the States."* With the advent of national planning from 1951 onwards, the educational statistics were found inadequate for planning purposes. A number of revisions in "Form A" have, therefore, taken place to make more statistics available.

(*vii*) *University Grants Commission* (*UGC*). The University Grants Commission (UGC) started collection of educational statistics from the academic session 1961-62. It collects information from the universities and colleges affiliated to them. The data collected relate to enrolment, hostel facilities, library facilities, courses offered, staff position, post graduate education (subjectwise enrolment of M.A./M.Sc. and Ph.D. in Arts and Science subjects). These statistics relate to August 15, of every year and are published in "University Development in India—Basic Facts and Figures."

(*viii*) *Directorate General of Employment and Trainning* (*DGE & T*). The DGE & T constitutes the central headquarters of the National

*Education in the States discontinued since 1962-63.

Employment Service as well as of the craftsmen training scheme of the Ministry of Labour and Employment. The collection of statistics relating to training facilities was taken up at the instance of the working group on manpower studies of the Planning Commission. The first publication (1954) on training facilities was issued in February 1955 under the title "Hand Book on Training Facilities." The publication has two volumes—one dealing with the institutional training facilities and the other with the implant training facilities. Besides, the DGE & T regularly collects data under the employment market information programme. It also collects statistics from industrial training institutions, the state apprenticeship advisors, and occasionally through some field investigators.

The data collected by the DGE & T suffer from a number of limitations. The EMI programme does not cover agriculture, small establishments and the self employed. The basic frame of establishments used by many employment exchanges is not updated. There is always some non-response, especially on educational details of employees working in small private sector establishments. The data on the live register suffer from non-registration, multiple registration and registration of employed persons as unemployed. There is also an undue time-lag in processing and publishing the data.

(*ix*) *Labour Bureau, Simla.* The Labour Bureau was set up 1946 to assist the Government in framing labour policies based on reliable statistics. Through administrative reports and legislative acts such as Workmen's Commensation Act, 1923, the Payment of Wages Act, 1936, the Factories Act, 1948, and the State Maternity Benefit Acts, state governments collect and summarise the data and forward them to the Labour Bureau. The Labour Bureau revises these data and supplements them by undertaking surveys on certain topics not covered by the States. All these data are then published in Indian Labour Statistics, Indian Labour Journal, Indian Labour Year Book and Pocket Book of Labour Statistics.

Besides the above mentioned sources, there are a number of other professional organizations and agencies which collect, compile and publish manpower statistics. It is difficult to list all of them here and give a detailed description of each. Some of the important ones are given below:

(*a*) *Central Bureau of Health Intelligence* (*Directorate of Health Services*). This agency collects and maintains statistics regarding medical colleges, medical teaching manpower, post-graduate medical education and para-medical institutions. The Bureau regularly brings out the directories of: (1) medical colleges in India; (2) medical teaching manpower in India; (3) para medical institutions; and (4) post graduate medical education.

(*b*) *Professional Bodies on Health Manpower*. Under this category we have: (1) the Medical Council; (2) Indian Nursing Council; (3) Dental Council of India; and (4) Pharmacy Council of India.

(*c*) *National Council of Educational Research and Training* (*NCERT*). The NCERT was set up in 1961 and since then it has initiated several significant programmes in educational research, training and extension. The Council, besides the qualitative assessments, has also undertaken some statistical compilations which contain data useful for manpower planning. Important among these are Year books, Monographs on Educational Expenditure and the All-India Educational Surveys.

(*d*) *The Indian Council of Agricultural Research* (*ICAR*). Maintains statistics regarding agricultural and veterniary education. The Council does not bring out any publication and the data are available in the cyclostyled form:

Gaps and Suggestions for Improvement

There is no doubt that India has fairly adequate statistics for its manpower planning exercises. Nevertheless, the position is not very satisfactory. We propose here to indicate some significant gaps in existing manpower statistics and suggest what improvements could be made.

One of the main defects of manpower statistics is that there is no single agency charged with the task of collecting and processing them. At present these statistics are collected by a number of organizations, for their specific individual needs and not from the point of view of total human resource development. The result is that the data collected are not only incomparable, as these agencies adopt varying concepts and definitions, but also, sometimes, they cannot be used as they refer to different reference periods. In short, they overlap. It is, therefore, necessary that all these agencies sit together, rationalise definitions and concepts, improve classifications and tabulations and decide on uniform reference periods. They should also pay attention to the poor quality of data. Data collected at the national and state levels should be reconciled before they are published so that readers are not confused with divergent sets of statistics.

Data collection agencies should also strictly follow the time schedule. At present there is an unusual delay in collection and publication of educational statistics. Some time-lag can be avoided if the different agencies collecting manpower data divide the work among them rather than duplicate it. The publication of statistical data by some agencies has not been regular. This should be attended to and all publications brought out regularly at fixed frequency.

In many cases the amount of data collected from the field is more than what is ultimately processed and published. Generally what is collected is not wholly processed, and what is processed is not fully published. This results in an expensive operation and loss of valuable information. In short, there is an urgent need of an effective coordination for collection, tabulation and publication of manpower statistics, both at the national and state levels.

Information on the current stock of various categories of manpower is hardly available. Different agencies, such as the Planning Commission, Institute of Applied Manpower, state governments, etc., have made *ad hoc* exercices for a few categories of manpower only. Stocks for all important categories of manpower in terms of education/training, industries, occupations and areas should be worked out at regular intervals by applying a standard methodology.

On the supply side, the statistics on the flow of statistics and training from the educational/training institutions suffer from a number of limitations. The data on intake and enrolment in higher education are inadequate is so far as information is not available separately on fresh entrants, repeaters and dropouts. Out-turn statistics are weak in more than one respect. The out-turn data at graduate and post-graduate levels are not classified by subjects and specialities. Although institutions and enrolment data are available separately for rural and urban areas, similar separate break-up of out-turn for rural and urban areas is not available. Some portion of the institutional out-turn involves double and multiple counting as many students take their masters degrees more than once.

There is no precise accounting for Indian students leaving for abroad for further or higher education. Similarly, 'Brain Drain' statistics are not complete and up-to-date. Its exact magnitude remains only a guess. There is no information available on the occupational paths the internal migrans take when they generally come from rural areas to urban areas.

The labour market information at present is inadequate in many respects. There is virtually no data on the number and size of establishments in terms of total employment and investment. Hiring and recruitment policies of the employing agencies are also not known. There is no information on wage differentials. With respect to wages, it will be useful to isolate the differentials between sectors of activity, between sizes of firms and between public and private sector firms.

Data Needs for Higher Education

BIKAS C. SANYAL*

Economic, social and political factors have contributed to the rapid expansion of higher education in the developing countries during the last two decades. The urgent need to replace expatriates in the civil service and in a wide range of public and economic services, and the concept of investment in human beings as a powerful factor for economic growth, were the main economic factors. The view that education was a basic human right, and the special economic incentives, the prestige and power attached to jobs given to the educated, contributed to the social factors of educational expansion. The university or an institution of higher education as a status symbol of a country or a region within a country was the basic political factor for such expansion.

This rapid expansion has created as many problems as it has solved for a developing economy. Problems facing the institutions of higher education today in a developing country can be listed as (*i*) the irrelevance of the education in content and method with respect to the national needs because of its being based on foreign models; (*ii*) extremely high cost per student and per graduate; (*iii*) increased regional and social disparity in respect of educational opportunities; (*iv*) alienation of the education system from the key production sectors of the economy; (*v*) increased mismatch between the output of the educational system in quantity and quality with respect to needs of the society; (*vi*) the rural exodus caused by the higher education system; (*vii*) the failure of higher education to create employment, inhibiting enterpreneurial spirit and self-employment; and (*viii*) increase

*The author is an Associate Staff Member of the International Institute for Educational Planning (Unesco), Paris, and the Head of the Research Project on Higher Education and Employment.

of expectations among the students which often remain unmet resulting in political and social crises.

The problems facing the labour market are (*i*) the difficulties in estimating the needs for skills in quantitative and qualitative terms for the economy; (*ii*) the identification of the right kind of education for any type of job; (*iii*) the occupational mobility – horizontal and vertical, the role of attitudes of the students and graduates towards conditions of work in this mobility; and (*iv*) the changing participation rates of the educational output among different social and regional groups.

Although our special emphasis is on higher education, these problems are affecting to no less a degree the other levels of education. It is, however, the higher education system which provides guidance for the whole educational sector in a developing country, and any defect in this system creeps into the other levels very quickly. It is the higher education system which produces the leaders of a developing society. One cannot expect strong leadership to come out of a bad education system.

No educational policy can solve the above-mentioned problems if it is not an integral part of the general development strategy of the country. However, in this world of interdependence, institutions of higher education have some and they must use this to reduce the intensity of the problems. Before they can act, they must have knowledge about the relationship between higher education and the labour market based on clear analysis and correct interpretation.

A properly planned education system will take into account the stock of natural, physical, financial and human resources at national and regional level. It would take into account the degree of exploitation and indigenous processing of raw materials. This should have as objectives not only to develop the available resources but also to affect the operation of the economy, generate new employment and reduce regional disparity in economic well-being. The system should generate skills and aptitudes needed for the exploitation of the resuorces. Information is therefore needed on the estimates of skills in quantitative and qualitative terms.

This would involve identifying factors that affect occupational mobility—the role of salary structures, conditions of work, career guidance, recruitment and promotion practices, and an analysis of the relevance of the education with the needs of the job, growth of earnings and promotion of the employed graduates. Knowledge about the credential requirements for certain kinds of jobs are also necessary. The analysis of the role of social, economic and educational background of the unemployed, the self-employed and employed graduates could furnish important guidelines in order to develop different modes of employment. Employability of the different types of graduates should be a useful criterion for the development of higher education in any country or region.

Information is also needed on the job descriptions for any role in the society so that content and methods of instruction could be developed to meet those needs. Users of higher education have a role to play here. The ill-effects that higher education has generated in our society could be rectified if we knew what are the right attitudes and values that should be instilled through our educational programmes at a particular point in time. The sandwich programmes and need for work experience before University entrance are some experiments going on around the world and whose effects are to be followed with care.

In addition to the educational flow statistics by year of study over a period of time, the adequacy of the pre-tertiary level of education and the existing examination system calls for investigation. The evaluation of a student should be done more precisely *on the job* rather than in the examination hall. The role and importance of the determinants of the demand for higher education call for in-depth analysis not only to adjust the intake to different specializations but also to channel the students to areas where they are needed for the economy.

The above types of analysis requires the selection of suitable cohorts of students and collection of information on them through suitably designed sampling techniques. The students can then be followed up periodically after they have graduated to form the basis of the graduate survey. In the initial stage, the above aspects of the operation of the labour market and the system of higher education can be analysed through sample surveys of students, graduates and employers. These analysis would need continuous revision because most of the characteristics are sensitive to time.

REFERENCE

SANYAL, BIKAS C., and EL SAMMANI A. YACOUB, *Higher Education and Employment in the Sudan*, Paris, IIEP, 1975.

SANYAL, BIKAS C. CASE, JOHN, *et al.*, *Higher Education and the Labour Market in Zambia –Expectations and Performance,* Paris: The Unesco Press and the University of Zambia, 1976.

SANYAL, BIKAS C., and KINUNDA, MICHAEL J., *Higher Education for Self-Reliance --The Tanzanian Experience,* (in preparation).

SANYAL, BIKAS C., *Higher Education and Labour Market Needs in Developing Countries*; Paper presented at the International Round Table on 'Factors determining school achievement' at the University of Dijon (France), 10-11 June 1976.

—— *The Role of Non-Formal Higher Educatiou to Meet Labour Market Needs*; Paper presented at the Latin American and Caribbean Meeting on New Forms of Post-Secondary Education held in Caracas, 20-30 September 1976.

Statistical Needs for Educational Planning

H.N. PANDIT*

Educational planning in India during the last 25 years has been broadly guided by the "Manpower requirement approach" with respect to scientific, technical and professional education and "individual demand for places approach" for the elementary and secondary stages of school education and general higher education. Application of "manpower approach" implies that one of the most important functions of educational system is to provide the economy with right amount of different types and levels of qualified manpower. The "demand for places approach" starts with the assumption that the educational plans should be prepared in such a way that educational facilities are made available to all who wish and are able to benefit from them. The technique is also used in the formulation of positive policies like provision of educational facilities to weaker sections of society, such as, scheduled castes and scheduled tribes. In actual practice, use has been made of both the approaches in working out the educational plans to meet the needs of the economy and to democratize the educational facilities in the country. Furthermore, the working out of resource implications pose various conceptual difficulties. In recent years, some attempts have been made to apply social/private cost-benefit analysis to education to improve the knowledge about the resource allocation within education on the one hand and education and other sectors on the other hand. Another aspect of educational planning in India is mobilization and management of resources by the central and state governments, district board (in rural areas), municipal boards (in urban areas) and private organizations interested in education.

Educational system in the country has expanded considerably from

*Professor, National Council of Educational Research & Trainning.

25 million enrolment in 1950-51 to 100 million enrolment in 1975-76. In terms of allocation of resources, the share of education in relation to GNP has increased from 1.2 to 2.9 per cent during the same period. It is clear that education industry has become very important in the socio-economic life of the country. Particularly, responsibility of the central and state governments in the management and financing of education has increased considerably. Thus, there is the need for collection of comprehensive statistics for the preparation of short, medium and long term plans for the further developments of education in the country. In general socio-economic data are expensive to obtain. In the present paper analysis is limited to the needs for primary statistics relating to *institutions*, *pupils*, *teachers*, *building*, *educational expenditure*, etc. Besides these statistics, there is also need for a large body of supplementary data required by the educational planners for calculation of forecasting and planning coefficients within the educational system. These include demographic, economic and social data. These are not covered here, except, where (*i*) they are of great importance for educational forecasting, e.g. data by age of school going children; and (*ii*) statistics in the required form but unlikely to be collected for purposes other than educational planning, e.g. the tabulation of labour force data by educational characteristics, occupations, and industries or age education-earning profiles of the working force. These data are not likely be tabulated except to meet the needs of educational planners.

In the present paper, discussion is organized in following manner: In the second section attempt has been made to give the mechanism of organizations mainly responsible for collection and publication of information on the working of national educational system. In the third section the scope of main publications has been given. Fourth section gives main gaps and inconsistencies in data on *enrolment, costs of education*, and classification of labour force data by socio-economic characteristics etc. Appendix I gives the scope of different forms used by the Ministry of Education and the UGC for collection of data from the institutions.

ORGANIZATION OF EDUCATIONAL STATISTICAL SYSTEM

The main sources of time series data on *pupils, teachers, buildings* and *equipment* and *expenditure on education by sources and management* are the annual publications brought out by the Statistical Unit of the

Ministry of Education, Government of India and the University Grants Commission.[1] Data on enrolment and teachers by various stage school education have been collected through three *All India Educational Surveys*, in 1957, 1965 and 1973 by the Ministry of Education and the National Council of Educational Research and Training. In fact, the Third Survey was widened in scope by also collecting data on higher education by the UGC, vocational education by the IAMR, educational administration by the National Staff College for Educational Planners and Administrators and Cultural statistics by the Department of Culture of the Ministry of Education. Information on literacy and educational levels of population are published by the Registrar General of India through the decennial census reports for 1951, 1961 and 1971. Information on training facilities both institutional and inplant with respect to craftsmen has been published by the Directorate General of Employment and Training since 1955. The Association of Indian Universities also brings out a hand out about university-wise institutional facilities in India. About educational and training statistics like in-take and out-turn of institution in medical and para-medical fields are collected and published by the Medical Council of India, Dental Council of India, and Indian Nursing Council and Pharmacy Council of India. Indian Council of Agricultural Research maintains statistics regarding the in-take capacity and out of turn the agricultural and allied institutions/colleges. It may also be added that the National Sample Surveys (NSS) also provide a lot of information about educational level of population and private expenditure on education as a part of family budget surveys. Information about age, education and earnings of working population are available in consumer expenditure and income surveys organized by the National Council of Applied Economics Research and City Surveys of Delhi, Bombay, Hyderabad and now of Bangalore by ISEC. The CSIR also maintains information about the educational profile of the scientific and technical manpower in India. Institute of Applied Manpower Research also publishes line series and cross section data on stock and flow data by various educational categories in the Fact Book on Manpower.

[1]Historical statistics with respect to education are available in the *Quinquennial Review of the Progress of Education in India* for 1886, 1891-92, 1897-98, 1901-02, 1906-07, 1911-12, 1916-17, 1920-21, 1926-27, 1931-32 and 1936-37. *The Decennial Review of Education in India* (1937-47) gives annual statistics for the period. Since 1913-14, annual statistics were also collected and published upto 1947.

Ministry of Education

It is seen from the preceding section that the Ministry of Education is the principal source of annual statistics on education. For collection of comprehensive data on education from institutions, *Form A* was introduced by the Ministry of Education in 1949-50. In fact, the educational data have to flow through a long channel from the institution to the Ministry of Education. The primary and the Middle Schools send their returns to the tehsil/taluk offices, from where these are forwarded to the district education officers. The district offices are also responsible for collection of returns for high/higher secondary schools, teacher training schools, vocational and technical schools and special education schools. Apart from receiving district returns, the State Headquarters collect returns from colleges and other departments of the state Governments. In order to collect more data, system of collection of data through Form A, was revised in 1963-64. From 1964-65, data on education have been collected in the revised *Form A*. In this revision some of the useful information like contribution by endowments in financing of institutions has been merged into other sources and the Central Government contribution is put with that of State Governments and shown together under Government. Institutional classification has become more detailed. Since 1964-65 pay scales of teachers, problems of wastage and stagnation and scheduled castes and scheduled tribes are collected through Forms A-1 and A-2.

The Ministry of Education has also collected separate educational statistics of Universities and their affiliated colleagues for the *Education in Universities in India* through Forms B and B-1. Data in Form B-3 (cyclostyled) relating to Evening Colleges is collected directly by the Ministry of Education. Statistics of Boards of Education is also collected by the Ministry in Form B-4 (cyclostyled), introduced from 1968-69. However the collection of university-wise data is now to be done by the University Grants Commission.

The factors responsible for delays in the collection of data were reviewed in the Sixth All India Conference on Educational Statistics held in 1975. As a result of the recommendations of this conference, major changes have been made by the Ministry of Education in the collection of data. Now it has been decided to publish data collected on the basis of *Form A* in the combined volumes of I and II in *Education in India* on the existing pattern upto 1970-71. In order to make data comparable with the first year (1968-69) of the Fourth Plan, data on education will be collected on the existing pattern for

1973-74, with certain modifications in terms of mode of collection of data at the state level. It has been recommended to utilise the *Third All India Survey* (1973) for the school level and financial data from the budget books etc. for this purpose.

For remaining years i.e. 1971-72, 1972-73 and 1975-76 the arrears were to be cleared by collecting data in a simplified proforma designed by the Working Group set up at the Sixth Conference. The form is known as *Arrear Form*. The arrears of collection of educational data from 1970-71 to 1974-75 were supposed to have been cleared by end of September, 1976.

Further the main reason of time lag in collection of data was the comprehensiveness of Forms A, A-1 and A-2 designed in 1964-65. On the basis of the recommendation of the Sixth Conference on Educational Statistics held in August 1975, the existing forms have been simplified and split into four forms. These are:

(*i*) *Form ES-I Numerical Data*. It gives information on institutions, pupils and teachers as on 30th September. Form F-IV collects information about students and teachers from SC/ST.

(*ii*) *Form ES-II Financial Data*. It gives data on income by sources and expenditure by items for the financial year ending on 31st March.

(*iii*) *Form ES-III Examination Results*. It reports both annual and supplementary results in terms of the number appeared and number passed. For example, the annual examination results for 1976-77 will state examination declared in 1976-77. Further details about the information to be collected through these forms is given in the *Manual of Instruction for Filling Forms of Educational Statistics*, 1976 of the Ministry of Education.

A note on the various types of Forms mentioned in this section is given in the appendix. Further the collection of data in the proforma with respect elementary education will be done at the bloc level and the data will be consolidated at the district level, along with data relating to secondary education. The statistical units at the state headquarters will collect and consolidate data relating to affiliated and non-affiliated institutions in addition to data received from the district.

University Grants Commission

The University Grants Commission started in 1961-62 collection of educational statistics from universities and colleges affiliated to them. The statistics pertains to courses for which the minimum qualification for admission is matriculation or school leaving certificate examination irrespective of the fact whether the course is affiliated to university or to a Board or is recognized by the government, provided it is conducted in a college affiliated to University. These statistics are published since 1961-62 in *University Development in India Basic Facts and Figures.* It has been decided that the UGC will stop collection of information in Form B-I from 1975-76. However the UGC will continue to collect data in their on Form B-4. Incidentally, it may be mentioned that the present coverage of data collection by the UGC not only leaves out non-affiliated institutions but also it does not cover certain institutions of national importance. Further, the UGC will be collecting data on institutions enrolment and teacher as on September 30 as against 15 August as it is being done now and financial data at the end of each financial year on a separate proforma.

National Council of Educational Research and Training

During the last two decades three All India Educational Surveys have been conducted to study the problems of school mapping. In fact, the need for these surveys owes its origin to the "Universal Declaration of Human Rights" adopted at the third session of the U.N. General Assembly in 1948. In Article 26(i), it is stated, "Every one has the right to education. Education shall be free, at the elementary and fundamental stages. Elementary education shall be compulsory." The fulfilment of these goals required a careful study of the existing situation in educational development in every country so as to provide the base line data which would be needed to plan educational development.

The first All India Educational Survey was conducted by the Ministry of Education in 1957. The main aim of the survey was to plan the creation of schools on a national basis and to correct the existing uneven distribution of schools in the states. The survey collected a very useful data on the following items:

(*i*) Habitations where the schools were located.

(*ii*) Number of habitation survey by each school.

(*iii*) The population served by the existing schools, the enrolment in each school, etc.

This information helped in the location of new school.

The second All India Educational Survey was organized by the NCERT in 1965 more or less on the same lines. The main objectives of the survey were stated as:

(*i*) To revise the data of the first survey in terms of the distribution and size of habitations and delimitation of school areas of existing primary, middle and high schools and to collect data required for the preparation of district plans for educational development.

(*ii*) To undertake intensive studies regarding the existing conditions in educational institutions etc.

Unlike first and second surveys, the Third All India Educational Survey in 1973 was more comprehensive and covered all institutions at all stages of education. The responsibility for surveying higher education was with the UGC, technical and vocational education with IAMR, of educational administration and inspection with the National Staff College for Educational Planners and Administrators and that of cultural statistics with Department of Culture of the Ministry of Education. The NCERT was incharge of the survey of school education and coordinated the work of all surveys. The objectives of the third survey were similar to those of the preceding surveys. Further, it was, designed to help in the formulation of the Fifth Five Year Plan.[2] It was also to make intensive study of facilities like library, audio-visual aids, laboratories, age distribution of final attrition rates and other qualitative aspects of education. The results of the three surveys are available in three reports brought out by the organising agencies.

MAIN SOURCES OF EDUCATION STATISTICS

Table 1 p. 343 gives main educational statistical publications, their periodicity and other details.

It is seen from the Table that the Ministry of Education in the past has been bringing out publications, combining data on many aspects of the education. This has its advantages but it also leads to delays because the non-finalisation of even one category of data holds up the publications as a whole. Under the near system to be introduced from 1976-77, it has been decided to bring out separate publications entitled

[2]The survey took considerably long time to complete. The Third All India Educational Survey: Some Provisional Statistics on School Education (1975) were released in 1975 and these were utilised in the Fifth Plan Document which was finalised only in October, 1976.

Annual Statistics of School Education (General), Annual Statistics of Vocational Educational and Special Education and *Annual Statistics of Higher Education* (*outside the UGC*) by the Ministry of Education. The UGC will bring out Annual Statistics of Higher Education (UGC). This replaces the present publication on *Education in Universities in India.*

TABLE 1 *Latest Position of Publications brought out by the Ministry of Education, UGC and NCERT.*

Organization title	*Petriodicity*	*Year of Ist issue*	*Year of latest available issue*
1	2	3	4
A. *Ministry of Education*			
(*i*) Education in India	Annual	1949-50	1970-71
(*ii*) Education in Universities in India*	Annual	1947-48	1966-67
(*iii*) Education in the states	Annual	1949-50	1962-63**
(*iv*) Directory of Institutions for Higher Education	Bienniel	1959	1973-74
(*v*) Educational Statistics in District Wise	Five Years	1960-61	1965-66
(*vi*) Educational Statistics at glance	Yearly	1970-71	1975-76
(*vii*) Report of the All India Educational Surveys	No Fixed	1960***	—
(*viii*) Analysis of Educational Expenditure as shown in the budget Estimates of the State Governments	Annual	1967-68	1976-77
B. *University Grants Commission*			
University Development in India some basic facts and figures	Annual	1961-62	1972-73
C. *National Council of Educational Research and Training*			
(*i*) Indian Year books of Education	No Fixed	1961	1972
(*ii*) Second All India Educational Survey	No Fixed	1960***	1967
(*iii*) Third All India Educational Survey: Some provisional Statistics on School Education	No Fixed	1960	1975

*For 1969-70 and onwards the UGC will bring it out.

**Discontinued after 1962-63.

***First Survey was organized by the Ministry of Education.

The advisory Committee on Educational and Cultural Statistics set up by the Ministry of Education in its first meeting held in 1975 took following decisions:

(*a*) *Scales of Pay of School Teachers of Different Categories.* Information contained in this publication relates to 31st March of each year. It has now been suggested that the information should be collected as on 31st December of each year for this publication.

(*b*) *Organization of State Educational Departments.* The National Staff College should collect and publish information about the organization of the State Departments of Education as on 31st December of each year.

(*c*) *Universities in India.* This is not a continuation of the existing publication Education in the Universities. The UGC should annualy, beginning with 1974-75, collect and publish minimum essential university-wise statistics regarding institutions, enrolment, teachers, expenditure and other relevant items.

(*d*) *Education of Scheduled Castes and Scheduled Tribes.* This is to continue as at present.

(*e*) *Examination.* The Ministry of Education brings out results of examinations conducted by Boards of Secondary Education. A similar publication of University examinations should be brought out by the UGC.

(*f*) *Quinquennial Statistics of Education in Districts.* These publications have been brought by the Ministry of Education for 1960-61 and 1965-66. These publications for 1970-71 should be brought out by the Ministry.

Finally, the Committee suggested that the new publication on *Education in India* should be published every year by September. It will deal with principal events and developments in education and culture at the Centre and in all the States and Union Territories. It also suggested that Annual Digest of Educational Statistics should be brought out from 1974-75. This will give all available statistics as well as abstracts of importance statistics. The committee made one more important recommendation regarding publication of Year Book on the lines of the First Year Book of Education (1950-51 to 1960-61) brought out by the NCERT. This is to cover the educational developments during 1966-67 to 1973-74.

The Advisory Committee also made recommendation to collect data on following items on the basis of sample and not on census basis as it is being done now.

(*i*) Data on school teacher regarding age, employment, qualifications and subjects taught; and number retired, resigned or died during the year for determining attrition rate.

(*ii*) Study of wastage and stagnation by collecting details about the composition of students at the beginning of the year bifurcating it into fresh admission and repeaters and at the end of the year into continuing from the same class, in-migrants, out-migrants, drop-outs, deaths, etc.

(*iii*) Class-wise examination results.

(*iv*) Average daily attendance.

(*v*) Age data of students: (i) In case of schools for general education, this data is proposed to be collected class wise while in the case of other categories, the age data is proposed to be collected non-class wise but for broad categories, i.e. for Arts/Science/Commerce Colleges, for colleges of professional and other education and for school of vocational technical and special education.

(*vi*) Distribution of classes/sections according to number of pupils and teachers per section.

(*vii*) Data on multipurpose schools.

Detailed statistics about various categories of professional and vocational institutions.

Sample Statistics will be published separately by the agencies collecting them. Further, the committee has recommended to drop the collection of information on examination results (being collected at present in Form A) and number of villages not served by schools (being at present collected on Form A-2).

These recommendations when implemented will reduce delays and remove duplication existing, at present, in the collection and publication of statistics on education.

Data Needs for Educational Planning

Accurate and up-to-date statistics are needed for analysis and appraisals of plans; formulation of proposals, projection, programming and allocation of projects; costing, feasibility testing and choice of alternatives; and implementation and evaluation of educational plans. A brief analysis of types of data for these purposes is given below.

Students. The most important statistics in the field of education is the information about the pupils enrolled and their characteristics.

There are two basic sources of information relating to enrolment in educational system in India. The first source of information is the institutions themselves and the second source is the households. Another way of looking at this is to say that the suppliers (i.e. the educational authorities) and the demanders (i.e. the households) at the lowest stages constitute the two sources. The Union Ministry of Education, NCERT and the UGC and other agencies publish data collected from the institutions. The census on the other hand publishes data collected from the households. Fulltime students constitute one of the sub-groups of non-working population. But the data on student population from the two sources do not tally. For example, in 1961, *Education in India*, of the Ministry of Education showed that number of students was of the order of about 48 million as against 41.4 million shown by the Census. There was a deficit of 6.6 million students between the two sources. Further, it is disturbing to note that enrolment data published even by the Ministry of Education and NCERT are not the same. At the elementary stage alone in 1973, the Ministry of Education and the NCERT sources showed a difference of 4.2 million students. It is, thus, clear that there is certain amount of 'bogus' enrolment as published in the two sources. This problem was officially recognised even in *Progress of Education in India*, 1917-22 Vol. I (1921, p. 104). It is suspected that over reporting in enrolment mainly exist at the Elementary stage of Education. This is due to existence of compulsory enrolment laws and some times government assistance and subsidy for expansion of elementary education given on the basis of progress of enrolment. It is suggested that existing mechanism for collection of enrolment data may be reviewed so that enrolment data by sex and rural and urban location on accurate basis is collected to establish a sound basis for planning education in the country. Some of other types of data required for planning purposes about pupils is listed below:

(*i*) Sex wise number of students at various stages of education in relation to population in relevant age groups.

(*ii*) Progress of education of weaker sections of particularly with respect to scheduled Caste/Tribes, rural poor and those living in urban slums.

(*iii*) Information about employment status, social characteristics, educational level etc. of non-attending children of school going age group.

(*iv*) Regional inequalities measured in terms of stock (literacy rates) and flow (enrolment ratios by sex etc.) indicators.

Further, information on ability (income per capita) and willingness (share of state resources allocated to educated) to support education will help in deciding the extent of the Central help to be given to weaker states:

(*i*) Socio-economic background of new entrants, enrolled pupils and graduates by types and stages of education.

(*ii*) Information on parental status (father's and mother's occupation and education size and type of community, income and size of family, caste/religion etc., personal status (age, sex intelligence, birth order in family) and behaviour in school (grades obtained in examinations) types of specializations.

(*iii*) Private cost of education of children by sex, and parental status.

(*iv*) Socio-economic background of beneficiaries of scholarships and grants.

(*v*) Wastage (drop out and stagnation) rates by level and types of education and socio-economic background of the drop outs.

(*vi*) Transition proportions and flow rates into different courses over a period of time.

Teachers. The information about teachers needed for planning falls into two main categories: (*i*) stock; and (*ii*) Mobility. In addition, the quantitative relationship between students and teachers is needed in the form of: (*iii*) student teacher ratio. In this connection, annual statistics about stocks, qualifications and flow of teachers by sex and marital status are to be analyzed so that the growth and changes in the structure of teaching force and mobility rates can be traced as a basis for projection of future needs and supply of teachers. Following types of data are needed for this purpose.

(*i*) Analysis of shortages and surpluses in the demand and supply of teaching manpower by stages of education and specializations.

(*ii*) Information about non-active teaching force is also useful for mobilization of their services for formal and non-formal types of programmes.

(*iii*) It is necessary to have information about the graduates of teacher training colleges/schools who join teaching forces and other services.

(*iv*) Knowledge about the qualificational improvement through in-service training programme is necessary for working out the training needs of fresh entrents into teaching profession and for working out gains/losses in each category of teachers.

(*v*) For working out losses from the teaching force information about deaths and withdrawal rates by age, sex, qualifications and category is needed. Similarly, gains to teaching profession due to re-entry to teaching force to work out the net loss to the stock over time.

(*vi*) Information about student/teacher ratio involves knowlege about full-time equivalent teachers. For example, if more than one shift of children is taught by the same group of teachers, the number of teachers is to be divided by the number of shifts per day to get full day equivalents. In other words, while working out pupil/teacher ratio necessary account of *teaching load* has to be taken into consideration.

(*vii*) Analysis of data on administrators and inspectors of educational services are required to find out (*a*) quantitative relationship between educational services and those whom they control; and (*b*) the number of teachers who will move from active services into administration and inspection services and have to be replaced.

(*viii*) Information about non-teaching staff employed in the education industry by occupational groups and qualifications and sex is needed for planning growth of this sector manpower needs.

Expenditure and Costs of Education. Education represents a major claim on scarce resources of the economy. The expenditure on this sector must, therefore, be assessed against expenditures on other priority areas. This is done by relating total expenditure on education either to national income or to public expenditure on all sectors. Educational expenditure data, as published by the Ministry of Education, do not include expenditure incurred by unrecognized institutions, pensions paid to retired teaching and non-teaching staff, administrative expenditures of Ministry of Education, UGC and NCERT. It also does not include non-tuition private costs of education, earnings foregone by non-attending students. The classification of expenditure into "direct" and "in-direct" types used in the past is misleading. It did not give a clear picture of stage wise allocation of expenditure on education. Furthermore, government expenditure is classified into "revenue" and "capital" expenditures. Education is lumped into revenue expenditure. This creates great difficulty in working out the investment effects of educational expenditure. Another aspect of educational expenditure is its classification into current and capital expenditures. At present, data does not permit the estimation of the capital formation in the educational sector. Again it is only after many adjustments in expenditure data that it is possible to examine educational expenditure in relation to total resources of the economy. At the state level income estimates are not prepared on the basis of common methodology. It is, therefore, difficult to work out state wise ratio of educational expenditure in relation to state income on a comparable basis.

Unit Costs of Education

At present the knowledge of social institutional and private unit costs is grossly inadequate. In this connection, information about private non-tuition costs, earnings forgone, and capital costs has to be collected through surveys and studies to fillup major gaps existing in estimation of unit costs of education.

Financing of Education. Another aspect of the problem is the financing and management of educational expenditure by the central, state, local bodies and private organizations. Resources flow from the Central Government to states through the grants given by the Planning Commission and the Finance Commission. In the absence of data on financial transfers, it is difficult to know the contribution of the Central and State Governments separately. There are also grants from the State Governments to local bodies. It is not possible to know the extent of the transfer of funds from States to local bodies. In the context of the 44th Amendement in the Constitution of India the informantion about the sources of income and items of expenditure of institutions managed by the private enterprise will be useful for nationalisation of education industry in full. Another important gap in expenditure statistics is the knowledge about the structure of fee income of the institutions.

Preparation of Performance Budgets. The conventional budgets on education give broad heads of expenditure, such as, pay of officers, establishment, etc. This gives idea about what government buys and not what it does. It does not help management to control and appraise performance of various programmes, projects of schemes, nor it serves as a basis for informal decision making and management. In order to help in the effective management of educational sector, performance budget showing expenditure according to the classifications based on activities, objects and sources has to be evolved. These will also involve presentation of budget on basis of cost per unit of output, performance etc.

Cost-Benefit Analysis. In order to study resource effectiveness in the sector of education, information has to be collected about the following items:

(*i*) Working force classified by age, education and earnings.

(*ii*) Death rates, non-participation rates and unemployment rates by educational level and sex.

(*iii*) Influence of non-education earning determining variables on earnings of educated labour force.

(*iv*) Non tuition costs on books and stationery and additional living, cost of transportation, etc.

Manpower Demand Data. Following data are required for the application of manpower demand approach to educational planning:

(*i*) Classification working force by occupations, industries and educational levels;

(*ii*) Utilisation levels of educated manpower by rural and urban sectors;

(*iii*) Education and occupation/industry-wise out-put norms;

(*iv*) Mobility of working force by levels of education;

(*v*) Average waiting period before first employment;

(*vi*) District-wise information about emerging, declining, stagnant and growing occupational families to help in the identification of vocational courses for vocationalisation of secondary stage of education.

(*vii*) Cohortwise flow charts of educational output by sex according to occupation and industry and by various branches of specialization.

(*viii*) Wastage rates and transition proportions by levels and types of education.

School Mapping. At present sufficient attention is not being paid to collection of data about location of institutions. As a result, there are large number of un-economic institutions and sick universities. These Educational Surveys mentioned earlier collected some data about "habitations" with and without schooling facilities but no attempt seems to have been made to involve urban and rural geographers in the preparation of school maps. Data about transportation, distance travelled, etc have to be collected. Information about level of utilisation of school buildings by types and location does not exist.

APPENDIX

A BRIEF NOTE ON FORMS USED FOR COLLECTION OF DATA UP TO 1970-71 AND THOSE PROPOSED AFTER 1976-77

Main forms used to collect data are Forms A and B. Other forms used for the purpose are Forms A-1, A-2, A-3, B-3 and B-4. Primary proforma for collection of statistics from school level institutions by the respective State/Territory Government are also designed. Forms B-1, and A-4 are used as primary forms for collection of data from individual colleges and university teaching departments/Non-affiliated Institutions for Higher Education. Details of the information being collected in different forms are given below:

FORM-A

(*i*) *Number of institutions by type and management*, number, type and standards of attached classes to different types of institutions and number of attached hostels by type of institutions separately for boys and girls.

(*ii*) *Enrolment in institutions by type of institution* and management, number of students in attached classes by type and level of Education and number of residents in attached hostels separately for boys and girls.

(*iii*) *Enrolment by stages*. Number of students receiving collegiate education (General Education, Professional and other Education) by courses and stages as well as by age groups for boys and girls separately; number of students receiving General school education class-wise, age-wise and sex-wise, number of students studying general Science, Elective Science and Hindi at secondary level and number of students receiving Vocational, Professional, Special and other Education and by age groups.

(*iv*) *Number of teachers in different types of institutions*, number of trained and untrained teachers in schools for general education by types of institution, by stages of school education and management separately for men and women and number of teachers (men and women) separately with different qualification in different types of institution and different stages of education in schools for general education.

(*v*) *Scholarships, stipends, freeships and other financial* concessions, awarded to students in different types of institutions; also gives information regarding number of students in institutions where education is free.

(*vi*) *Expenditure on educational institutions.* Direct expenditure by Management—source-wise and for each type, presented separately for institutions' for Boys and Girls; distribution of Direct Expenditure on salaries of (*a*) Teachers and (*b*) other staff, as well as on 'Equipment, and other appliances' and other items, source wise distribution of indirect Expenditure on Direction and Inspection, Buildings, Hostels, Scholarships, stipends and other financial concession, 'Equipment and other appliances' and for other items.

(*vii*) *Education in rural areas.* Details of institutions in rural areas by type of institution—public and private institutions their number, enrolment therein and Total Direct Expenditure (separately from Government funds and Indirect expenditure) on Buildings, Equipment and Appliances (Non-Recurring), on Scholarships and stipend, on other financial concessions and on hostels; as also Number of Teachers in the Public and Private institutions.

(*viii*) *Examination results.* Both annual and supplementary giving number of boys and girls appeared and passed the various examinations from recognised institutions and as private candidates.

The data collected in this form is published in the annual report Education in India. Vol. I. This publication gives the descriptive account of the progress made in the various fields of education in different States along with the write up on the statistical tables included in the publication. Education in India—Vol. II gives all India consolidated picture without any State-wise break up or any write-up.

Form A-1

(*i*) The number of students enrolled by type of institution and by sex, separately for Scheduled Castes and Scheduled Tribes (*ii*) Enrolment of Scheduled Castes and Scheduled Tribes separately by type of education and stage (*iii*) The number of Scheduled Castes and Scheduled Tribes students, benefitting from scholarship, stipends and other financial concessions and also the amount disbursed to them by type of institutions in broad categories, (*iv*) Number of attached hostel meant for these communities and the number of students of these communities residing in them. The form was introduced from the year 1964-65 to collect annualy separate data on Scheduled Castes and Scheduled Tribes. Some of the important data collected in this form forms the basis of chapter IX of *Education in India* Vol. I. However a separate report on the progress of Education of Scheduled Castes and Scheduled Tribes has also been brought on the basis of this data.

FORM A-2

(*i*) Distribution of primary sections/classes by number of teachers and enrolment groups and by States. Similar data are avilable for middle school classes and also high school classes.

(*ii*) The enrolment in classes I-VIII distributed by the duration for which the students are attending those classes, e.g. for the first time, for the second time, etc. (stagnation) by states.

(*iii*) Age distribution of teachers in primary and middle, high/higher secondary stage by States, sex and whether trained or untrained.

(*iv*) Distribution of teachers in primary stage, middle stage and high/higher secondary stage by emoluments and management of institutions.

This form was also introduced from the year 1964-65. The data collected in this form can be utilised for special studies on these selected topics of school education.

FORM A-3

District wise statistics are collected in this form every five years starting from 1960-61 and are published in the publication Educational Statistics—District wise. District-wise statistics bring out the regional disprities existing within different areas of the State. Data collected in this form relates to a variety of items including educational as well as related aspects viz. area and population, age group population (age groups 6-11, 11-14, 14-17 and 17-23), literacy rate, number of institutions, pupils, teachers and expenditure, enrolment of scheduled castes and scheduled tribes in different classes. Number of teacher training, vocational and technical schools and number of institutions and enrolment relating to higher education.

FORM-B

(*i*) University including University Teaching Departments, Year of foundation, Type of University, Territorial limit or jurisdiction; Dates of commencement and end of terms; Minimum age of admission to the Univerisity; Hostels managed as well as approved, giving total living area and details of facilities like Reading rooms, Common rooms, Play grounds and Medical facilities, etc. New courses started; Medium of Instruction Examination; Tutorial system; Seminar system; Physical Education, Classification of University teachers by designation and scale of pay and allowances.

(*ii*) University/Constituent Colleges and Affiliated/Associated Colleges—Hostels managed and approved giving total living area, details of facilities and number of residents of different categories and number of residents of different categories and Tutorial and seminar systems as well as classification of teachers by designations and salary scales.

(*iii*) Comparative information for the current as well as the previous year, on number of Institutions and Enrolment—University Teaching Departments and Colleges (Separately for General, Professional and other Education), Students from Rural areas and those belonging to Scheduled Castes and Scheduled Tribes and those from foreign countries; Teaching and Research staff and number of Teachers from foreign countries; Expenditure on University and on Colleges for 'General Education', Professional Education and 'other Education'.

(*iv*) Subjects offered for Degrees, Diplomas and Certificates by faculties giving minimum admission qualifications required and the duration of each course, year of foundation and affiliation, management and Degree/Diplomas/Certificates provided at different Departments/Colleges, year wise enrolment in University Teaching Departments and colleges for Pre-University Intermediate (Arts, Science, Home Science and others), Graduates (Arts, Science, Home Science and others); Post Graduates (Arts, Science, Home Science and others), Doctorate (Arts, Science, Home Science and others) and diploma/certificate at under-Graduate and post-Graduate levels for General Education and for Pre-professional, Intermediate, Graduate, post-Graduate, Doctorate and Diploma/Certificate levels in various type of professional Education. Other education courses at under-Graduate, Graduate and post-Graduate Levels, Statistics of admission to Professional and other education courses, giving the intake capacity and the number admitted.

(*v*) Country wise statistics of foreign students—Government's scholarship holder, other scholarship holder and private by type of education and by sex.

(*vi*) Classified details of teachers by their qualifications, designations and salary groups for various types of education. Honorary and part-time teachers to be specified separately.

(*vii*) Details of examination results—showing number of passes giving their division or class and those who passed as regular students or privately as well as those belonging to scheduled castes/ scheduled tribes.

(*viii*) Scholarships, stipends, other financial assistance and free studentships given by various agencies including Central Government, University Grants Commission, State Government, Universities, College and others to all student beneficiaries and separately for scheduled castes and scheduled tribes studying (*a*) General, (*b*) professional, and (*c*) other education.

(*ix*) Details of Income and Expenditure—for Universities Recurring-Grant from Central Government, University Grants Commission, State Government and Local Bodies plus fees, 'endowments' and 'other sources', Non-recurring grants from Central Government, University Grants Commission and State Governments and contributions by other sources. The recurring expenditure on (*a*) Salaries paid to research guiding and teaching staff and administrative and other staff; (*b*) Grants to colleges; (*c*) Equipment and stipends, Library, Games and sports, conduct of examinations, maintenance of hostels and repair of buildings etc. and the non-recurring expenditure on library buildings, equipments and other items. Details of income and expenditure separately for the constituent and affiliated colleges. Statistics of libraries giving details of book, periodicals, manuscripts and other volumes at the beginning and end of the year in the University as well as constituent/affiliated college libraries. Details of recurring and non-recurring expenditure on various items.

The data collected in Form 'B' is published in "Education in Universities in India" The statistics in Form 'B' relating up to the year 1968-69 are to be collected and published by the Ministry of Education and Social Welfare. As recommended by the committee on the reorganisation of the statistical unit, work for the later years has been entrusted to the University Grants Commission.

Form B-3

Statistics of Evening College (Courses) (*i*) General information such as name of the institution, university to which affiliated; year of affiliation, Degree/Diploma/Certificate for which instructions provided.

(*ii*) Number of teachers by sex for General Education, Professional education and other education.

(*iii*) Number of students in General Educrtion at different stages separately for Arts, Science and other subjects.

(*iv*) Number of students in Professional and other Education at different stages for different courses.

(*v*) Intake capacity, number applied for admission and number admitted for General Education and Professional Education at different stages.

Form B-4

Statistics of Boards of Education (*i*) General information, number of institutions of different type recognised by the Board, income by sources and expenditure by items.

(*ii*) Number of students registered for different examinations, number appeared by sex and number passed by sex and division.

Forms to be used for collection of data after 1976-77 are given below:

Form ES-I

It has four tables. Table I collects information on the number of institutions according to management. Table II gives enrolment in institutions by rural and urban location. Table III is divided into five sections. The first section gives enrolment in General (higher) Education levels. Second section deals with enrolment in professional and other (higher) education by levels. Third Section gives enrolment in post-matric courses (General education but below degree level). Fourth section gives enrolment in General (school) education. Fifth section gives professional, vocational, special and other (school) education. Table IV gives the number of trained and untrained teachers in institutions for general education (below degree level).

FORM ES-II

Table I gives the financial data by sources of income corresponding to all types of institutions in Table II of the Form ES-I. Similarly Table III gives break up of expenditure in terms of recurring and non-recurring instead of 'direct' and indirect expenditure as was done previously unto 1975-76. Source of income included in Table I are the Central Government, State Government, UGC, University, Local bodies, Tuition fees, Hospital fees and other fees, endowments and other sources. Main items of recurring expenditure mentioned in the Table II are: salaries and allowances of teaching staff and non-teaching staff separately, maintenance of buildings, furniture and equipment, consumable forms, libraries, stipends and scholarships, games and reports, hostels and other items. Items of non-recurring expenditure include libraries, buildings, equipments, furniture other items.

FORM ES-III

This form gives number appeared and passes in the annual and supplementary examination by sex.

The results are grouped as under:

1. Degrees and diplomas equivalent to degrees.
2. Diploma/Certificate—post-graduate.
3. Intermediate/pre-degree/pre-University certificate.
4. Post-Matriculation Diploma not leading to degree.
5. Post-Matric certificate not leading to degree.
6. School Examination Certificate.

FORM ES-IV

It has three tables. Table I gives the number of students and teachers from ST/SC by types of institutions.

Table II gives enrolment in general, professional and other (Higher education by levels, general (school) education by level and vocational and professional (school) education.

Table III gives the number of trained and untrained teachers in institutions of general education (below degree).

Inter-State Disparities in Per Capita Expenditure on Education and Medicine in India

BINA ROY*

The purpose of this paper is to explore the possibility of studying the disparities in per capita household expenditure on education and medicine with the help of National Sample Survey (NSS) data as well as the distribution of the aggregate expenditure on these two items by the size-group of population by level of living within each state and in all-India between urban and rural areas. The present study also seeks to investigate the disparities in the distribution of the aggregate all India expenditure on these two items namely, education and medicine among different states in India.

It is increasingly realized in developing economies that improvement in educational and health services plays an important part in the process of economic development. It is an indisputable fact that improved educational and health services can influence economic growth in a positive manner. For example, improved health services can, by raising the general health standard of the people, make them more capable of productive work. Similarly, improved and even distribution of educational facilities may affect in a positive way, not only the productivity of an economy but also may favourably affect the demographic conditions of a country like India with a high rate of population growth. An even distribution of educational and health facilities between rural and urban areas would certainly exert suitable influence in reducing the size of the family according to the laws of population growth.

But developing countries are characteristically marked by a high degree of inequality in distribution of income, wealth and other amenities needed to raise the skill for productive work. Yet, it is a fact that through the process of planned development, certain amount of

*Indian Statistical Institute, Calcutta.

aggregate growth has also been achieved not only in total income and consumption expenditure but also in health and educational services.

The central question now is: Who are the actual beneficieries of these aggregate achievements? It is a redeeming point that scholars and scientists at different levels are already searching for an answer to this question. As a result, numerous attempts have been made to investigate the trends in the distributions of income, consumption expenditure and wealth in the country. It is needless here to cite the volume of work already accomplished in this field as it is well known to the scholars concerned.

Nevertheless, all these studies are mainly related, by and large, to the distributions of total consumption expenditure on food items and also income and wealth. The point however is that a better level of living for all the sections of population implies something more. A rise in the standard of living does not mean only the increase in the per capita income and per capita consumption expenditure; it also depends on how this increased volume of income per head is spent. Improvement in the standard of living should also mean the increase in per head expenditure on the average enjoyable quantity of educational, medical, social-cultural amenities with an even distribution over the total population.

It is perhaps necessary at this point to comment on the possibility of a fruitful investigation into these aspects of the problem with the data base now provided through official statistics. The Ministry of Education and the Directorate of Health Services are regularly publishing statistics of education and health conditions of the total population. But these data are not sufficient for an investigation of the cross-section distributions of these two services, namely, education and health. It is needless to say that this could only be undertaken through extensive surveys in the level of living of different sections of the population. The consumption expenditure surveys conducted by the NSSO have already thrown up information in this direction which could be used to measure the disparities in distributions by states and inequalities in distributions of these two items over different points of time.

One way of measuring the extent of inequalities in the distribution of education and health services is by calculating the shares of these two items in the per capita total monthly consumption expenditure by the size-distributions of population by level of living of all states and also of total India. The present undertaking is a preliminary attempt in this direction. This study is based on the data available from a special tabulation of the 18th round survey of the NSSO covering the period from February 1963 to January 1964 for all the 16 major states for rural areas and for all India, extending to the areas of both rural and urban. The two items chosen for the present study are the per capita household monthly expenditure on education and medicine.

The size distributions of population by per capita expenditure by states are available by quintal groups and are different from the all-India distributions which are available by decile groups. The relevant data are available for the following states: Andhra Pradesh, Bihar, Gujarat, Himachal Pradesh, Jammu and Kashmir, Kerala, Madras (Tamil Nadu), Maharastra, Mysore (Karnataka), Madhya Pradesh, Orissa, Punjab, Rajasthan, Tripura-Manipur-Assam, Uttar Pradesh and West Bengal. Among these 16 states, Himachal Pradesh could not be included in the calculations as data for this state are not available consistently for all the sub-samples.

Methods followed in calculating the disparities in distributions by the size-group of population and by states are the same as adopted in measuring inequalities in the distributions of consumption expenditure in India. First, specific concentration coefficients have been calculated to find out the disparities in distributions of the aggregate expenditure on education and medicine within each of these 15 states by the size-group of population by level of living. Secondly, to study the inter-state disparities in the distributions of the aggregate all-India expenditure on these two items, the states have been ranked in ascending order to actual per capita expenditure on education and medicine by size-group of population. And then, specific concentration coefficients have also been calculated. Lastly, specific concentration coefficients have also been calculated to study the disparities in the distributions of the aggregate all-India expenditure on education and medicine between different size-groups of population by level of living both in rural and urban areas separately. Attempt has also been made to find out the urban-rural disparities in monthly capita household expenditure on these two items by different size-groups of population.

The result of all these calculations are presented in a summarised form in the following sections.

Share of per capita expenditure by size-groups of population

In Tables 1 and 2, the figures of monthly per capita household expenditure and the percentage share of expenditure on education and medicine are presented respectively by size-groups of population. The figures in the tables clearly indicate the trends in the percentage share of household expenditure on education and medicine. However, only the trends of the share of expenditure to top 20 per cent, bottom 20 per cent and the average share of general population are explained below.

Three kinds of trends of the share of expenditure on these two items may be noted from Table 2 in the bottom 20 per cent of population in different states. In the case of Andhra Pradesh, Orissa and Rajasthan, the share of expenditure on education and medicine is equal, while in Karnataka, Punjab and Tripura-Manipur-Assam, the share of expenditure on education is higher than the share on medicine. Third trend is that the share of expenditure on medicine on this size-class is higher than on education. And this trend is noted in the case of all the other states except the above mentioned states.

One may notice a somewhat trend from the share of expenditure on education and medicine in the case of top 20 per cent of population. Except in Tripura-Manipur-Assam, the share of expenditure on mediciue is higher in all the states than the share of expenditure on education. In Tripura-Manipur-Assam, the share of expenditure on education is higher than on medicine in all the size-groups of population.

The trend in the group—0-100 or average for total population is almost similar to what is reflected by the trend in the top 20 per cent group. Besides, there is a general trend of the share of expenditure on medicine being higer than the share of expenditure on education in all the size-groups of population. The tendency of increase in the share of expenditure per capita on both education and medicine in higher expenditure groups is marked in the case of all states. Among the states, Kerala has the highest share of per capita expenditure on both education and medicine though per capita total consumption expenditure is lowest in this state.

The results of the calculations of disparities in distributions of aggregate expenditure on education and medicine within each state over different size-groups of population are presented in Tables 3 and 4. It is evident from Table 3 that there is sufficient amount of disparities in the percentage share of aggregate expenditure on education and medicine by different size groups of population by level of living. Share of expenditure on education varies from 1 per cent to 7 per cent over different states in the case of bottom 20 per cent of population; it

TABLE 1—*Average per capita per household consumer expenditure on all items in Rs per 30 days in rural areas: NSS 18th round: rural: February 1963-January 1964.*

quintal groups	*sub-sample*	*Andhra Pradesh*	*Bihar*	*Gujarat*	*Himachal Pradesh*	*Jammu & Kashmir*	*Kerala*	*Madras*	*Maha-rashtra*	*My-sore*	*Madhya Pradesh*	*Orissa*	*Punjab*	*Rajasthan*	*Tripura Manipur-Assam*	*Uttar Pra-desh*	*West Bengal*	*all-India*
1	*2*	*3*	*4*	*5*	*6*	*7*	*8*	*9*	*10*	*11*	*12*	*13*	*14*	*15*	*16*	*17*	*18*	*19*
0-20	1	9.60	9.30	11.24	14.48	13.60	9.25	10.26	10.05	9.49	9.33	8.49	12.38	10.64	14.68	9.89	11.91	9.95
	c	9.72	9.97	9.90	14.49	15.01	8.86	10.11	10.62	9.54	9.18	9.03	12.49	9.44	14.35	9.23	11.87	9.92
	2	9.59	9.61	10.45	15.46	14.64	9.09	10.24	10.24	9.60	9.22	9.05	12.36	9.91	14.66	9.51	11.73	9.90
	1	13.87	13.93	15.47	27.58	18.96	13.39	15.36	14.20	13.43	14.17	12.63	18.53	14.66	18.70	14.29	16.04	14.69
10-40	c	13.67	14.31	14.63	15.36	20.29	12.96	14.73	14.46	13.51	13.78	12.95	19.73	14.54	19.56	13.71	16.80	14.58
	2	13.46	14.29	15.23	20.12	19.44	13.11	14.91	14.36	13.48	14.09	12.98	18.80	14.38	19.10	13.83	16.55	14.50
	1	17.07	17.88	19.30	16.81	24.86	16.86	20.47	18.13	17.35	18.19	17.22	24.09	19.56	21.78	18.21	19.97	18.78
40-60	c	17.06	27.94	18.21	30.56	25.34	16.97	18.45	18.14	16 65	18.26	16.49	25.06	18.44	25.00	17.63	21.38	18.76
	2	17.03	17.92	18.65	19.28	24.67	17.02	19.29	18.32	17.30	18.34	16.57	24.59	19.22	23.30	17.96	20.71	18.68
	1	21.78	22.91	23.77	12.23	32.23	21.56	26.77	23.16	21.86	24.55	21.96	32.38	26.48	26.58	23.74	25.23	24.38
60-80	c	22.26	22.84	23.44	15.21	30.27	22.92	24.62	23.29	21.50	23.84	21.40	31.89	25.76	30.23	22.35	27.18	24.42
	2	22.20	23.07	23.89	26.04	31.39	22.86	25.85	23.18	21.33	24.36	21.96	32.19	26.49	24.48	23.66	24.94	24.38
	1	39.78	40.58	45.64	57.51	49.58	41.28	48.35	40.01	36.83	54.76	36.83	50.92	47.90	41.46	41.77	40.34	43.75
80-100	c	44.12	42.24	44.34	36.70	48.73	39.79	45.56	44.74	42.90	45.13	36.50	54.84	44.52	44.95	41.67	46.78	44.02
	2	41.93	41.22	44.82	41.78	49.04	39.97	46.96	42.50	39.94	49.97	36.52	56.97	45.73	43.63	41.67	44.93	44.21
0-100	1	20.42	20.92	23.09	25.72	27.85	20.47	24.24	21.11	19.79	24.20	19.43	29.26	23.85	25.64	21.58	22.70	22.31
	e	21.37	21.46	22.11	22.45	27.93	20.30	22.70	22.31	20.82	22.04	19.27	28.80	22.54	26.82	21.12	24.80	22.32
	2	20.84	21.22	22.61	24.54	27.83	20.41	23.44	21.72	20.33	23.20	19.42	28.98	23.15	25.83	21.32	23.77	22.33

TABLE 2—*Percentage share of education and medicine in total house-hold expenditure on all items, by states and quintal groups: NSS 18th round: rural: February 1963-January 1964, combined sample.*

States	percentage share of education & medicine by quintal groups (percentage)											
	0-20		20-40		40-60		60-80		80-100		General Population	
	Education	Medicine	Education	Medicine	Education	Medicine	E	M	E	M	E	M
1	2	3	4	5	6	7	8	9	10	11	12	13
Andhra Pradesh	0.10	0.10	0.15	0.22	0.12	0.59	0.40	0.85	1.09	2.43	0.56	1.31
Bihar	0.10	0.40	0.28	0.84	0.28	1.23	0.78	1.18	1.49	3.29	0.84	1.91
Gujarat	0.10	0.20	—	0.55	0.16	0.60	0.51	0.68	1.01	1.87	0.54	1.09
Himachal Pradesh	—	—	—	5.34	0.13	—	0.26	0.72	0.03	0.90	0.09	0.76
Jammu & Kashmir	0.13	0.40	0.44	1.08	0.32	0.87	0.40	1.68	0.82	2 98	0.54	1.75
Kerala	0.54	1.73	0.93	2.62	1.53	3.65	1.35	2.71	2.14	4.65	1.58	3.50
Madras	0.20	0.49	0.41	0.41	0.57	0.76	0 89	1.58	1.40	2 24	0.93	1.45
Maharashtra	0.09	0.56	0.41	0.69	0.39	0.65	0.86	1.46	0.92	3.69	0.67	2.06
Mysore	0.21	0.10	0.07	0.37	0.18	0.24	0.28	0.56	0.79	1.63	0.43	0.91
Madhya Pradesh	0.11	0.33	0.15	0.58	0.22	1.15	0.38	1.34	0.31	2.26	0.36	1.50
Orissa	0.22	0.22	0.08	0.23	0.73	0.91	0.65	1.40	1.04	2.49	0.67	1.45
Punjab	1.04	0.48	1.22	0.71	1.00	1.56	1.03	2.51	1.51	2.77	1.25	2.81
Rajasthan	0.11	0.11	0.14	0.48	0.38	0.98	0.63	1.09	0.34	2.85	0.35	1.60
Tripura-Manipur-Assam	0.56	0.28	0.31	0.20	0.72	0.48	1.29	0.46	1.31	1.07	0.97	0.63
Uttar Pradesh	0.22	0.65	0.29	1.17	0.28	1.59	0.60	1.76	0.94	2.47	0.62	1.85
West Bengal	0.25	0.34	0.18	0.54	0.65	0.94	1.10	1.18	1.65	2.84	1.05	1.61
All-India	0.19	0.53	0.34	0.79	0.42	1.01	0.66	1.41	1.12	2.63	0.76	1.70

TABLE 3—*Percentage distribution of aggregate expenditure on education and medicine by quintal groups, separately by states: NSS 18th round: rural: February 1963-January 1964, combined sample.*

States	*average monthly total per capita expenditure in Rs of total population*	*quintal group percentages* 0-20 (*percentage distribution of expenditure per quintal group on*)		20-40		40-60		60-80 (*percentage distribution of expenditure per quintal group on*)		80-100	
		Education	*Medicine*	*Education*	*Medicine*	*Education*	*Medicine*	*Education*	*Medicine*	*Education*	*Medicine*
1	2	3	4	5	6	7	8	9	10	11	12
Andhra Pradesh	21.37	1.92	0.66	3.03	2.14	2.78	7.18	14.67	13.77	77.60	76.25
Bihar	21.46	1.02	2.01	3.97	6.09	5.06	10.50	20.36	13.39	69.59	68.02
Gujarat	22.11	1.00	1.70	0.55	6.63	4.70	9.49	19.79	13.05	74.05	69.13
Himachal Pradesh	22.45	—	—	0.99	4.39	47.52	—	43.23	12.90	8.25	38.71
Jammu & Kashmir	27.93	3.41	2.54	12.63	8.98	11.59	8.82	16.69	20.89	55.68	58.76
Kerala	20.30	3 00	3.79	7.75	9.60	16.37	17.35	19.59	17.37	53.29	51.89
Madras	22.70	1.70	2 83	5.68	3.65	9.71	8.32	21.15	23.33	61.76	61.78
Maharashtra	22.31	1.54	2.77	8.14	4.56	8.73	5.11	26.55	15.13	55.03	72.43
Mysore	20.82	3.36	1.43	1.40	5.13	6.24	4.74	14.28	13.11	74.72	75.59
Madhya Pradesh	22.04	3.08	1.51	5.52	4.72	9.31	12.63	23.82	19.61	58.26	61.52
Orissa	19.27	2.53	1.60	2.03	1.96	17.70	10.85	20.39	21.16	57.36	64.43
Punjab	28.80	7.33	2.19	13.28	4.70	14.19	13.16	18.57	27.63	46.63	52.32
Rajasthan	22.54	2.63	0.72	5.79	3.93	17.11	9.86	39.07	15.28	35.40	70.21
Tripura-Manipur-Assam	26.82	6.32	5.27	4.84	5.27	13.50	14.06	30.00	17.21	45.34	58.20
Uttar Pradesh	21.12	2.91	2.94	6.77	8.32	8.26	14.36	22.05	21.02	60.01	53.36
West Bengal	24.80	2.47	1.79	2.69	4.78	10.92	9.92	23.42	16.39	60.50	67.12
All-India	24.80	2.47	1.79	2.69	4.78	—	—	—	—	—	—

varies from as much as 35 to 77 per cent in the case of top 20 per cent. In the case of the share of expenditure on medicine, almost similar trends may be noted; the share varies from 1 per cent to 5 per cent in the bottom as against 52 to 76 per cent in the case of top 20 per cent of population over the states.

It may be noted from the results of the calculations of specific contentration coefficients of the distributions that in the case of the distributions of aggregate expenditure on education, high concentration in upper consumer expenditure group is noted in the states—Mysore, Gujarat, Maharashtra, Madras, Madhya Pradesh, Bihar, Uttar Pradesh, Andhra Pradesh, Orissa and West Bengal. Medium concentration in the distributions is noted in the states—Kerala, Tripura-Manipur-Assam and Jammu and Kashmir. Lowest concentration is noted in the states—Rajasthan and Punjab. Trends in the distributions of the share of aggregate expenditure on medicine are noted here. Higher concentration in the distribution of this item is noted in the states—Mysore Gujarat, Maharashtra, Madras, Madhya pradesh, Bihar, Andhra

TABLE 4—*Specific concentration coefficient of the distribution of population by aggregate expenditure on education and medicine by states and all-India for rural areas: NSS 18th round: February 1963-January 1964.*

States	*Education*			*Medicine*		
	s.s. 1	*s.s. 2*	*Comb.*	*s.s. 1*	*s.s. 2*	*Comb.*
1	*2*	*3*	*4*	*5*	*6*	*7*
Andhra Pradesh	.6000	.6770	.6520	.6323	.6695	.6512
Bihar	.5995	.6295	.6141	.5347	.5794	.5574
Gujarat	.5932	.7434	.6610	.5403	.5515	.5651
Jammu & Kashmir	.4223	.4754	.4344	.4993	.4820	.4975
Kerala	.4021	.4738	.4497	.4298	.3914	.4159
Madras	.5546	.5544	.5424	.5463	.5722	.5510
Maharashtra	.5044	.4850	.5016	.7064	.5908	.5996
Mysore	.6094	.6275	.6224	.5869	.6391	.6252
Madhya Pradesh	.5335	.4353	.5147	.5098	.5733	.5397
Orissa	.5770	.4145	.5120	.6236	.5772	.5794
Punjab	.3606	.2986	.3356	.5085	.4652	.4928
Rajasthan	.3868	.3943	.3953	.6647	.5294	.6013
Tripura-Manipur-Assam	.3273	.4265	.4128	.3241	.5453	.4712
Uttar Pradesh	.5149	.5268	.5179	.4882	.4228	.4542
West Bengal	.5508	.5708	.5472	.4951	.6154	.5691
All-India	.5544	.5623	.5707	.5557	.5638	.5709

Pradesh, Orissa, West Bengal and Rajasthan. Concentration is medium in the states—Kerala, Uttar Pradesh, Tripura-Manipur-Assam, Jammu and Kashmir and Punjab.

The results of the calculation of specific concentration coefficients to find out the disparities in the distributions of the aggregate all-India expenditure on education and medicine among the different states included in this study are presented at this stage. First, the states have been ranked in ascending order of actual per capita monthly household expenditure on these two items. To save space, only the results of calculations of selected quintal groups are mentioned, namely —0-20, 80-100 and also 0-100 by all the samples. The ranks of states are presented in Tables 5 and 6. Using these figures of per capita expenditure on education and medicine, ranked in ascending order and total rural population for each of these states, the figures of aggregate expenditures by quintal group in each state have been estimated. Next the specific concentration coefficients of the distributions of all-India aggregate expenditure by states on education and medicine have been

TABLE 5—*Ranking of States in ascending order of monthly per capita household expenditure on* **education** *by selected quintal groups of population in rural areas: NSS 18th Round: February 1963-January 1964.*

States	*quintal groups*								
	0-20			*80-100*			*0-100*		
	S.1	*S.2*	*Comb.*	*S.1*	*S.2*	*Comb.*	*S.1*	*S.2*	*Comb.*
1	*2*	*3*	*4*	*5*	*6*	*7*	*8*	*9*	*10*
Andhra Pradesh	3	7	4	2	11	9	2	9	5
Bihar	8	4	6	10	12	11	10	11	10
Gujarat	5	5	2	6	9	8	5	4	4
Jammu & Kashmir	4	9	7	4	7	6	7	8	8
Kerala	13	14	13	13	15	15	14	15	14
Madras	2	11	10	14	13	12	11	10	11
Maharashtra	7	3	5	7	6	7	9	7	9
Mysore	12	2	9	9	3	3	6	1	3
Madhya Pradesh	6	6	3	3	2	2	3	2	2
Orissa	1	10	8	5	5	4	4	6	6
Punjab	15	15	15	15	10	14	15	14	15
Rajasthan	9	1	1	1	1	1	1	3	1
Tripura-Manipur-Assam	14	13	14	11	8	10	12	13	12
Uttar Pradesh	11	8	11	8	4	5	8	5	7
West Bengal	10	12	12	14	14	13	13	12	13

TABLE 6—*Ranking of States in ascending order of monthly per capita household expenditure on* **medicine** *by selected quintal groups of population in rural areas: NSS 18th Round: February 1963-January 1964:*

States	*quintal groups*								
	0-20			*80-100*			*0-100 (total population)*		
	S.1	*S.2*	*Comb.*	*S.1*	*S.2*	*Comb.*	*S.1*	*S.2*	*Comb.*
1	*2*	*3*	*4*	*5*	*6*	*7*	*8*	*9*	*10*
Andhra Pradesh	3	2	3	6	9	8	4	7	5
Bihar	13	9	9	11	12	11	10	11	11
Gujarat	7	4	5	5	2	3	3	3	3
Jammu & Kashmir	9	11	11	12	10	12	13	10	13
Kerala	15	15	15	15	13	15	15	15	15
Madras	14	8	10	9	5	6	9	4	7
Maharashtra	6	14	13	10	15	14	7	14	12
Mysore	4	1	2	2	3	2	2	2	2
Madhya Pradesh	5	5	6	7	7	5	8	5	6
Orissa	1	10	4	8	8	4	5	6	4
Punjab	12	12	12	14	11	13	14	13	14
Rajasthan	2	3	1	13	6	9	12	8	8
Tripura-Manipur-Assam	11	7	7	1	1	1	1	1	1
Uttar Pradesh	8	13	14	8	4	7	11	9	9
West Bengal	10	6	8	4	14	10	6	12	10

calculated using the proportionate share of each state in the aggregate expenditure and total population.

Interesting patterns emerge from the ranking of states in respect of their monthly per capita household expenditure on education and medicine. Punjab, Kerala and West Bengal may be ranked as the first three states in respect of per capita expenditure on education. In West Bengal, the existence of a slight elasticity is noted in the upper expenditure group which is almost absent in the case of Kerala and Punjab. In some states, the divergence in rank by sub-samples is high. In the case of expenditure on medicine, the ranks of states are slightly different. In this case, states of Kerala, Punjab and Jammu & Kashmir may be noted as the first three states.

However, this ranking of states in respect of their monthly per capita household expenditure gives only a rough idea about the situation. To have a precise picture of real happenings in this respect, an examination of expenditures on these items by other agencies is essential. In the case of education, for example, the expenditure on this item from Government sources plays no less a vital role. It is however gratifying to note that the ranking by NSS data in this study reflects, to some extent, the trend of assessment of per capita expenditure on education by the Ministry of Education, Government of India. Of course, as the number of states is not the same in their case as in this study, some differences are by no means unnatural.

Official statistics give the figure of per capita expenditure on education at all-India level as Rs. 10.2 for 1963-64 (annual). The maximum per capita expenditure among state was in Nagaland (Rs 18.8) followed by Kerala (Rs 14.8) and Maharashtra (Rs 14.7), Madras (Rs 13.0) and West Bengal (Rs 12.7). The lowest per capita expenditure was in the state of Bihar (Rs 5.6) and Uttar Pradesh (Rs 6.9). In all the states and Union Territories, about 60 per cent or more of the total expenditure on education was government funds.

The following are the figures of specific concentration coefficients of inter-state disparities in the distribution of aggregate all-India expenditure on education and medicine:

Quintal group	*Sub-sample*	*Education*	*Medicine*
1	*2*	*3*	*4*
0-20	1	0.5661	0.3558
	2	0.3647	0.3808
	comb.	0.4031	0.3145
80-100	1	0.2112	0.1841
	2	0.2765	0.2794
	comb.	0.2401	0.1514
0-100	1	0.2450	0.1886
	2	0.2494	0.1845
	comb.	0.2415	0.1606

It may be noted from the above figures that inter-state disparities in the distribution of aggregate expenditure on education and medicine are greater among the bottom 20 per cent of the population than those in the top 20 per cent with higher per capita expenditure. Further, disparities in distribution are higher in education than in medicine. Graphical representations of the trends of the concentration of the distribution by the size group of population by states are presented in Figures 1, 2 and 3 below.

Trends of average all-India rural-urban figures

The percentage shares of monthly per capita expenditure on education and medicine by size-groups of population for all-India rural and urban areas and the specific concentration coefficients of the distributions of the aggregate all-India expenditure on these two items are presented. It may be noted from the table that the percentage share of per capita monthly household expenditure on education of the bottom 10 per cent of population is only 0.12 as against 1.33 per cent in top 10 per cent of population. Rural figures clearly indicate gradual rise in the expenditure on education in the size-group with higher per capita consumer expenditure. The figures of the share of

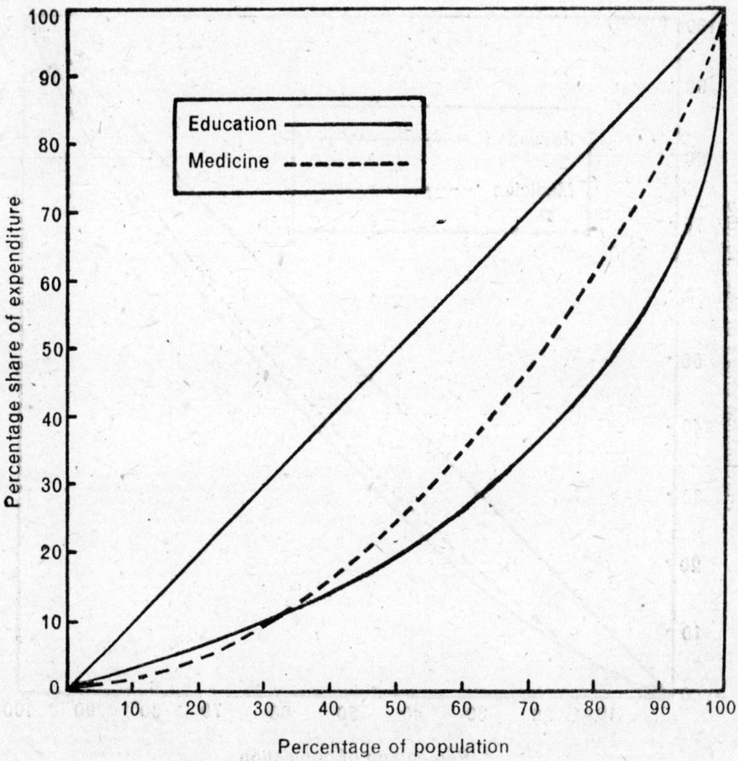

Fig. 1. Figure showing the distribution of expenditure on education and medicine by states in rural areas in the bottom 20 percent size-group of population : combined sample.

expenditure on medicine indicate similar trends. Further, the share of expenditure on medicine is generally higher than the share of expenditure on education in rural areas in all the size-group of population with exceptions in one or two size-groups.

The figures for urban areas indicate somewhat different trends than those for rural areas. The rise in the shares of expenditure on education and medicine in the higher expenditure classes is rapid in urban than that in rural areas. And from the decile groups 50-60 per cent of population to the top most group namely, 90-100 with higher monthly per capita consumer expenditure, the share of expenditure on education is higher than that on medicine.

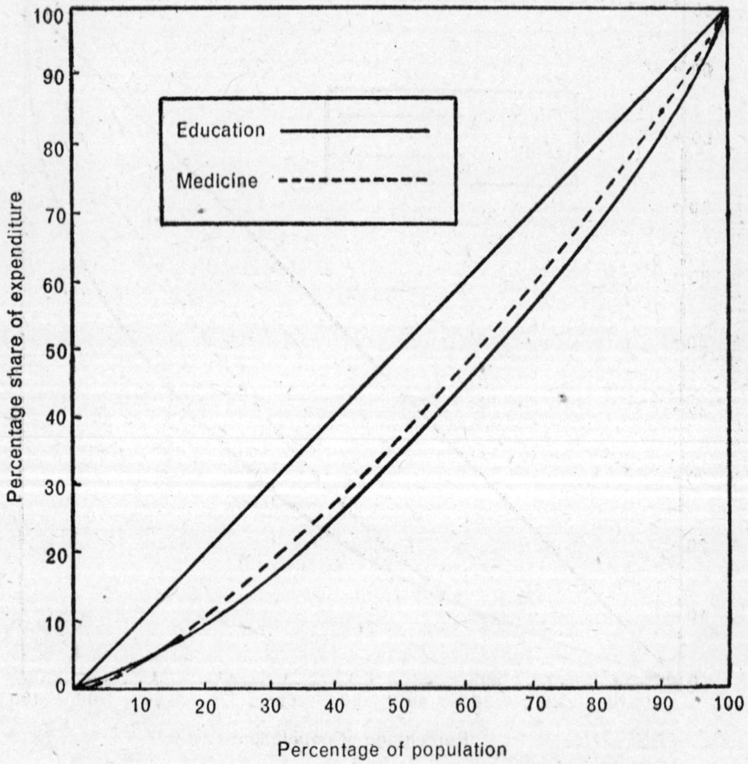

Fig. 2. Figure showing the distribution of expenditure on education and medicine by states in rural areas in the top 20 percent size-group of population: combined sample.

Interesting results emerge from the calculations of urban-rural disparties in actual monthly household per capita expenditure in all-India figures. It is noted that the disparities in the expenditure on education by size-groups by level of living are higher in higher expenditure groups than in lower expenditure groups. Rural per capita expenditure on education varies from 20 to 29 per cent of urban expenditure which decreases further in the higher expenditure groups and varies from 10 to 20 per cent. In the case of expenditure on medicine, the rural per capita expenditure varies from 50 to 60 per cent upto to the decile group 30-40 percent from the bottom. The disparity widens

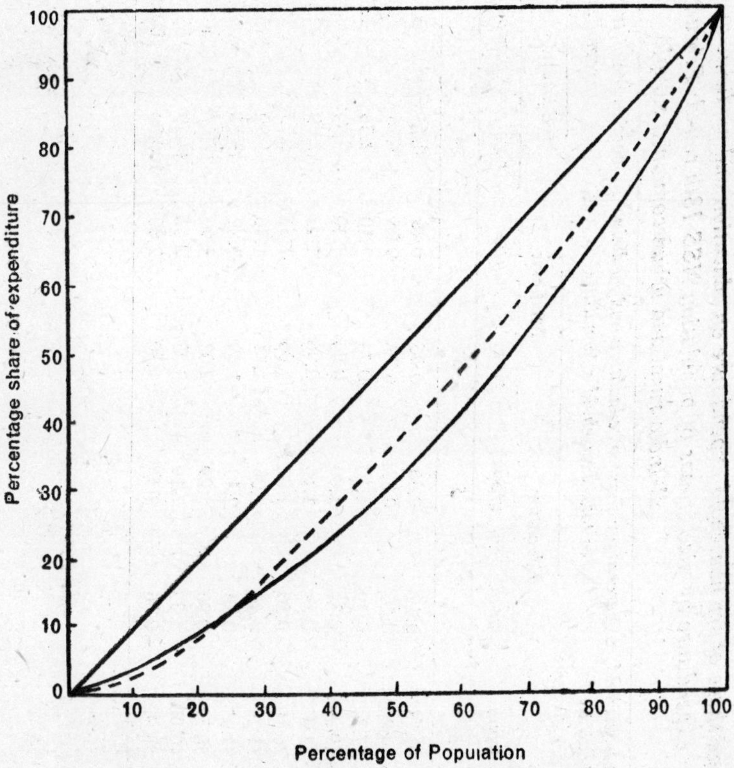

Fig. 3. Figure showing the distribution of expenditure on education and medicine by states in rural areas of average total population (0-100): combined sample.

TABLE 7—*Percentage share of per household expenditure on education and medicine as well as the distribution of the aggregate expenditure by size groups of population NSS 18th round: February 1963-January 1964: all-India rural and urban combined sample.*

Decile groups	average per capita household consumption expenditure in all items in Rs. per 30 days		percentage share of education and medicine in total household expenditure				percentage distribution of aggregate expenditure on-				urban-rural disparities in monthly per capita household expenditure	
			Education		Medicine		Education		Medicine			
	rural	urban	rural	urban	rural	urban	rural	urban	rural	urban	Education	Medicine
1	2	3	4	5	6	7	8	9	10	11	12	13
0-10	8.34	10.78	0.12	0.46	0.36	0.46	0.74	0.42	0.78	0.80	20.00	60.00
10-20	11.49	14.80	0.26	0.88	0.70	0.95	1.76	1.10	1.99	2.03	23.08	57·14
20-30	13.69	17.29	0.29	1.10	0.73	1.10	2.36	1.60	2.49	2.74	21.05	52.63
30-40	15.47	19.99	0·39	1.00	0.84	1.30	3.79	1.69	3.35	3.80	30.00	50.00
40-50	17.74	22.85	0.34	1.14	0.96	1.93	3.79	2.15	4.37	6.40	23.08	38.64
50-60	19.81	26.40	0.50	1.82	1.06	1.63	5.73	3.97	5.43	6.27	20.83	48.84
60-70	22.58	31.29	0.44	2.05	1.33	1.76	5.99	5.35	7.79	8.06	15.62	54.55
70-80	26.26	37.97	0.88	2.13	1.49	1.82	13.58	6.71	10.12	10.11	28.40	56.52
80-90	32.23	50.79	0.90	3.29	2.02	2.90	17.67	13.89	16.88	20.17	17.37	47.45
90-100	55.81	107.00	1.33	7.10	3.23	2.52	44.59	63.12	46.80	39.62	9.74	66.67
0-100	22.32	33.92	0.76	3.54	1.70	2.00	100.00	100.00	100.00	100.00	14.17	55.88

further in the groups 40-50 and 50-60 decile groups. Then again the percentages increase in the top decile groups from 60-70 to 90-100.

The calculations of specific concentration coefficients of the distributions of aggregate expenditure on education and medicine by size-groups of population by level of living in total rural and urban areas may be noted from the following Figures:

Sub-sample	*Rural*		*Urban*	
	Ed.	*Med.*	*Ed.*	*Med*
1	*2*	*3*	*4*	*5*
1	.5544	.5557	.6178	.5326
2	.5623	.5638	.6582	.5298
comb.	.5707	.5709	.6922	.5259

It may be noted that the concentration coefficients of the distributions for both urban and rural are high. Figures for rural areas indicate that concentration in the distributions of expenditure on both education and medicine is almost similar. But for urban areas, the concentration coefficients of the distributions of aggregate expenditure on education over different size-groups of population are higher than that of expenditure on medicine. Graphical representations of the concentration of the distributions in rural and urban areas are presented in Figures 4 and 5 given on pages 374 & 375.

CONCLUDING REMARKS

It may be concluded from the findings of the present study that percentages of household monthly per capita expenditure on education and medicine are still negligible in the bottom size-group of population by level of living in both rural and urban areas. There is a clear indication of the existence of elasticity of expenditure on education and medicine with higher total monthly per capita expenditure in both rural and urban areas and in all the states included here. In general, expenditure on education is lower than the expenditure on medicine in almost all the size-groups of population in rural areas in all the states and in all-India. But in urban areas, the expenditure on education is higher than that on medicine from the size-groups—50-60 to 90-100 with higher monthly total per capita expenditure.

Ranking of states indicates existence of sufficient degree of disparities between states in this respect. In respect of education, the first four states are, Kerala, Punjab, West Bengal and Tripura-Manipur-Assam. In the case of expenditure on medicine, the first four states are, Kerala, Maharashtra, Punjab and Bihar. Government and other agencies play an important role in respect of education and health services. So the findings of the present study have to be judged in that light.

Specific concentration coefficients of the distributions of the aggregate expenditures on these two services within each state indicate high degrees of disparities between the top and bottom size-groups of population in almost all the states in their rural areas as well as in all-India both in rural and urban areas. But the coefficients of distributions of all-India aggregate expenditure on these two items between

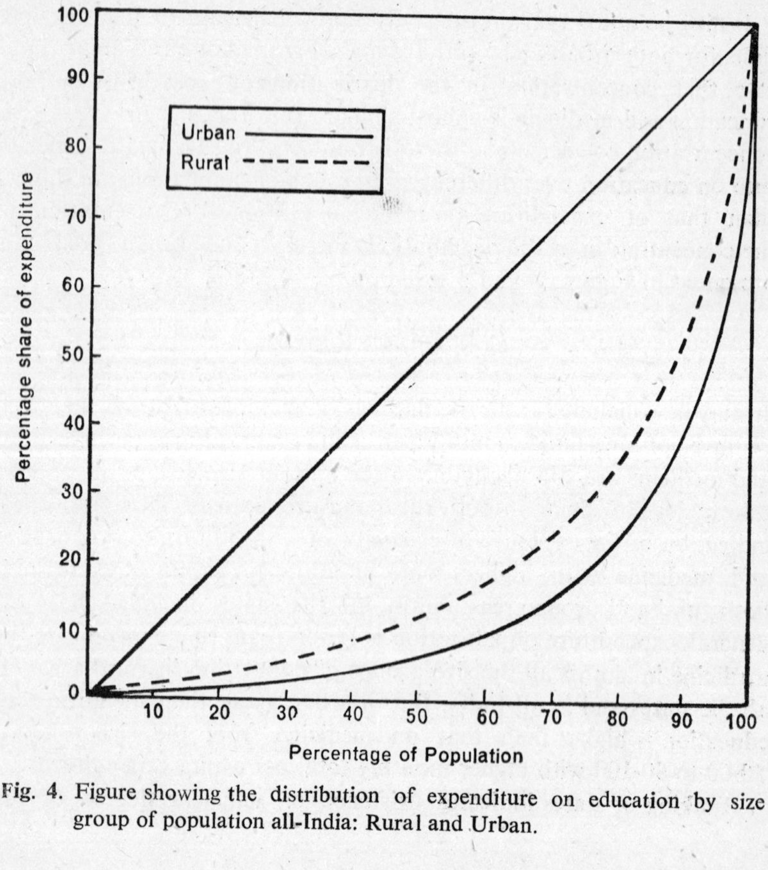

Fig. 4. Figure showing the distribution of expenditure on education by size group of population all-India: Rural and Urban.

states are not so high as within each state over different size-groups of population by level of living.

There is high degree of disparity between urban and rural areas in respect of monthly per capita expenditure on education and medicine in all size-groups of population.

As already mentioned at the outset, the purpose of this study has been to examine the possibility of studying the disparities in the distributions of expenditure on education and medicine. It is a matter of regret that more up-to-date data could not be used to determine the changes in the distributions over time. However, more extensive surveys in future may help scholars to undertake more fruitful probes in this direction.

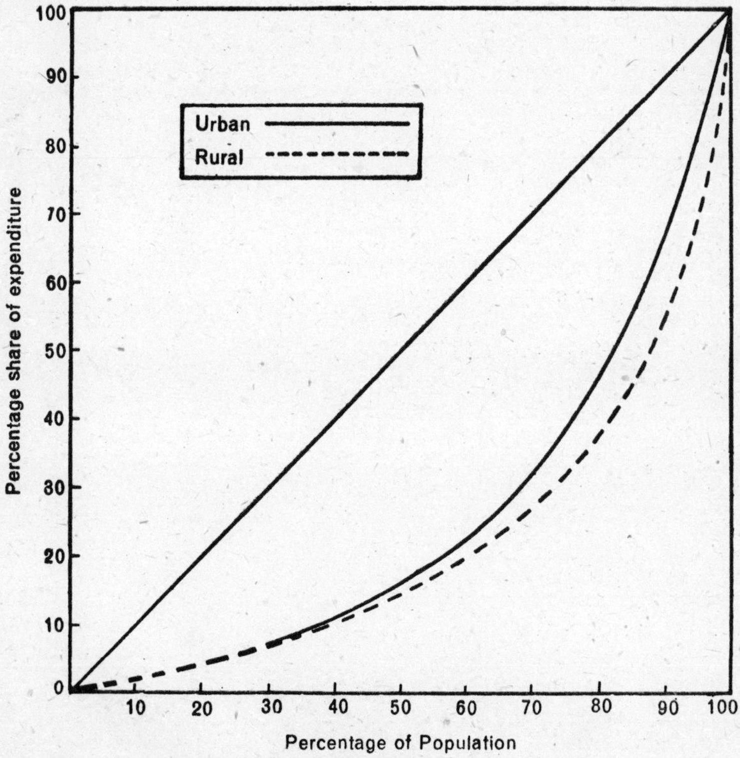

Fig. 5. Figure showing the distribution of expenditure on medicine by size group of population all-India: Rural and Urban.